BIRTHING A SLAVE

BIRTHING A SLAVE

Motherhood and Medicine

in the Antebellum South

Marie Jenkins Schwartz

Harvard University Press
Cambridge, Massachusetts
London, England
2006

Library of Congress Cataloging-in-Publication Data

Schwartz, Marie Jenkins, 1946–
    Birthing a slave : motherhood and medicine in the antebellum South/
Marie Jenkins Schwartz.
        p. cm.
    Includes bibliographical references and index.
    ISBN 0-674-02202-5 (alk. paper)
        1. Childbirth—Southern States—History—19th century.
    2. Obstetrics—Southern States—History—19th century.
    3. Gynecology—Southern States—History—19th century.
    4. Motherhood—Southern States—History—19th century.
    5. Reproductive health—Southern States—History—19th century.
    6. Women slaves—Health and hygiene—Southern States—History—
    19th century.
    7. Women slaves—Medical care—Southern States—History—19th century.
    8. African American women—Health and hygiene—Southern States—
    History—19th century.
    9. African American women—Medical care—Southern States—History—
    19th century.
    10. Medicine—Southern States—History—19th century.
    I. Title

RG518.U5S34 2006
618.20089'96075—dc22   2005044861

Contents

Acknowledgments

FINANCIAL SUPPORT FOR THIS BOOK CAME IN PART FROM THE American College of Obstetricians and Gynecologists and the Ortho Pharmaceutical Corporation, whose jointly sponsored fellowship in the History of American Obstetrics and Gynecology allowed me to begin the research. The American Historical Association's award of an Albert J. Beveridge Research Grant provided funds for the completion of research on the final chapter. The University of Rhode Island's Center for the Humanities provided money to purchase microfilmed documents. The University of Rhode Island granted a semester of sabbatical leave at an early stage of the book's development.

Ira Berlin, Sharla M. Fett, Deborah Kuhn McGregor, Andrea Rusnock, Todd L. Savitt, and Steven M. Stowe read the entire manuscript and offered words of encouragement along with practical advice on how to make the book better. Mara Berkley, Nancy Cook, Lynne Derbyshire, Rae Ferguson, Valerie Karno, Karen Markin, Helen Mederer, Libby Miles, Cat Sama, Eve Sterne, and Kathleen Torrens offered camaraderie along with valuable advice for improving several chapters. Janet Billson offered helpful commentary on one chapter.

I presented parts of the research at professional forums sponsored by the Organization of American Historians, the American Association for the History of Medicine, the Institute of the History of Medicine at Johns Hopkins University, the John Nicholas Brown

Center for the Study of American Civilization at Brown University, and the University of Rhode Island Women's Studies program. I am grateful for formal comments offered at these meetings by Stephanie Shaw and Steven M. Stowe, written remarks by Harry Marks, and numerous suggestions from other participants.

Archivists and others at various repositories named in the notes helped secure sources without which this book would not have been possible. I am especially grateful to the editors of the Freedmen and Southern Society Project at the University of Maryland, College Park, who generously granted me access to the project's files. Steven F. Miller was particularly helpful in aiding my efforts to locate pertinent material. Emily Greene at the University of Rhode Island has been diligent in finding books, articles, and pamphlets, some of them quite obscure.

I am fortunate to have worked with Harvard University Press's senior editor Joyce Seltzer, who supported this project from the first day she heard about it.

I am thankful for the help I have received from these many individuals and institutions. Any shortcomings and errors, are, of course, entirely my own.

I have enjoyed the encouragement of numerous family members. I dedicate this book to them, especially to Ron, who has listened to me talk about *Birthing a Slave* from its inception.

Editorial Note

Q<small>UOTATIONS HAVE BEEN REPRODUCED VERBATIM FROM THE</small> sources, along with any unusual spellings, without the notation *sic*. People who interviewed former slaves, often decades after the end of slavery, frequently and deliberately inserted misspellings into written records of oral interviews such as those published under the editorship of George P. Rawick as *The American Slave: A Composite Autobiography*.

Throughout this book I refer to adults after first mention by their surnames if known, except when doing so would create confusion, as in the case of spouses using the same surname. Many sources list slaves by only first name, however. Thus I sometimes refer to enslaved adults by first name only.

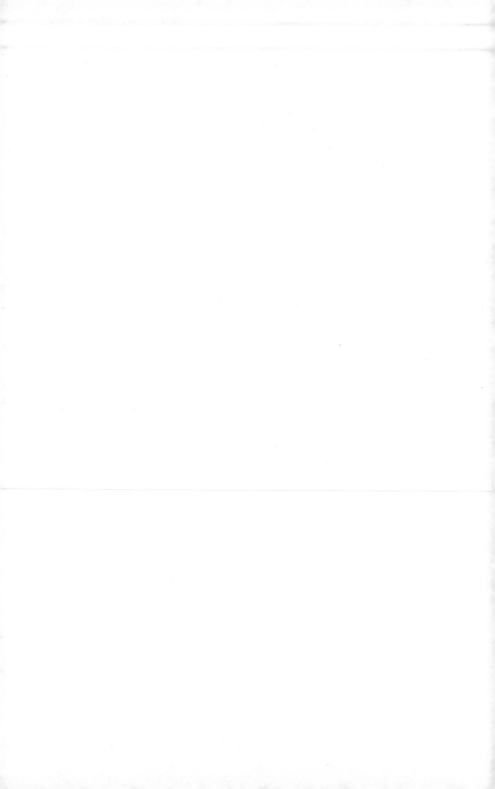

BIRTHING A SLAVE

Introduction

SLAVEHOLDERS MAINTAINED A KEEN INTEREST IN THE BIRTH OF slaves in the decades before the Civil War. After the United States stopped importing slaves in 1808, slavery and the southern way of life could continue only if children were born in bondage. This state of affairs enhanced the importance of enslaved women in the eyes of southern planters, who hoped to exploit their capacity for bearing children along with their ability to perform productive labor. The vested interests of slaveholders in enslaved women's childbearing encouraged owners to take measures, some coercive, to ensure that they had the opportunity to conceive and bring a baby to term.

By the mid-nineteenth century, slaveholders had become aware of increased professionalism among medical doctors, who were deeply immersed in the study of "Woman" in general. Priding themselves on their modern attitudes and scientific approach to plantation management, owners sought physician assistance in increasing fertility among slaves. Doctors responded, putting themselves forward as scientific caregivers who were uniquely to be trusted with African American women's ailments. Medical intervention began with puberty and followed women throughout their reproductive years. Slaveholders and doctors alike considered the slaveholder's willingness to provide this medical care as evidence of a benevolent concern for a slave woman's well-being.

Southern doctors embraced the goals of their slaveholding clients as well as their declarations of compassion, but they had reasons

1

of their own for collaborating with slave owners in treating reproductive ailments of enslaved women: they sought financial security
and professional status. In a region where the largest number of potential patients were enslaved, doctors could ill afford to ignore the
inhabitants of the slave quarter. Although obstetric cases were not
very lucrative, they offered southern practitioners the opportunity
to ingratiate themselves with planters who might request other
services. Obstetric cases also allowed doctors to participate in important medical debates about women's health that were occurring
in Europe and in the United States generally. However much enslaved and free women might be set apart by status, their anatomy
did not appreciably differ.

The needs of slaveholders (who summoned medical attention for
slaves and who paid the bills) thus meshed with the interests of physicians; together they served as an incentive for antebellum doctors to
intervene to a greater or lesser degree across the entire spectrum of
slave women's reproductive health. Physicians attempted to manage
pregnancy and childbirth (most often when events took a turn for
the worse), but they also treated infertility, menstrual disorders,
cancers, and gynecological complaints stemming from complications of childbirth. The practitioners followed "heroic" medical traditions that emphasized boldness and recourse to extreme measures,
an approach to healing that was not peculiar to the South but that
took a unique form in the region.

Patients in the slave quarter were steeped in a different tradition
of birthing and healing from that of the doctor, one that emphasized
the powers of roots and herbs and the importance of social relations
(both those among slaves and those that cut across class lines). Black
women were distrustful of white doctors, who not only practiced a
peculiar form of medicine but also served as the agents of the slaveholders. They considered doctors ignorant of practices important for
ensuring the well-being of mother and child and much preferred
their own ways of birthing and handling women's illnesses—methods

that left matters in the hands of women rather than men. Like patients today, they wanted attendants who understood and respected their social circumstances and values, their fears, aspirations, joys, and sorrows. When doctors intervened, the women were instead tended by people who misunderstood or dismissed their traditions and anxieties and established goals for care based on slaveholders' and their own professional wishes. Women found themselves struggling to control their own bodies in a society that did not define control of one's body as a fundamental right of slaves. As white men intervened more and more in birthing and healing during the antebellum era, enslaved women were forced to keep secret certain of their own customs for ensuring women's health. The situation helped create a shared intimacy among women—a sense of community that at times extended to male slaves.[1]

A dual approach to the management of women's health developed on southern plantations as both black women and white men sought to enhance women's reproductive health in different ways and for different reasons.[2] Whenever feasible, bondwomen relied on one another for assistance with childbearing and other health matters rather than on the slaveholder's medical man. They put faith in the wisdom of elder women, pleaded for the amelioration of slavery's worst features, and trusted their own knowledge of the body to see them through pregnancy, childbirth, and aftercare. The doctors, in contrast, tended to reject or ignore time-honored customs of their patients, empathize with slaveholding clients, and emphasize their own heroic interventions. Whereas enslaved women's approach to well-being led them to seek changes in the material conditions of living and social relations as well as to administer medicinal teas and other preparations, doctors focused more narrowly on identifying a physiological problem (diagnosis) and its therapeutic correction (cure). Only rarely did doctors examine critically the social circumstances in which the women lived and in which they practiced medicine. Instead, they operated within the context of slave society to ensure that a black woman's reproductive behavior satisfied her owner—in other words, that she gave birth to children. When doctors joined with slaveholders to exercise control over enslaved women's health, medical practice became entwined with the cause of slavery's continuance. Simultaneously, slavery helped to further the medicalization of childbirth and the professionalization of medicine.

Childbirth is a biological, social, and cultural process,[3] as the encounters between black women and white men made clear; but doctors typically conceived of pregnancy and childbirth only as a naturally occurring biological process. They attempted to use biological science and learning to uphold power relations in the South, and they asserted their professional status by classifying as ignorant the folkways of slaves and black women's knowledge of their own bodies. By intervening socially and culturally, they transmuted pregnancy and childbirth into a series of unfolding events that reflected the choices made by physicians and their slaveholder clients. All the while, slave women had their own ideas of what was fitting and effective.

Neither doctors nor slaves were able or willing to bridge the social and cultural gap that separated physician and patient; each judged his or her own methods to be superior. Doctors claimed scientific sureness based on reason and knowledge acquired through literacy and professional associations. Enslaved women, in contrast, cited their own traditions wherein knowledge was gained through revelation, study of the natural environment, and scrutiny of social relationships. Although neither doctors nor slave women produced consistently positive outcomes, both claimed cultural certainty about how women's health should be managed.

Women's health is a particularly rich place to study efforts by the slaveholding class to exercise hegemonic sway over enslaved people.[4] While the ideal in plantation management called for owners to exercise mastery over the labor force, in actuality owners understood that they could not maintain total control over slaves and that many issues were up for negotiation. They limited their exercise of authority to matters deemed of particular interest. Their choice to focus on fertility and childbearing reflected the importance of human reproduction to the future of slavery.

The peculiarly intrusive nature of nineteenth-century medical therapies marked important new ways in which the material and emotional terrain of slavery expanded through the antebellum era. Slavery shaped even the most intimate of human acts—the conception and birthing of a baby. Women found themselves struggling in the most basic physical terms for control over fertility and childbearing and over health generally. Slaveholders acknowledged few constraints on their ability to intervene. Limits to medical knowledge posed one barrier, resistance by enslaved women another, but each was viewed more as an obstacle to be overcome than as an absolute boundary beyond which an owner's authority could not extend.

Encounters between enslaved women and slaveholders' doctors endow the themes familiar in the historical literature on slavery—white dominance and brutality, black resistance and community—with stark immediacy. The importance of their wombs and breasts for the future of slavery meant that the struggle for domination centered on women's bodies. The women suffered a peculiar form of violence as slaveholders and doctors exploited female anatomy for their own purposes. Thus women experienced slavery differently from men precisely because of their childbearing experiences.[5]

It is impossible to know what percentage of enslaved women encountered the slaveholder's doctor in conjunction with pregnancy, childbirth, or reproductive ailments. Southern doctors were expected to know about and treat the many different medical problems that arose in their clientele, including enslaved women. Numerous medical publications, southern agricultural journals, letters and diaries of slaveholders, and testimonies of former slaves make it clear that doctors were called upon regularly to attend to enslaved women in the late antebellum years, particularly for problem pregnancies. It seems likely, as one scholar of southern medicine has noted, that beginning doctors frequently witnessed their first case of childbirth in the slave quarter.[6] Menstrual problems, which resulted in days lost from labor as well as in infertility, also prompted planters to seek medical cures from professionals. Numerous other gynecological problems added to the number of enslaved women treated by physicians. The regular appearance of enslaved women as patients in published case histories on women's health suggests an important role for bondwomen in the development and discussion of medical practice related to human reproduction. Obstetrics and gynecology would not emerge as specialties until after the Civil War; meanwhile general practitioners did what they could when called upon, gaining experience and helping to shape standard obstetric and gynecologic practice in the process.

Birthing a Slave examines encounters between black mothers and white doctors in the South during the decades leading up to and immediately after the Civil War. The pages that follow focus on the contest that evolved between physicians, slaveholders, and enslaved women as each attempted to manage human reproduction for his or her own purpose and according to a different understanding of how best to ensure woman's health and the perpetuation of a people in bondage. The text is organized thematically around a woman's reproductive life: fertility, pregnancy, childbirth, postnatal complications, gynecological disorders, and the related topic of cancer and other tumors. The final chapter explores how encounters between black women and white doctors changed after emancipation and thus elucidates slavery's importance for shaping medical practice.

The main body of evidence lies in the published writings of physicians, the records of slaveholders, and accounts by former slaves and their descendants. Doctors wrote case histories and other sorts of articles for publication and kept records related to their medical practices. Medical journals, many of which originated in the antebellum era, allowed physicians to share the benefit of their growing knowledge with colleagues, to solicit reaction to or refinement of new medical treatment from peers, and to call attention to their individual command of the healing art. They regularly included the proceedings of medical societies and associations, and in this way the journals managed to encapsulate the ideas and experiences of physicians who for lack of time or inclination never wrote letters and essays for publication.[7] Slaveholders also recorded events related to women's health in farm books, business papers, and correspondence. Agricultural journals flourished in the antebellum South; these frequently addressed the management of slaves. Former slaves related their own version of events, sometimes in memoirs but also in oral interviews, the most ambitious of which were conducted by U.S. officials during the 1930s as part of the Federal Writers' Project of the Works Progress Administration (WPA). Some recounted their own experiences with pregnancy, childbirth, and other health matters; others shared the experiences of loved ones either witnessed firsthand or as told to them by friends or relatives, particularly parents. Their voices tell the story of medicine as part of the history of slavery.

1

Procreation

WHEN IN THE 1930S LULU WILSON WAS INTERVIEWED ABOUT HER life before the Civil War, she described herself as an "old time slavery woman." She had "plenty to say about slavery" and why it should never be brought back. She had been born about 1841 near the Mammoth Cave in Barren County, Kentucky, to an enslaved woman and a free man of color on a plantation belonging to the Wash Hodges family. After Lulu's birth, "some time passed" but no other children were born of her parent's union. Believing that Lulu's father "was too old and wore out for breedin'," the Hodges used dogs to "run him away from the place." Lulu never saw him again. Her mother, who soon took up with a new man, said he had left for a free state. The Hodges were pleased because Lulu's mother gave birth to sixteen more children who lived to adulthood.[1]

Lulu lived a hard life as a child. Sorely missing her father, she soon found herself living apart from her mother in the owner's house, where she learned to wash, iron, clean house, and milk cows to please her mistress. She cried for her mother, "but I had to work," she explained. She grew up hearing about such atrocities as a black man whose legs were nearly eaten off by dogs when he tried to escape slavery. She endured punishments that included having her hands tied and snuff rubbed in her eyes. When she was about thirteen or fourteen, her mistress told her she "ought to marry." Arrangements were soon made to pair her with an enslaved man belonging to the master's nephew. Wash Hodges read a passage from the Bible to mark the occasion. Not long afterward the mistress engaged a doctor to attend the bride. He "told me that less'n I had a baby, old as I was and married, I'd start in on spasms," the former slave recalled. "So it twan't long 'til I had a baby." Lulu apparently yielded to the advice of mistress and doctor, although it remains unclear whether she meant she became sexually active, took action to enhance her fertility, or abandoned efforts to prevent pregnancy. She gave birth to a son. Shortly after, the Civil War brought about a general emancipation of slaves. "I left the Hodges and felt like it was a fine good riddance," she said.

Family was important to Lulu. After her first husband died (soon after the war), she remarried. Her only son grew to adulthood, but he, too, died young, though not before having a child of his own. Her grandson, who became the father of four children, was the light of Lulu's life. "I'm crazy 'bout that boy," she told an interviewer in the 1930s who was collecting stories as part of a government effort to interview former slaves. She also told of a lifetime spent as a nurse waiting on sick people. Nurturing others extended beyond her immediate family.

These sketchy details hint at an important aspect of slavery that has been all too often ignored: slaveholders expected to appropriate and exploit the reproductive lives of enslaved women. Control of one's body was not a fundamental right of slaves. Emboldened by law and custom to do with human chattels as they wished, the Hodges family and other owners felt entitled to intervene in even the most intimate of matters. Women's childbearing capacity became a commodity that could be traded in the market for profit.

During the antebellum era the expectation increased among members of the owning class that enslaved women would contribute to the economic success of the plantation not only through productive labor but also through procreation. The idea was at once both powerful and seductive and shaped the way women experienced enslavement, the way owners thought about the future of slave society, and the way doctors practiced medicine.[2] Bondwomen who did not achieve motherhood because they could not become pregnant, carry an infant to term, or keep a child alive came to be viewed as a problem in need of correction. Slaveholders tried a variety of means to boost the number of children born to enslaved mothers, including medical treatment. As slaveholders called upon their services, doctors were increasingly drawn into the drama of slavery's perpetuation. They held out hope that the female deficiency known as barrenness might be cured.

Enslaved people, like slave owners, valued motherhood. They cherished children for reasons of their own. Family life offered a welcome respite from the dehumanizing slave regime. Children especially represented a chance to love and be loved in return. On a practical level, daughters and sons also performed tasks that helped establish an economic foundation for family life that would otherwise have been more vulnerable to the manipulation of slaveholders. While parents labored as the slaveholder demanded in the field or at another worksite, young children could fish, trap animals, gather fruit and nuts, and otherwise secure food for the family table. Their efforts supplemented the owner's food allotments, generally doled out to families once each week, and rendered the slave family less dependent on an owner for sustenance. Everyone knew that owners might (and sometimes did) withhold food rations as a means of forcing compliance with their rules. Contributions of food by children assured the family that they might cope at least for a while under these conditions.[3]

Children also could be counted upon to assist with cleaning, cooking, and caring for younger siblings. They gathered chips and wood for fuel and herbs for making medicine. At times they lent a hand to parents in completing chores dictated by owners. For example, some women were expected to card (comb the seeds from) a specific amount of cotton after they finished cultivating the crop in the field. Children could help with this chore and free up a mother's time to perform another activity of benefit to her family. Working together, family members might card not only the owner's cotton but also additional fiber for the family's use. If the children completed much of this work, the mother might find time to spin the extra fiber into thread, weave the thread into cloth, and sew the cloth into garments. Such activities helped define the slave family as a meaningful unit of production.

Except on the smallest and most isolated slaveholdings, enslaved families were part of a larger community of enslaved people. Some of these communities were specific to the property of one slaveholder, but others extended beyond the boundaries of a particular owner's estate to encompass enslaved people living on neighboring plantations. Although slaveholders attempted to restrict movement of bondmen and women across property lines, in practice many enslaved people moved around the countryside and town with and without an owner's permission. The business interests of owners sometimes brought slaves together, as when owners gathered workers from more than one holding to harvest a crop or when individual slaveholders sent slaves to market to purchase or sell commodities. In addition, slaves used time off from work to visit neighboring slaves in secret. Generally slaves worked for owners from sunup to sundown six days a week, but they considered the time from sunset to sunrise their own. Communal activities, some of which were carried out with the owner's knowledge, included but were not limited to hunting, fishing, storytelling, music making, and dancing. The need for midwives and healers also brought slaves together. Lulu Wilson played an active role in the provision of health care to the black community through her role as nurse.

When the slaveholder's physician came to the quarter at the slaveholder's request, he encountered not only the patient but also members of a community. Some had a claim to the calling of midwife or healer that superseded his own. At times slaves cooperated with the slaveholder's physician in managing women's health, but at others they acted out of the sight of whites, to ensure the well-being of individual women as well as the enslaved community. Procreation of the enslaved population was not the exclusive domain of either the slaveholder or the slaveholder's physician.

———

Southern slave owners paid increased attention to the birth of slave children as the nation expanded westward and cotton planting grew in importance. By the 1820s planters and would-be planters were moving in large numbers to places previously unavailable for settlement and growing the fiber for sale in Europe and New England, where a textile industry was beginning to thrive. The extension of the so-called Cotton Kingdom required new laborers. As of 1808, when Congress ended the nation's participation in the international slave trade, planters could no longer import additional slaves from Africa or the West Indies; the only practical way of increasing the number of slave laborers was through new births. If enslaved mothers did not bear sufficient numbers of children to take the place of aged and dying workers, the South could not continue as a slave society.

Women entering their childbearing years—especially those who had proven their fertility through the birth of a baby—sold easily and for a high price. Former slave Boston Blackwell, who witnessed the sale of two women in Memphis, Tennessee, reported that a girl of fifteen who had no children sold for $800, but a "breeding woman" sold for $1,500. Robert Williams, who was sold in a slave mart alongside a female, reported that she brought "a big price" because the purchaser believed she would "bring in good children." Millie Williams, a former slave whose owner sold her at auction, maintained that men usually sold for more than women, but exceptions occurred for a woman who had birthed a lot of children. The size of her family indicated that she was "a good breeder."[4]

Human reproduction was so important to the continuation of slavery that members of the South's ruling class willed their heirs the unborn children of slaves as well as living people. Anna Matilda King of Georgia assured her daughter that she would inherit not only the enslaved Christiann but also "her child & future children." "If it was not for my children I would not care what became of the negros," Elizabeth Scott Neblett wrote her absent husband during the Civil War. Left to work the Neblett plantation on her own and plagued by a less-than-competent overseer, a shortage of goods, and illness among the enslaved farmhands, Neblett maintained that she would gladly do without slaves to save the bother of managing them, but for her children's sake she could not let them go.[5] This wish to benefit future generations of slaveholding families pressed owners to look for ways of ensuring that enslaved mothers bore plenty of children. Barren women were cause for concern.

The "problem" of slavery's perpetuation was exacerbated throughout the antebellum era by politics. Successive acquisitions of territory extended the country westward, beyond the Mississippi into Texas and finally to the Pacific. Americans understood that eventually this territory would be populated, and its people would request admission to the Union as separate states. Would these states enter as slave states, enhancing the power of the South within the national government? Or would the new states bar slavery and bolster the interests of the North in national politics? California, acquired as a result of war with Mexico, entered the Union in 1850 with a constitution that banned slavery, but it was possible that Texas and other territory in the Southwest might be carved into states more sympathetic to the extension of the southern institution.

Some Americans were eager to see the nation's boundaries pushed farther southward, into Cuba or Central America. In 1848 President James K. Polk offered Spain $100 million for the island of Cuba, and similar offers were made repeatedly (but unsuccessfully) over the next decade. If the nation extended into Cuba, where would the slaves be found to work Cuba's sugar plantations? Its slave population historically had been unable to sustain itself except through the ongoing importation of enslaved Africans.[6] Advocates of slavery's extension could hold out little hope that the United States would reauthorize participation in the international slave trade. Rather, slaves would have to be obtained through the interregional slave trade, and this trade depended on the birth and survival of bonded infants in older regions of the South. With so much at stake, black women's reproductive role became politically, as well as economically, decisive.

Southern slaveholders' perceived need for additional slaves did not play out solely as abstract political or economic rhetoric. It helped to justify increased emphasis on the birth of children in the slave quarter. Every woman of an appropriate age needed to bear children. Most did for reasons similar to those of other nineteenth-century parents: they cherished children but also counted on them to help out around the house and yard when they grew old enough. In addition, sexual relationships usually resulted in pregnancy in the days before effective birth control was known. Women who did not readily become mothers were subjected to scrutiny and possible action.

Early in the nineteenth century, slaveholders looked to both heaven and earth for answers to why a childless woman had not given birth. They were willing to attribute a role to providence, but they also scrutinized the behavior of the woman herself and the circumstances in which she lived. Generally, owners adhered to a racist assumption that all black women were fecund—more so than whites—and would breed if given the chance.[7] Most provided an opportunity for a woman to become a mother by ensuring that she had access to a mate, even if it meant tolerating the visits of an enslaved man living on another plantation or purchasing additional slaves.

Purchases of slaves could be calculated to ensure that a planter had a sufficient number of women "of breeding age" and that each woman had a suitable sexual partner at hand. North Carolina planter

Jessup Powell went to Richmond specifically "to buy good breeders," according to one of his former slaves. Another North Carolina master became wealthy as the result of purchasing two women of child-bearing age. One of them, Long Peggy, was particularly prolific and reportedly gave birth to twenty-five babies. After purchasing Fanny from Virginia and Jim from Louisiana, Mississippi master Bill Gordon arranged for them to live together, which they did. Fanny gave birth to five children before slavery ended. Georgia slaveholder David Ferguson purchased Jacob Gilbert specifically as a husband for an enslaved woman. Planter Bill Alford of Mississippi first purchased Jacob Dickerson. Shortly after, he bought Sally. When he brought Sally home he said to Jacob, "I brung you a good woman, take her an' live wid her." The couple consented, and according to their son lived contentedly thereafter.[8]

Not all slaves accepted planter matchmaking docilely, but the willingness of some couples to mate under such circumstances is not hard to understand given that the majority of enslaved people wanted to marry and have families. The constraints that enslavement placed upon a man's or woman's ability to choose a spouse rendered marriage difficult. In an effort to exert mastery in plantation management, owners restricted movement off the plantation and withheld resources from couples who mated without their approval. Only those couples who gained an owner's consent for marriage obtained separate housing with furnishings, patches of land for growing foodstuff, passes to visit one another if husband and wife lived on separate plantations, and other accouterments of married life. Any couple who did not have the approval of an owner might be denied access to material resources as well as the owner's assistance in maintaining family ties.[9] Although no slave couple could be certain that they would be allowed to remain together, everyone knew that an owner was more likely to respect a union that had been approved. For these reasons, a woman or man would have thought long and hard before rejecting a spouse proposed by the owner.

Not all owners purchased spouses specifically for particular slaves. Those who did not might hurry women to have children in other ways. Many exploited an attraction that already existed by encouraging or insisting on marriage. Jacob Thomas married Phoebe the year the Civil War began. Their courtship lasted only a brief time, Jacob later recalled, because the master gave his permission for marriage "'fore I axes fer hit." Georgina Gibbs testified that her Virginia master "would marry" any couple he saw spending time together. She apparently meant that he would press the pair to live together as husband and wife. For youths experiencing the glow of first love and sexual attraction, mild pressure often proved effectual.[10]

An owner who suspected a couple of courting might persuade the man and woman to set up a household by offering a variety of inducements. These could consist of not only separate housing, small patches of land, and passes but also chickens or other animals and time to perform domestic tasks. Rewards for motherhood followed the birth of children. These included "extra clothing," exemption from harsh punishment, even (rarely) freedom. Lula Cottonham Walker had to work hard as a slave in Alabama, according to her later testimony, but the mother of eight children was never beaten. If the master had a sow that gave birth to a litter of pigs each year, he would not take a stick and beat it. It was the same with his slaves, she offered by way of explanation. Betsey Calcote Cotten's Mississippi master promised her freedom if she bore ten children. He kept his word in 1833 after the birth of Cotten's tenth child. Her children remained enslaved.[11]

Some women were able to avoid field or other arduous labor as the result of bearing children. A woman with six living children on one plantation had Saturday to herself, presumably to care for them. Jane Cash did not have to work hard, her granddaughter maintained, because "she was a good breeder." The slave woman Eliza had so many children that she was considered an asset to the plantation as a result of this alone. She did no more work than she wished to do for her own (and presumably her family's) benefit. Rhody Jones also was taken out of the field because she had a lot of children, according to her daughter Annie Coley. The mother of twelve did not avoid work altogether: she was expected to weave ten yards of cloth a day. Her owner excused her from more taxing labor, however. "A 'breeder' always fared better than the majority of female slaves," former slave Douglas Parish observed.[12]

Slaves considered rewards for motherhood a customary right and acted proactively to secure them from the owner. Although slaveholders could command obedience by law, by custom slaves sometimes negotiated better treatment by bargaining. Owners knew only too well that slaves could work slowly, poorly, or not at all when confronted with intolerable conditions. Because such outcomes entailed a financial cost as well as a breach of the owner's prerogative to command, most owners preferred to avoid a direct confrontation by allowing slaves a degree of latitude to negotiate their work and living conditions. Discussions were not between equals; the slaveholders always held the upper hand. They could (and frequently did) resort to violence to get their way. Yet the practice whereby slaveholders and slaves came to an understanding about the terms of servitude made room for slaves to protest the most egregious terms of bondage and served as a way of preventing other, more vigorous forms of dissent. Jane Brown of Arkansas was "a fast breeder," but she was unable to keep up with the work expected of her. Because it was common for slaves to be whipped when they failed to complete assigned chores, Jane and her husband William ran away. While hiding in a thicket of canes, Jane gave birth to their child. The Browns returned to the Woodlawn plantation after extracting from owners David and Ann Hunt a pledge that Jane's work would consist solely of taking care of the children. In return the couple would not run away again. Altogether the Browns had ten children, including three sets of twins.[13]

Childless women could not expect any of the rewards or concessions available to mothers. Single women without children lived with parents or other enslaved families, dependent on them not only for shelter but also for a share of the family's food, clothing, and other resources. If they took husbands, their situation remained much the same until the birth of a child, particularly in the upper South, where slaveholdings tended to be relatively small and husbands and wives frequently lived apart because they belonged to different owners. Their work regimens were similar to those of men. Mandy Buford did the same work as the men on her Arkansas plantation because, according to her niece, "she wasn't no multiplying woman." The disparity between men's and women's work could be considerable. In the case of cotton picking, the difference could be measured by the pound. On the Bertrand estate in Jefferson County, Arkansas, the men were expected to pick 300 pounds, women 200. Agricultural tasks also might be measured by the row. In Alabama on George Walker's plantation, men were expected to hoe each day seventy rows, seventy yards long; women had to hoe only sixty rows. Childless women could be pressed to do as much as a man.[14]

There were other repercussions for barrenness. Young women who had not demonstrated fertility faced the possibility of separation from family as well as additional labor, as the story of Lulu Wilson's mother illustrates. If a married couple lived together for long without having a baby, North Carolina planter Joe Fevors Cutt would force both husband and wife to choose new partners. Former slave Henry Bobbitt maintained that many marriages did not last longer than five years because if no children were born within that period, husbands and wives were expected to find other spouses.[15]

More commonly, childless women were sold. If a woman did not "breed," in the parlance of the slaveholder, she was put on the market, explained Henry Banner, who experienced slavery firsthand in both Virginia and Tennessee. "You better have them whitefolks

some babies iffen you didn't wanta be sold," former Tennessee slave
Alice Douglass recalled. Mary Grayson, enslaved in the Oklahoma
territory, was sold twice for infertility. Her Creek Indian owner—believing her "too young to breed"—sold her to another, who waited a
while before deciding she was not a "good breeder" and selling her
again.[16]

The emotional pain of losing family members in this way is
impossible for postslavery generations to fathom. Marriages were
broken up, siblings split apart, older children separated from parents.
Much of the selling occurred in states of the upper South, where
there was a surplus of labor. Planters in the cotton-growing region of
the lower South were eager to have whatever laborers the interre-
gional slave trade could provide. The memories of three freed people
of their time in Virginia capture some of the sense of loss. Fannie
Berry, who witnessed sales near her home, still shuddered decades
later to think of cotton country. "I ain't never seen dar an' I don't
wanta!" she cried. Anna Harris maintained in the 1930s that she had
never allowed a white person to enter her house. They sold "my sister
Kate," she told a black interviewer sent by the federal government
to collect the stories of former slaves. Some "folks say white folks is
all right dese days," she admitted. "Maybe dey is, maybe dey isn't.
But I can't stand to see 'em. Not on my place." Samuel Walter
Chilton also told of slave sales to the deep South. It "was a sad
partin' time," he recalled.[17]

The fact that a woman proved a poor breeder did not necessarily
mean she was infertile. Slaveholders were often poor judges of
whether a woman could bear children. Because Miny had never
given birth, her Virginia owner sold her to a man named Taylor.
Along came eleven children, much to the delight of her descendants,
who enjoyed telling the story. When an enslaved woman called
Minerva was badly burned and scarred, her owners were "disappointed because before the accident they had thought she would be a
good breeder." It is unclear whether they feared she would be unable

to attract a mate, conceive, or bring a baby to term, or perhaps all three; but their assessment proved wrong. Minerva gave birth to more than one child, including her namesake, Minerva Davis, who related these facts years after slavery had ended. An Alabama planter traded a woman he thought could not have children, only to learn two months later that she "was heavy with child." When he tried to buy her back, her new owner refused, much to the original slaveholder's consternation.[18] The slaveholder's poor judgment in such cases reflected in part common misperceptions about the causes of infertility as well as the difficulty of enforcing particular sexual relations upon others. Owners did not know, for example, that to become pregnant a woman must have sex during ovulation. Even if they had known, they would not have been able to predict when a particular woman ovulated, nor would they have been able to police behavior in the slave quarter to ensure that each woman of childbearing age engaged in sex at an appropriate time.

Slaveholders were well aware that women who were sold because they did not bear children sometimes gave birth at a later date. Indeed, planter Addison (or Adubon) Hilliard of Louisiana unknowingly sold a woman who was pregnant to Sack P. Gee. Complications of pregnancy rendered her health unstable, and she may have been returned to her original owner. Her child, Isaac Adams, remained the property of her second owner, however. Such situations galled slaveholders, who evaluated the situation not only as an economic or disciplinary problem but also as evidence of their ability to manage a plantation, including the laborers who toiled on it. Southern white men staked their reputations on the mastery of others. There was no honor in misjudging slaves, particularly female slaves.[19]

Miscalculations such as these explain in part the efforts undertaken by some slaveholders to intervene directly in sexual relationships among slaves. They tried to orchestrate courting by insisting that couples obtain an owner's approval before seeing each other.

Some masters and mistresses went so far as to write love letters on behalf of slaves. Wedding ceremonies also required prior approval by the owner. On the Louisiana plantation where Jacob Aldrich was enslaved, the master not only insisted on sanctioning marriages between slave couples but also quizzed them the next morning about whether they had consummated the union. If not, the reluctant partner would receive fifty lashes.[20]

Forced pairings were uncommon, but slaveholders attempted them from time to time. Reverend Robert Barr, whose parents were enslaved in Mississippi, believed that masters would press slaves to marry "whether you liked it or didn't." Barr likened the procedure to breeding horses or cows. "If they told a woman to go to a man and she didn't, they would whip her," he maintained. In North Carolina, Ambrose Hilliard Douglass received "a sound beating" when he refused to mate with a woman his master had chosen for him. "Big Jim" McClean forced slaves to mate indiscriminately, according to two of his former slaves. If either one of the pair showed the slightest reluctance, he "would make them consummate this relationship in his presence." Former slave Virginia Davis testified that the master of her aunt, Eliza Williamson, "put her and her husband together." The degree of force used to pair this couple is unclear, but Davis' choice of words suggests at least some form of coercion. In North Carolina Rilla McCullough was told by her master that she had to take a strong black man living on a nearby plantation as her husband. Rilla, who was only sixteen at the time, acquiesced and eventually learned to love the man. Her adjustment may have been aided by the support of her mother, who had been "put to . . . several different men . . . just about the same as if she had been a cow or sow," according to one of her descendants.[21]

Slave women tended to have their first children between the ages of twenty and twenty-one, somewhat younger than southern white women at first birth.[22] This phenomenon may have been the result of owner interference. Individual women may have chosen partners and had children at an early age in the hope that doing so would deter owners from forcing unwanted partners upon them or putting them up for sale. However, clearly some women waited long enough to have children—possibly because they could not find partners to their own liking or because they simply could not get pregnant—that they were sold, victims of the slaveholder's desire for an increasing slave population.

Some former slaves charged that owners forcefully bred slaves not only to enlarge their workforce but also to "improve" their "stock." Henry H. Buttler claimed that his former owners in Virginia and Arkansas attempted to manipulate reproduction in the slave quarter to produce superior workers. Neither of his masters would approve a match unless they "considered it a proper mating," Buttler explained, and the only men and women who received permission were those the owner expected to produce offspring with "perfect physiques." A North Carolinian claimed firsthand knowledge of the practice whereby masters assigned "large, hale [and] hearty" men from other plantations as husbands to women and girls, some as young as twelve or thirteen, in an effort to produce slaves with desirable physical traits. Rose Williams recalled that she was paired against her wishes in Texas with a man named Rufus because both were portly. Citing his enslaved father as his source of information, J. F. Boone claimed that healthy men and women—those who had proven themselves capable of having children—would be "stalled up" and not even released for work until they had bred like horses and cattle. Judge Wilkerson of Florida "selected the strongest and best male and female slaves and mated them exclusively for breeding" because he "found it very profitable," according to one of his former slaves.[23]

Other informants spoke of "stockmen" assigned the role of stud. One former slave testified that a stockman would be locked in a room with women of childbearing age overnight. In the morning, he would be quizzed about what had happened. If he did not engage in sex (the women might resist him), his owner would not be paid for his services. Emma Barr of Arkansas reported her mother's allegation that one of her owners kept a "fine man" whose duty it was to impregnate the house women. The man performed no difficult labor, and the other slaves—both men and women—"hated him," an indication that any man who cooperated with such a scheme was despised by other slaves. One Louisiana planter with sizable slaveholdings, William Maddox, allowed the majority of slaves to choose spouses to their liking, except for about ten women, whom he bred to a large man. His goal was physically fit children who might be sold for a good price. Those planters who attempted to breed slaves generally relied on their own judgment in selecting women and men to mate. Maddox took no chances, however. He hired a doctor to examine both the women and the man to ensure that all were in good health before implementing his scheme.[24]

Wash Austin achieved a degree of notoriety as a "stud" in Texas shortly before the Civil War. He was sold as a slave eight times—his good looks and big muscles attracted buyers—but many an owner ended up disappointed if not downright angry when Austin proved an incompetent worker. One enterprising slaveholder—no doubt in an attempt to recoup his purchase price—began offering the slave to gullible and greedy neighbors who hoped not only to gain a working hand but also to improve their slave "stock" by having a seemingly strong and handsome man impregnate their bondwomen. When the new owners realized that Austin was not what he seemed, his former owner offered to buy him back at a reduced price.[25] It is possible that Austin continued for a time to secure money for his master in this fashion. More likely the scam came to an end as word spread that Austin's virility was more apparent than real.

The need to keep silent about certain sexual practices in the slave quarter fueled unrestrained speculation about paternal identity. If a child's parent was the master or another white man in the family or neighborhood, there might be repercussions for speaking this truth publicly, including the sale of the mother, child, or both. Similarly, some children were the sons or daughters of a forbidden relationship within the slave community. When a woman went against her owner's wishes and entered into a relationship forbidden by her owner, she might attempt to protect her child and the man by refusing to reveal his identity, even to the child. Children were (are) notorious tattletales, and some could not be entrusted with the name of a father, at least until they were old enough to keep it secret. A small number of children were parted at an early age from both parents by sale or death. The situation in which the paternity of a child was known only to two or a few people was uncommon, but it arose often enough to fuel whispered gossip concerning stud men. The enslaved Sam Jones Washington growing up in Texas never knew his father. Years later he speculated that his owner hired the man from another slaveholder to impregnate his mother. Such a man was called a "travelin' nigger," Washington explained. They came, performed a service, and then returned to their owner's home.[26]

Not many planters tried to breed slaves through forced pairings. Given the predisposition of slaves to become parents, they were needless. As one Mississippi slaveholder maintained, no studs were necessary, because slaves formed sexual relationships on their own. Yet slaveholders did nothing to dissuade slaves from believing that force might be used. This potential threat frightened slaves and helps explain why so many former slaves remembered stories about forced pairing on a nearby plantation if not their own. The anxiety produced by the possibility of forced breeding was real and prevalent.[27] For this reason, perhaps, slaves enjoyed passing along stories of a man like Austin who managed to fool owners about his virility.

Nancy and Tip managed to thwart their Louisiana master's plan to pair them. When the master first decided that the two should mate, Tip was willing to go along. Nancy resisted, however, and received a whipping as a result. Feeling sorry for Nancy, Tip suggested that they live together without establishing a sexual relationship.

After several months the master, frustrated at the lack of a visible pregnancy, agreed to let Nancy remarry, this time to a man of her own choosing. The change of heart had a happy ending as far as the master was concerned: a child born every year until the Civil War ended the couple's enslavement. Nancy, too, was pleased at the outcome, and Tip was presumably free to find a partner who would love him in return. Such tales resembled the trickster tales enjoyed by slaves wherein the weak and powerless overcame the strong and powerful through wit and cunning.[28]

Stories about slaves who managed to manipulate to their own advantage an owner's desire to mate particular slaves had credibility because of the difficulty inherent in forcing men and women to establish intimate relationships against their will. Former slave Willie Blackwell acknowledged that some owners deliberately chose big and powerful men as partners for their female slaves, but he also observed that they had difficulty getting couples to cooperate. Considerable visiting went on between dark and morning no matter what owners wanted. If an owner wanted to pair a "comely wench" with a particular man, he had no choice but to sell any other man who maintained an interest in her. But even this step might not resolve the problem of policing the relationship. The man might manage somehow to visit her despite the distance separating the couple. Only if he was sold "a thousand miles away" could an owner keep a man apart from the woman he loved, Blackwell observed. Family feelings could stay strong for many years, and a couple might remain devoted to each other across space and time. Enslaved couples had their own ideas of whom they wished to marry, and they generally did not yield readily to the dictates of owners in this facet of life.[29]

More common than forced pairings among slaves were forced sexual encounters between white men and black women. Potential sexual partners of enslaved women included the master, his sons, neighboring planters, visitors of the slaveholding family, traveling salesmen, and hired workers. Although some relationships were less coercive than others, rape occurred and was discussed privately if not publicly throughout the region. When Virginia physician William G. Craghead examined a sixteen-year-old slave who was suffering from vaginal pain, he immediately suspected rape as the cause. Charles A. Hentz recorded a case of sexual abuse in his autobiography. The young physician was boarding at a home in Florida when one of the house servants, Celia, bore the child of the householder's son. Testimony from former slaves provides further evidence of the widespread nature of rape and other forms of sexual exploitation by whites. One Kentucky slave observed her master's practice of fathering the first child of each woman enslaved on his plantation. It is not clear that sexual exploitation occurred with the idea of expanding the size of a particular slaveholding, but slaves understood this as the end result of rape and other types of coerced sex, since children inherited the slave status of the mother. In their minds, forced sex, population growth, and the perpetuation of slavery were inextricably linked.[30]

Although slaveholders intervened with human reproduction in the slave quarter in a variety of ways, they did not always find the results satisfactory. Time and again, their efforts were foiled by the determination of slaves to keep reproductive matters under their own control. To help achieve the goal of increasing the size of the slave population, some slaveholders, like Lulu Wilson's owner, turned to medical men.

Slaveholders placed increased emphasis on the importance of slave women's reproductive role as male midwifery was starting to gain acceptance in Europe and the United States and as doctors were becoming immersed in the study of "Woman" generally. South Carolina–born D. Warren Brickell, who went on to become a noted gynecologist in New Orleans, made gynecology a subject of special study when he attended the University of Pennsylvania in the 1840s. Moses M. Pallen, who studied medicine at the University of Virginia and served as a professor at the St. Louis Medical College

during the late antebellum period, was said to have shared with his
students "every detail of the lying-in period." By 1854 Warren Stone
could remark in the pages of the *New Orleans Medical News and
Hospital Gazette* that "the diseases of the uterus have, of late years,
engaged the special attention of many men eminent in the profession."[31] Medical texts increasingly elaborated on the subject.
Through the antebellum era, owners more and more turned to medical men, who they hoped would identify the cause of barrenness and
provide a cure, help ensure that enslaved women would bring a pregnancy to term, assist at the childbed in difficult cases, treat complications from childbirth, surgically repair reproductive organs, treat
cancerous and other tumors, and provide advice and assistance for all
the diseases of women. By securing the aid of physicians, owners
hoped to extend their mastery over slaves to include not only social
relations but also bodily functions related to human reproduction.
Doing so would ensure not only a well-ordered plantation for the
present but also a secure future for generations of slaveholders to
come.

For their part, physicians argued that it behooved planters—
some of whom attempted to treat slave health problems by consulting medical manuals published for home use—to seek advice from
physicians skilled in midwifery. Chronic health conditions that affected the "procreative relationship" warranted attention, since "the
raising . . . of young negroes on a plantation is an important item of
interest on our capital," one doctor observed. Another expressed a
belief (opposite that of prevailing wisdom) that infertility occurred
more commonly among black than white women.[32] The dissemination of such statements by medical men both reinforced and helped
create concern among slaveholders about their ability to maintain or
expand an enslaved labor force. They encouraged slave owners to
seek medical assistance in overcoming the "problem" of expanding
slavery into western territories and into future generations.

The subject of infertility led doctors to investigate issues of sex and sexuality, matters not generally discussed publicly. Research by W. Tyler Smith, for example, concluded that women reached orgasm during sex but that orgasm was not essential for conception. Such frank discussions of sexuality seemed scandalous at first, even to physicians. When a copy of *The Causes and Curative Treatment of Sterility, with a Preliminary Statement of the Physiology of Generation* arrived, evidently for review, at the offices of the *Atlanta Medical and Surgical Journal,* the editors pronounced it marred by "a touch of obscenity." An advertisement for the book that appeared in the *New York Tribune* and the *Western Lancet* was even worse—downright indecent, in part because it was intended "for the public eye."[33] Yet such research was seen as directly relevant to the problem of infertility.

In the South, rhetoric surrounding barrenness took a peculiar turn. The focus was on enslaved women in general and on the reproductive history of specific women. The topic came up in everyday conversations related to the profitability of plantations, the management of labor, and the monetary worth of individual slaves. These conversations, as one historian has pointed out, did much to foster notions of the black woman as "Jezebel," a woman governed by her libido. "People accustomed to speaking and writing about the bondwoman's reproductive abilities could hardly help associating her with licentious behavior," writes Deborah Gray White.[34] Both medical discourse and treatment regimens reflected and reinforced this stereotype, which served to dehumanize black women at the very time that they were engaging in the most human of acts—birthing a child. The frank discourse concerning a slave woman's reproductive capacity encouraged slaveholders and doctors to extend the conversation to ways of promoting fertility.

Enslaved women and men resisted efforts by slaveholders and their physician allies to define human reproduction in the slave quarter as a medical problem and to exert control over this aspect of life. Enslaved people were appalled by owners' insistence that only they or their physician representatives could determine acceptable patterns of fertility, positive or negative outcomes from pregnancy, appropriate procedures for childbirth, and effective means of curing or coping with gynecological disorders. Slaves were convinced that the events surrounding fertility, pregnancy, and childbirth specifically and women's health generally fell under their purview. Human reproduction was an unfolding series of events that held meaning only insofar as they were understood within the narrative of the lives of the mother, other relatives, and members of the surrounding enslaved community.

———

By the late antebellum years, slaveholders were regularly eliciting the assistance of physicians in treating slave women's health problems. Medicine was emerging as a profession, and new ideas were evolving about who should do what and how with regard to medical treatment. Medical journals increased in number, and southern doctors who took to writing for them frequently focused on the case narrative, in which they played the part of hero. As a historian of southern medicine has observed, the case narrative was "the story of something gone wrong, and of the doctor's attempt to restore what had been lost."[35] In the case of enslaved women, one thing that could go wrong was barrenness. Southern doctors with their new interest in women's health seemed situated to assist with this medical problem.

The involvement of doctors with enslaved women's reproductive health represented an expansion of the slaveholder's domain—an intrusion into an area of life that had once been under the purview of the slave. Encroachment into the private lives of slaves had begun in the eighteenth century, when a plantation economy began to characterize the South. Planters, who had once been satisfied to have slaves feed and clothe themselves, began issuing rations and allotting clothing in an attempt to rationalize plantation operations and thereby increase the time slaves spent cultivating the cash crop. By the middle of the nineteenth century, planters were rationalizing sick care in an effort to improve both production and reproduction. As with their provision of food and clothing, planters cited their oversight of sick care as evidence of their compassion.[36] They gradually extended this concern to women's reproductive health. From the standpoint of enslaved women, the slave owner's foray into the scientific management of their bodies represented something beyond benevolence. It was an effort to decrease the importance of women's community and to substitute the ways of white men for those of black women. The women struggled to assert their own customs. Rather than acquiescing in slaveholders' demands that they bear as many children as possible, enslaved women attempted to regulate childbearing to accord with their own notions of the proper timing and frequency of motherhood. In resisting the dominion of white men in this regard, black women cast themselves as central actors in the unfolding drama that constituted slave life and culture in the antebellum South.

2

Healers

IN 1838 AN ALABAMA SLAVE WOMAN WHO HAD RECENTLY GIVEN birth developed a chill, followed by a fever, prompting her owner to request the assistance of physician J. Y. Bassett. To relieve her symptoms, the doctor tried quinine and calomel (mercurous chloride, widely used to evacuate the bowels in the days before it was known to be toxic), but later that day, she appeared "hot, dry, and restless; her pulse fluctuating, and mind wandering. I *poured* over her *slowly* two buckets of cold water," the doctor later recalled. By morning the fever had abated, but the physician continued treating her with quinine, unaware that her master and mistress were each doing the same. None of the three realized what the others were doing. By midday, the woman's skin had turned damp and clammy. She could neither see nor hear nor feel nor speak, according to the physician's later account. "Candles and pistols were flashed and shot about her head, and pins stuck in her" to test her sensibilities; the doctor threw three more buckets of water on her. After being wrapped in a warm blanket, she came finally to her senses.[1]

The medical encounter of this anonymous slave woman and doctor illustrates important features of southern medical practice before the Civil War. First, antebellum medical therapies tended toward the heroic, that is, toward proactive and visible (modern Americans would say reckless) treatment, involving bleeding, blistering, purging, perspiring, vomiting, and prescribing heavy doses of drugs for patients. The aim was to promote a physical response. A doctor whose treatment left no symptomatic trace was considered the equivalent of no doctor at all.[2] Second, when a physician attended an enslaved woman, he did so at the invitation of her owner, who claimed the right to orchestrate the delivery of medical care and who often began treatment before the physician's arrival. The patient or the patient's family might not be consulted or even informed about the course of treatment. Bassett mentions no discussion with them. This raises an important third point about antebellum southern medicine: the physician considered the owner, not the patient, his client. Doctors identified with and empathized with slaveholders, not slaves. To be sure, physicians also attempted to help patients—including enslaved patients—improve their health. This was a professional imperative. But they did so within a society that regarded racial slavery as right.

The brief account of the case written by Bassett obscures an important facet of southern medicine. Slaves practiced their own form of healing. Although they sometimes accepted or even sought medical care from slaveholders or their physicians, most favored remedies that differed from "scientific" medical practices. Whereas physicians preferred bold treatments intended to induce drastic change in physical functioning, enslaved healers paid attention to a broader range of symptoms and worked to create harmony between the patient's physical condition and the human environment. Slaves did not draw sharp distinctions between matters involving the body and the spirit, between physical and emotional well-being. Sickness might be viewed on the one hand as something gone wrong with bodily processes or on the other as the result of supernatural powers either deliberately or inadvertently inflicted. Certain therapies evoked a change in body function, others a change in social situation. One charm could ward off disease, another make someone fall in love.[3]

Doctors (the so-called regulars or orthodox practitioners) tended to view medicine and spirituality as separate fields of study and practice, although their clients—free as well as enslaved—did not. Physician treatments and procedures were grounded not so much in knowledge revealed by faith as in facts learned through a combination of abstract study and an applied apprenticeship. Doctors considered themselves men of science and modernity, for they formulated protocols that could be proven true case by case for particular health conditions. There was much that they did not understand with regard to disease and well-being, which left a role for providence despite the secularized focus of the profession. Doctors dealt with negative outcomes by citing God's will, for example. An editorialist in the *New Orleans Medical News and Hospital Gazette* reminded readers that no one could live longer than providence intended; doctors could not perform miracles. But generally physicians separated the secular and the sacred. Their patients continued in contrast to place much trust in God or other supernatural powers to cure disease or to ensure a healthy outcome from pregnancy.[4] For most southerners, the secular and sacred were compatible.

Antebellum Americans North and South did not confine their search for medical cure to consultations with the regulars. Most accepted a wide range of trained practitioners. Homeopaths were popular in the South after 1840. Homeopathic medicine employed minute dosages of drugs, in the belief that the symptoms the drug induced in a healthy person were those it would eliminate in a sick one. Eclectics freely borrowed whatever therapies appeared to work from other practitioners. Other approaches by "irregular" physicians involved a reliance on botanicals. Samuel Thomson enjoyed success following the publication in 1822 of his *New Guide to Health; or Botanic Family Physician*. Thomson assumed that the origins of disease lay in cold and its cure in heat. He and his followers restored heat through the use of such "hot" botanicals as cayenne pepper and steam baths. Later Thomson added botanic substances to induce vomiting, evacuation of the bowels, increased urination, and sweating, but he spurned bloodletting and blistering and mercury and arsenic, all commonly prescribed by regulars. Although Thomson intended his system to be used by laypeople, his followers founded medical schools that taught the approach to doctors in training.[5]

Most laypeople did not draw too much distinction between regularly trained physicians, practitioners of alternative therapies, and self-styled healers who purported to know time-tested home remedies. For one thing, training varied considerably in the antebellum period even for regulars. They usually attended some type of medical school, though of varying quality. Typically the doctor had a high school education and had attended two terms of medical lectures lasting four or five months (each covered the same material as the other). An apprenticeship of one to five years supplemented this formal training. Some physicians had no formal training at all, however—only experience as an apprentice. A survey of Virginia physicians conducted in 1847 indicated that at least one-quarter of the doctors had no medical degree. Doctors in states west of the Appalachian Mountains were even less likely to have had a formal education. A survey in 1850 of practicing physicians in eastern Tennessee suggested that more than half of all physicians had never attended any medical lectures.[6]

As they struggled for professional status in the antebellum years, orthodox doctors tried to distinguish their services from those of other types of healers. When it came to women's health, the orthodox physician's biggest competitor was the midwife. In the South, most midwives were enslaved blacks with no formal training, especially in the country, where the majority of slaves lived. No one expected midwives to cease serving enslaved women at childbirth, but doctors were exhibiting an increased interest in the subject and claiming that they could improve chances for a successful outcome when complications developed. By the 1840s obstetrics was receiving a separate emphasis. It had its own textbooks and had become part of the core curriculum of southern medical schools, although often it was taught as a part of a general course on the diseases of women and children. Increased emphasis on women's ailments encouraged medical students to write M.D. theses on the subject.[7]

Despite this increased emphasis, medical education in the antebellum South tended to be pragmatic. Even regulars who had attended formal lectures at medical colleges or departments were expected to learn the most about medicine through practical experience following school. Trial and error was grounded in a combination of reading of pertinent medical literature and consulting with other doctors. "Medicine was not an exact science," J. Marion Sims observed, but rather "wholly empirical."[8]

When it came to women's health, the knowledge of doctors entering practice was if anything more limited than other fields of study. Most had never witnessed a live birth or treated gynecological problems. Because elite women spurned inexperienced doctors, the majority of medical men in all likelihood attended their first case or cases of childbirth in the slave quarter, thus according black women an important role in the furthering of medical knowledge. Neither physicians nor members of the ruling class considered this practice inappropriate. It was generally assumed that race did not matter in obstetrics; black and white women would benefit from the same medical practices.[9]

The background of physicians varied not only as to medical training but also as to class. Some came from well-to-do families and enjoyed elite status; in contrast and more typical were the many physicians who struggled financially and socially to gain upward mobility. Physicians of the "better sort" sought to convince others that they might recognize a good doctor by his social graces. Laypersons could not be expected to recognize sound medical knowledge, but they might sort out legitimate practitioners from quacks by noting who was punctual, courteous, well mannered, urbane, educated in subjects other than medicine, and of good character. In other words, only those who exhibited behavior associated with the elite could be trusted. This genteel image was particularly important in the South, where only men of wealth and standing were apt to hire physicians with any frequency.[10]

Physicians who insinuated themselves into planter-class society could look forward to lucrative fees and a high social standing, perhaps even to becoming slaveholders themselves. Consequently, doctors tried to look and act like the men whose interests they served. Louisiana physician David Raymond Fox found it necessary to change his trousers, vest, and shirt every day and underwear once or twice a week in order to appear genteel before his slaveholding clients. A South Carolina doctor attending the sickbed of a white infant who died in 1861 stayed for tea and peppered the hostess with questions about her return home after a long absence, apparently in the belief that the two shared social standing—much to the consternation of the mistress. J. Marion Sims readily admitted that part of his appeal as a doctor came from "my gentlemanly deportment and kindly manner." When it came to treating slaves, elite doctors who were accustomed to interacting with slaves had an advantage over poorer practitioners. The air of authority they assumed around enslaved patients helped to reassure the slaveholder—if not the slave—that medical matters were being managed appropriately.[11]

A substantial part of a southern physician's income could come from treating slaves. They accounted for more than two-thirds of physician Arthur B. Flagg's practice in South Carolina. When a medical college opened a hospital for slaves in Charleston, an advertisement boasted that it would offer students an opportunity to acquaint "themselves with the diseases peculiarly incident to a class from which the majority must expect to derive their largest number of patients."[12]

In the decades before the Civil War, the number of physicians increased faster in the South than in the North, especially in newly established states where the population was booming. Where slavery flourished, it was said, medical practitioners stood a chance of making a good living. Statistics gathered in 1850 from four Alabama counties demonstrate the attraction of areas with large plantations. The ratio of physicians to persons residing in the counties ranged from one for every 600 people to one for every 4,160: the greater the number of slaves living in a county, the greater the number of doctors. Physicians flocked in large numbers to areas with sizable slaveholdings. Richard D. Arnold, a New Englander by birth who practiced medicine in Georgia, contrasted opportunities for physicians in the South with those in the North. In 1836 he wrote of the South, "*Here* he stands some chance of making his bread while he has teeth to chew it." Physician Charles A. Hentz of Florida similarly noted that men with large slaveholdings hired doctors to attend slaves and, just as important, were good for the bill. When Robert C. Henry in 1819 decided to relocate from Kentucky to the less settled Arkansas territory, he expressed optimism about his financial future: "the time will surely come, when to be the first physician or lawyer of Arkansas will be no mean station." As one former slave observed, "The success of the master depended on the health of his slaves." Consequently, owners were reluctant to forgo medical treatment when a slave was very ill.[13]

Doctors might be retained to treat all plantation slaves for the year, or they might be paid to treat an individual slave for a particular condition. Medical societies frowned upon the practice of contracting on a yearly basis with slaveholders to attend all slaves for one annual fee: an epidemic or other unusual medical need could tax the labor of the physician so obligated. When yellow fever struck Warren County, North Carolina, a weary Ben Wilson no sooner got home than he was called again to doctor patients on the plantation he had just left. A Virginia medical journal likened doctors who hired by the year to slaves. Fifteen physicians in Powhatan County, Virginia, pledged not to enter into any such arrangements. Despite such admonishments and resolve, doctors routinely entered into yearly contracts, leaving themselves vulnerable to economic distress should they lose a large contract for any reason. Lucrative fees served as the lure. In Louisiana David Raymond Fox received $500 annually for attending a single plantation. When disease broke out in 1857, he was forced to spend considerable time dealing with the epidemic to avoid losing the planter's business when his contract came up for renewal. Having already lost one plantation's clientele to another practitioner, he was concerned about a further reduction in his income.[14]

Whether doctors were paid by the year or by the visit, a slaveholder's patronage could make or break a physician's practice. In Tyrrell and Washington counties, North Carolina, the Collinses and the Pettigrews assumed responsibility for providing the local physician with housing. The two families selected a doctor to practice in the area, and generally gave their business to that individual. In 1818, however, Charles Pettigrew fell out with physician J. H. Ellis over the latter's drinking habits and sought a new doctor for his people. In the 1840s Pettigrew suddenly withdrew his business from another physician. This time the anguished Hardy H. Hardison acted quickly to mend the rift, which may have been caused by Hardison's having paid more attention to the Collins than to the Pettigrew plantation. Pettigrew eventually returned some of his business to Hardison, apparently much to the doctor's relief. The incident underscores the importance of slaveholder patronage to the financial success of individual doctors and demonstrates that those who hoped to maintain a lucrative practice had to keep in mind the wishes of their slaveholding clients. Southern physicians had no real choice but to please the paying customer.[15]

Slaveholder and physician were not mutually exclusive occupations, and the tendency for doctors to combine planting with medical practice either simultaneously or sequentially contributed to physician identification with the slaveholding class. Some doctors practiced medicine only on their own plantations or treated only those slaves belonging to family members. One benefit of having a family member become a doctor was the avoidance of physician fees.

Robert F. W. Allston's mother advised him to study "Phisic" specifically to "save yourself the expence of Doctors Bill on your Plantation, and in your Family." In North Carolina, physician Ben Wilson tended the sick slaves on his brother-in-law's plantation. Former slave Lucius Cooper of South Carolina said his owner's uncle served as the plantation doctor. Wealthy Tennessee slaveholder James Hoggatt never practiced medicine outside his family, although he had trained as a physician. Instead he earned a livelihood from planting.[16]

Among physicians who turned to planting as a means to supplement an income from medicine, the linkage between slaveholders and doctors inevitably strengthened. Benjamin Fleet treated black and white patients in Virginia, where he farmed 3,000 acres with slave labor. Thomas Gale, who began medical practice in 1816, was by 1833 producing 150 bales of cotton each year with the help of slaves purchased with his income from doctoring. Some physicians made substantial investments in slaves. Spanish West Florida physician Louis Faure, for example, owned at his death 12 slaves valued at more than $4,000. At times doctors left the profession entirely in order to pursue profits from cotton and other crops associated with plantation agriculture. Edmund Revenel, who earned a medical degree from the University of Pennsylvania in 1819 and who taught chemistry at the Medical College of South Carolina for more than a decade, abandoned medicine and teaching in 1835 for life as a Cooper River planter whose slave force numbered more than 100. John Wesley Monette of Mississippi, who studied medicine at Transylvania University and practiced in the Natchez area, eventually gave up medicine and took up residence on a Louisiana cotton plantation peopled by 77 slaves. In Arkansas, doctoring regularly served as a pathway into the planter class.[17]

Although a small number of doctors acquired enough land and slaves to be classified among the South's greatest planters, more typically planter-physicians held only a small number of bonded people,

and others held no slaves at all. A. Davis Brasher of Arkansas, for
example, held real estate in 1860 valued at $20,000 and three slaves,
one of whom was a child.[18] Doctors who did not own slaves, however, generally aspired to slaveholding and the class status that came
with it. They shared the assumptions of slaveholders about proper
social order, and they behaved accordingly.

One obstacle to professional as well as financial success was the
tendency of people to rely on home cures. Self-help style medicine
prevailed in all population groups, and every man or woman acted at
times as physician. Literate planters, men and women alike, recorded
recipes for medical treatments, women most often in commonplace
books and men in farm journals. Some were learned by word of
mouth and others through reading. Written sources included gen-
eral-purpose periodicals, as well as agricultural journals and women's
magazines. Planters also purchased medical texts telling them how
to use pharmaceuticals and otherwise treat particular medical conditions. J. J. Richards, a "fancy store," located in Atlanta, advertised
that it always stocked a large supply of medical books. Patrons could
order by mail or shop in person. Some of these medical manuals
were specifically written by physicians for a lay audience. James
Ewell's *Planter's and Mariner's Medical Companion* was one such
book. This and other guides were not intended to replace the physician, yet they were promoted in remote areas where people sometimes had to do without regular doctoring. Of course, the existence
of the guides fostered medical self-help treatment even in areas
where physicians congregated in large numbers. So great was the
tendency to self-treat among laypeople that doctors sometimes read
self-help medical manuals to learn what laypeople knew (or thought
they knew) about medicine.[19]

At a time when medical theories and practice had not yet become uniform and standardized, people other than physicians wrote
health literature. Some of these writers were critical of the regulars;
other authors tried not to disagree with orthodox advice. John C.

Gunn's *Domestic Medicine* was highly popular in the South and did not contradict the prevailing beliefs behind orthodox practice. A. G. Goodlett's manual likewise did not question orthodox thinking. By the mid-nineteenth century, women were writing some of the literature, and they took special care not to present themselves as challenging medical experts. On the other hand, Samuel Thomson's system of alternative medicine disputed many assumptions behind "regular" medicine.[20]

Medical textbooks intended for the instruction of orthodox physicians were also consulted by the self-educated who wanted to save money on medical bills, lacked access to physicians, or hoped to expedite a cure without awaiting the doctor's arrival. Elizabeth Scott Neblett consulted "Beach"—a medical manual published by Wooster Beach—when one of her slaves—in this case a man—became ill and the doctor's remedy proved ineffective. Beach had been trained as an orthodox doctor, but he advocated a brand of medicine that relied on botanical remedies. Although Beach expressed general distrust of regular physicians, he did not intend his text to be used by nonprofessionals. Neblett nonetheless consulted the text in developing a treatment for her slave, as did many others in a quest for remedies.[21]

The practice of consulting medical books was widespread among elite planters. When one of her grandchildren became ill, Anna Matilda King "got doctor books & read of inflammation of bowels & bladder." Charles Pettigrew regularly consulted medical treatises. His library housed the latest works for laypersons and specialists, including homeopaths. Samuel Ashwell's *Practical Treatise on the Diseases Peculiar to Women*, published in Boston in 1843, was among the works he read. William Pettigrew, who like his father, Charles, had no medical training, ordered enough medicine in 1852 to treat seventy people. He told the New York doctor with whom he placed the order that he intended to follow *Beach's Family Physician* as a guide in prescribing the drugs although he also sought advice from the supplier.[22]

Doctors called the application of home remedies garnered from all sources "tampering." It occurred for a variety of reasons. The doctor, possibly attending other patients, might not be immediately available. Some planters were located at an inconvenient distance from medical aid and had no choice other than to begin treatment before consulting a physician. Others prided themselves on being self-reliant; a well-run plantation operated as independently as possible. Still others distrusted doctors or hoped to avoid costs associated with medical care. For many, home care was simply the logical first and often only step taken to restore health for themselves as well as for their slaves.[23]

Delay in calling a doctor to the slave quarter was especially common. At least one doctor believed that as a result disease encountered among slaves was "of a more unmanageable character and the mortality . . . greater" than among whites. In fact it was not unusual for a slaveholder to wait until a slave's life appeared to be in danger before summoning a physician. When William Mitchie in 1814 requested the services of physician Charles Brown in Albemarle County, Virginia, for a slave woman who had given birth two weeks earlier, he explained the urgency of the case: she was in "great dainger." Minoah Via waited two weeks to summon the same doctor for another bondwoman who had been suffering for two months with abdominal pains and a discharge of blood. Only when the discharge and abdominal disorder turned into "severe flooding and puking" did Via consider her condition serious enough to warrant Brown's attention. His enslaved woman had been sick for nine days before planter James Douglass concluded she was "in a very Dangerous Situation" and summoned Brown. When a doctor was called, everyone understood the situation as serious, or "right low," as Molly Finley, a former slave in Arkansas, phrased it. Everyone understood that home remedies had been tried and found wanting and that the doctor was the last resort.[24]

Not surprisingly, home treatment administered by members of the slaveholding class frequently resembled the therapies of regular physicians. Slaveholders who consulted books written by the "regulars" and who had access to their drugs and instruments tended to base their ideas of treatment on what they read and had available. During the nine days his woman lay ill, Douglass "bled her several times." Her situation apparently deteriorated, but the slave owner did not lose faith in the treatment. He hoped the doctor would tell him "which side is the proper to bleed." Before calling a doctor to visit a slave woman suffering with a sore throat, owner Charles R. Battaile "bled her . . . gave her a dose of Calomel and castor oil, also blistered" her. John W. Selden gave an enslaved woman salts, oil, and calomel before giving up on home remedies and turning to a doctor. Mistress Elizabeth Gordon treated an enslaved woman with "several doses of calomel[,] one dose of tartar & a good of of [sic] bark & stimulants" before asking the doctor "what we had better do with her & also what medicine you may think proper." Polly Fox had a slave woman bled and blistered and given a cathartic before inquiring of the doctor what should be done. William Jones described in a letter to the plantation physician an enslaved woman "very sick for five or six weeks with an almost constant flow of the menses, sometimes considerable" who also suffered from abdominal and back pain. "I have given her bark, vitiriol, and laudanum but she still continues to suffer very much," Jones added.[25]

Even when a doctor was consulted, he was not necessarily expected to come to the bedside of the patient. Jones did not expect the doctor to visit the woman suffering a menstrual disorder. Instead he asked him to "please send what you think will be of service." In a letter to family physician Edward Carmichael, planter Battaile diagnosed the complaint of a slave woman as well of his own child and simply requested medicine that the doctor thought appropriate. "Furnish me with medicine for a negro woman who has thrash, and

also for my youngest child who has the Bowel complaint," Battaile
wrote. N. Seddon specifically requested "a few drops of Laudanum"
on behalf of a slave women "vy much indisposed in her Bowels."
William Richardson asked the doctor to send medicine for a child
with bowel complaint—a black infant. Lucy Alexander asked the
family physician in a letter to send "four ounces of castor oil and two
of paregoric for a sick baby." George W. B. Spooner asked a doctor
to "send me something to raise [the] palate and cure [the] throat" of
one of his slave women who was suffering from "a very severe sore
throat." Spooner had already tried in vain to achieve a cure with the
administration of "pepper salt." Knowing that the doctor would be
calling at the home of her grown daughter, Anna Matilda King
wrote her a note describing, among other things, her house slave's
symptoms and pleading for the daughter to find out from the doctor
what should be done. Apparently King expected her daughter to
outline a plan of care in her next correspondence. When a young
woman belonging to Ann G. Patton became ill, the Virginia slaveholder sent a note to the doctor explaining that the servant was indisposed and inquiring whether "it would not be proper" to give her
the same pills the doctor had furnished before in a similar case. "If
so," the mistress wrote in a note, I "will thank you to send them by
the bearer" along with directions for their use. Planter William
Payne did not even bother to specify whom they were for when he
asked his family physician "to send me up a Box of your blue Pills."[26]

In the frontier conditions that prevailed in some areas of the
South, the scarcity of physicians encouraged doctors to prescribe by
letter. Alabama planter John Horry Dent secured medicines from a
physician for the enslaved woman Jane when she suffered from
painful menstruation. Dent dutifully administered the drugs prescribed by physician William H. Thornton, but four days later Dent
wrote that she "still continues down with pains in lower part of
belly," apparently in the expectation that Thornton would be forthcoming with additional recommendations for treatment.[27] But even

in populated areas where doctors were close by, planters asked doctors to prescribe for patients without seeing them. In their account books, doctors distinguished between visiting and prescribing for a patient, even when the two were accomplished simultaneously.

Lay practitioners had easy access to drugs of all types because they could be made at home, purchased without a prescription at apothecaries, or ordered through the mail. The firm Massey and Lansdell advertised "pure medicines, drugs, oils, and chemicals, brandy and wines for medicinal purposes" to "physicians, dealers, and farmers." Alexander Duvel, apothecary and druggist in Richmond, Virginia, kept on hand for "physicians and others" a "good assortment of fresh and unadulterated medicines," chemicals, surgical and dental instruments, alongside "paints, dye stuffs, window glass and putty, perfumery and fancy articles of various kinds." Hunnicutt and Taylor offered medicines in addition to paints, oils, window glass, and fancy goods at its Atlanta store on the corner of Catur and Peach Tree streets. Former Louisiana slave Rachel Bradley recalled her master purchasing medicines along with sugar, salt, whiskey, and flour when he went to trade cotton in New Orleans.[28]

Each plantation should have "a few common medicines, with plain and proper directions pasted on each bottle," opined a Georgia planter in the pages of the *Southern Cultivator,* advice that few slaveholders failed to heed. When slaves became sick on the North Carolina plantation of George and Betsy Herndon, they saw no need to call a doctor. They cared for the slaves themselves, using the "store medicine" they had purchased for this purpose. When Virginia planter N. Seddon sent an enslaved woman to the doctor for examination, he informed the physician that he did not need to supply her with a drug. "I have all the common Medicenes in the house," he explained. Anna Matilda King bought liver pills for use on Retreat Plantation. Unhappy with the quality of one manufacturer's product, she sought another source rather than abandon the practice of keeping boxes on hand. Charles Pettigrew ordered drugs regularly for his own use but also for the physicians who visited the plantation to care for its black and white inhabitants. Joseph Temple Jr. managed to accumulate enough medicine that its valuation was listed as part of his estate when the Virginian died in 1819. Physician G. W. Cocke of Tennessee lamented that no one sent for a doctor before trying the widely available patent medications and that their availability deterred planters from calling one. Cocke was financially insolvent in 1853 and blamed his financial woes on the widespread availability of medication.[29]

Owners were not the only ones to try home remedies on slaves. They expected overseers to know something about medicine, and "on large plantations . . . overseers became, from necessity, pretty good routinists." Overseers often received from the plantation owner books and medicines to help them handle the types of routine or emergency problems they might encounter in managing a plantation. They were told to avoid drastic measures (better left under the purview of the physician), but they were directed to employ simple, judicious home remedies and to follow directions left by a physician. A. B. Hughes's overseer, known in the records only as Moore, bragged of his abilities. During thirteen years of plantation management, "he had treated all cases of sickness with all Negroes under his charge" so successfully that he expected to manage without calling in a physician except in the most dangerous cases.[30]

In medical journals doctors vehemently protested against home care. New Orleans physician D. Warren Brickell in 1856 complained that the same planter or overseer who sent for a mechanic to repair a cart wheel because he lacked the skills to fix it himself thought nothing of "tampering with their sick negroes for one, two, or more days before applying for medical aid." Physician C. R. Harris of Virginia blamed deaths from puerperal fever in Augusta County on the custom of excluding doctors from childbirth cases until complications arose. By then, it was too late, he lamented. Such complaints generally had little effect, although at least one owner won a case in court against a person who, after hiring a slave's labor from the owner, failed to call a physician to treat her medical problem. The planter's overseer had not only administered medicines to the enslaved woman known as Adeline but also "bled her on Tuesday night and then applied mustard plasters to her wrists and stomach." The patient died, and the owner sued, arguing that the plantation manager had overestimated his skills. The Alabama Supreme Court (which took up the case upon appeal) agreed, ruling in favor of her owner; a prudent overseer would have known to call a doctor.[31] Yet planters routinely engaged in behavior similar to that of the overseer. The difference was that when they treated their own slaves no one had standing to sue.

Home care of slaves was not solely the calling of men, as some of the cases above attest. Slaveholding women, who often took an interest in the obstetric, gynecological, and other health needs of enslaved women, summoned physicians on their own—as did masters—and monitored the treatment afforded them. Former slave Winger Vanhook of Texas recalled that his mistress, a small, frail woman, doctored all the slaves on the plantation, summoning a physician only if home remedies failed to cure. Even on a plantation belonging to physician N. B. DeSaussure the mistress tended to the health needs of slaves. One doctor upon arriving to see an ailing seventeen-year-old enslaved girl was met by her mistress, who apprised him of both the girl's medical history and the home remedy that had been tried. According to his recollection, "the usual domestic medicines had been used . . . but with no effect."[32]

When summoned by mistresses to care for slaves, male physicians answered to white women in a curious reversal of the gendered roles normally associated with the patriarchal South. Doctors worked in a domestic environment—a feminine sphere—rather than in a public arena. Although they were consulted for their expertise, they nevertheless had to consider the wishes of the mistress in devising a plan of treatment. Perhaps this is the reason physicians writing in

southern medical journals more frequently criticized the mistress
than the master for tampering. Their complaints, however, did little
to stem mistresses' involvement.[33]

Generally doctors complied with requests from owners for specific medications whether they were communicating over distance or
at the patient's bedside. In deciding upon treatment they rarely
bothered to speak directly with enslaved patients. Case histories,
which were regarded as an important diagnostic tool, were more
often gathered from the master or mistress or overseer than from the
patient.[34] In this way, owners and physicians demonstrated their
tacit understanding of who controlled medical care in the South.
From time to time doctors might directly quiz the patient, or in obstetric cases an attending nurse or midwife, but they felt a special
aversion for doing so. Most considered blacks in general—black
midwives in particular—unreliable. They preferred to depend for information on other whites, whose word they more readily trusted.

By far, most of the healthcare in the quarter was carried out by
slaves. Physicians found the situation exceedingly worrisome. It
complicated medical treatment, and (more important perhaps) it
also challenged the doctor's authority. It was one thing to have one's
professional judgment called into question by men or even women of
standing. It was quite another to have one's diagnosis and treatment
contested by patients regarded by doctors as inferiors.

Slaves generally exhibited a healthy distrust of their owner's
medicine men, who clearly served the interests of their slaveholding
clients. Unfavorable outcomes from invasive measures further convinced many slaves that regular doctors were no more efficacious
than their own folk healers.[35] Finally, slaves had their own healing
traditions, which they were reluctant to change. In their view, it was
the slaveholder and the slaveholder's doctor who were guilty of tampering. In general they preferred their own indigenous ways of handling health and human reproduction.

When medical conditions were not urgent or desperate, owners preferred to place their trust in the slave's root-and-herb doctor or midwife, if only to save the expense of the physician's visit but also to save the trouble of imposing particular treatment that might meet resistance. Slaves and owners alike promoted the idea that plantations should be as self-sufficient as possible when it came to healthcare. Medicines could be made on the home place "from roots, herbs, flowers, and leaves," according to one Arkansas informant.[36] The fact that it was often difficult to obtain the services of a competent doctor encouraged the concept of self-sufficiency for both blacks and whites.

Particularly at the early onset of disease, during mild spells of illness, or in routine obstetric cases, owners left healing in the hands of slaves. Only when the initial treatment or treatments appeared ineffective and the patient's condition became grim was a physician called. By then, slaves were more willing to allow a role for the slaveholder's doctor. On a typical Tennessee plantation, "an old negro woman on the place" began treatment. Only if her concoctions of roots and herbs did not work would the master call in a white doctor who routinely treated the slaves following any failed attempts at curing with folk remedies. Often slaves were subject to the home remedies of blacks and whites alike before a doctor was called. By the time Virginia planter William Herndon consulted physician James Carmichael about the care of a young male slave with mumps, the plantation's "Doctriss," known as Isabella, had already "given him a Cathartick" and planned to provide him with flaxseed tea. Herndon, meanwhile, assured the doctor that "I shall bleed him today" in addition to administering whatever medicine the doctor might think proper to provide.[37]

After a doctor arrived on the scene, home remedies did not necessarily decrease in importance. Many enslaved patients were treated by slaves and physicians simultaneously as well as sequentially.

When the enslaved Peggy was confined to bed in Baton Rouge because of illness, her mistress worried that "she would never again be fit for anything" because she persisted in "counteracting the effect of medicine and careful nursing by" adhering to healing measures favored by blacks. On Augustus Foster's plantation in North Carolina, slaves saw a doctor when they were sick, "the same as . . . white folks," according to one of the enslaved men. But they simultaneously took "a lot of spring tonic an' such, made out of barks an' roots." The list of home remedies administered to an eighteen-month-old infant belonging to George Banks (calomel, oil, cedar apple, spirits of turpentine, and the juice of the Jerusalem plant) suggests that both slaveholders and slaves were involved in deciding the baby's care. In 1822 an enslaved eight-year-old girl belonging to William Jackson Jr. received salts, tarter, and calomel because she was feverish, sleepy, and suffering from a "violent pain in the head." Someone had administered "a dose [of] worm Seed oil" as well.[38]

Slaves' continuing reliance on home cures stood in direct contradiction to notions by whites that blacks must yield to their supposed superior knowledge. Once the physician was on the scene, he expected to be in charge. Like many others, Kentucky planter George Brady relied on an old black woman using such herbs as sassafras roots and cami weeds to treat sickness on his plantation. But when serious illness occurred, he summoned a doctor. At that point the black woman was expected to relinquish management of the case and wait on the patient according to the doctor's orders.[39] This ideal was not often realized.

Doctors expressed concern about the compliance of black patients and looked for ways to enforce their orders. They complained that slaves would not follow directions and described them as uncooperative. One doctor went so far as to threaten a slave with physical violence "if you don't take that medicine like I tell you." Virginia physician A. S. Helmick, who in 1854 ordered blisters applied to the pubis of a woman suffering from uterine problems, realized that "the blisters had been neglected." The doctor treating Amy for prolapsed (fallen) uterus became frustrated when she refused to wear consistently in her vagina the pessary he prescribed to keep her uterus in place. She said the device was uncomfortable, but he described her as "restive and intractable," behaving "obstinately." When John Walker's slave Eliza died in July 1834, the master blamed the patient. She would not cooperate with the doctor he had hired, but instead insisted on dosing herself with other, more favored remedies. Helmick and the mistress of the woman treated for uterine problems arranged for the patient to move temporarily from her cabin to her owner's home, where she would no longer have to climb stairs and they would not have to worry that the blisters would be removed. The tactic was not uncommon. Other owners sometimes removed a patient from the slave quarter to a hospital or other location where she or he might be attended more efficiently and closely supervised.[40]

Doctors who despaired of convincing slaves to follow orders encountered a similar problem with slaveholders. Owners were reluctant—at times downright unwilling—to concede authority, especially to men whom many regarded as inferior. Slaveholders were accustomed to command, especially slaves but also family members and nonelite neighbors. Educated slaveholders kept themselves informed about medical developments by consulting medical texts and even at times by reading medical journals. They frequently learned to diagnose disease (or so they claimed) and took an active role in treating the health problems of their slaves. They stood at the top of the southern hierarchy, and the fact that they paid the physicians' fees reinforced their notion of superiority with regard to the doctors. The subordinate status of physicians was understood clearly by the father of J. Marion Sims, when the South Carolinian (who eventually achieved a degree of fame for innovations in the field of gynecology) discussed his desire to study medicine. The elder Sims, a minor government official, scorned the idea: "There is no honor to be achieved in it; no reputation to be made."[41]

Physicians called in for particular problems already identified by owners found it difficult to contradict the original diagnosis. The case of the slave woman suffering complications of childbirth, cited earlier, may have been extreme in that both master and mistress continued their own course of treatment after the doctor's arrival. Yet time and again physicians had to contend with owners who thought they knew the best medical therapies. Bennet H. Barrow, who had no medical training, regularly criticized the doctors for their treatment of his slaves but also of himself, his wife, and children. When Barrow's young son died, he blamed the doctor for failing to vomit and blister the child soon enough. After the death of his daughter Caroline, he faulted the attending physician for failing to induce vomiting. As his wife Emily lay dying, Barrow got into a dispute with attending physician J. W. King over whether she should have been blistered. Upon hearing of the death of yet another family member, Barrow pronounced the work of the doctor "murder." The patient died, in his estimation, "for want of bleeding & a purge." Barrow was better satisfied with a Doctor McKelvey, who "sanctioned every thing I proposed." The patient died anyway, but in this case Barrow attributed the outcome to the fact that the child "was too far spent" rather than to the treatment he received.[42]

Steeped in the heroic tradition of medicine that aimed to produce a visible reaction in the patient, Barrow boasted that his own cure rate among the slave children who contracted scarlet fever on his place was better than that of the regular doctors of the region. Physicians objected to bleeding in the early stages of the disease because the pulse was weak, he observed, but his own efforts to bleed and purge the children of the quarter at the first sign of illness had spared them the worst of the disease. He held in disdain a doctor called to treat the six-year-old slave Marcus. "A more undecisive man I never saw," Barrow carped. He "made [a] great many attempts to bleed him, but failed & large veins at that." Marcus died that morning.[43]

Throughout the country, laypeople became so involved in medicine that at times they demanded specific treatment. James Henry Hammond of South Carolina grew so frustrated with the physicians he employed on his plantation that he vowed to eliminate use of them altogether. A plantation manual written for his Beach Island estate in about 1834 specified that only homeopathy should be used in treating the slaves. "There being no homeopathist convenient— each case has to be examined carefully by the master or overseer to ascertain the disease," the manual stipulated. In cases in which the diagnosis was uncertain, the owner or overseer should carry the planter's medical books "to the bed side," where he would conduct a thorough medical examination and peruse the books to ensure the best choice of medication. Although Hammond never attended medical lectures or completed an apprenticeship, he purchased a medicine chest and other materials used in medical practice, and he read texts and domestic manuals intended for physicians and laypersons. Hammond applied his eclectic medical treatment not only to slaves but also to his white neighbors.[44]

As Hammond's experience illustrates, southern planters could carry efforts to influence a doctor's practice to the extreme. One Alabama planter actually persuaded Gideon Lincecum, an orthodox practitioner, to abandon regular medicine in favor of the Thomsonian system. The slave owner overcame the doctor's initial reluctance to give up orthodox measures in favor of roots and herbs by pointing out the economic benefits of the arrangement: "You are struggling with a big family, and we want to help you." When Virginia farmer John Walker hired out his slave Daniel to Moses Robinson, the agreement specified that Robinson was to employ "only Tomsonian drs" in the event that Daniel became ill. Indeed, Walker went so far as to purchase a license to practice Thomsonian medicine himself, although he reverted to regular doctors—or even black folk practitioners—when Thomson's approach failed to bring the desired outcome. Planters like Walker could be quite eclectic in their approaches to healthcare. Walker employed both orthodox and Thomsonian health measures. He liked certain aspects of Thomson's system better than others, so he relied heavily on these. Even so, he did not follow Thomson's instructions to the letter. Rather than limit himself to the dosages recommended by Thomson, Walker generously increased the prescribed amount, reasoning that more would produce better results. In fact the Virginia planter ordered per annum more than four times the quantity of medicines recommended in Thomson's manual.[45] Faced with such determination among slaveholders, doctors probably felt they had to find some way to accommodate their recommendations or at least to present an argument that would change the slaveholder's mind. A different situation arose when slaves failed to follow the doctor's orders or engaged in treatment of their own devising.

Slaves were familiar with the therapies of the physicians. Knowledge of regular medicine among slaves stemmed from their involvement as patients, nurses, midwives, and servants. Lucretia Brown's Mississippi mistress specifically trained the slave girl to care for the sick, thereby exposing her to the medical practices of the white community. Lizzie Williams was sent as a girl to New Orleans to nurse the sick child of her mistress's sister. Sallie Carder, who nursed her Tennessee master, fed him, helped him get around, and no doubt observed any drug or other medical regimens prescribed for him. Steve Connally in Georgia accompanied his mistress when she sought medical treatment in town. She stayed about a month at a time, during which the young slave served as a waiting boy. James Monroe Abbot was only seven when he was called to the bedside of his dying master. He stayed on duty night and day for months, charged with keeping the flies off the dying man. He could not have helped observing his owner's ideas of proper care for a terminally ill man.[46]

Some doctors owned slaves who assisted in their medical practice. J. Douglass of South Carolina relied on a slave woman to assess the situation of a woman in labor and to summon him if the delivery took an unexpected turn for the worse. Moses Roper as a youth mixed medicines intended for use on the plantation by his owner, a physician and cotton planter. William Hutson accompanied his owner—another planter physician—on his rounds in Georgia, carrying the doctor's black bag and no doubt learning something of his practice. J. H. Curry's father served as waiting man for a physician who taught the enslaved man to read and write so that he could take messages while the doctor was out on rounds.[47]

Some slaves became so proficient at healing that they gained the confidence of free whites in the neighborhood. John Walker paid his slaves for medical services rendered in their off hours. Ten dollars went to the black doctor Lewis for medical care he provided the enslaved Jack and lesser sums to women who acted as midwives. Lewis also received three dollars for concocting a tea of soot and pine-tree root for the enslaved woman Eliza. A Virginia slave received freedom as a reward for curing a white man from painful disease in 1792. Residents of six Tennessee counties in the early 1830s petitioned the General Assembly to allow a slave known as Doctor Jack to continue his practice of medicine in the vicinity. Tennessee law stipulated that owners who allowed a slave to practice medicine would be fined and the slave subjected to as many as twenty-five lashes. The petitioners hoped to protect Jack and his owner from punishment.[48]

Such healers represented a very real breach in the power relations idealized by white southerners. When slaves followed doctors' orders or even when they practiced the healing art out of sight of the ruling class, the authority of owners, doctors, and other members of the ruling class appeared intact. But when slaves became known for their knowledge of medicine within a particular white community, a contradiction was revealed that challenged the existence of slavery. By any measure, successful healers commanded knowledge or a spiritual gift or both. Such men and women could hardly be regarded as brutes incapable of any but physical labor. Their ability to restore health (and by implication impede it) represented knowledge and power that might—slaveholders feared—be turned against the slave system. It is little wonder that one by one, slave states moved to ban black practitioners from medical practice, even as individual owners relied on them to attend not only slaves but also at times members of the slaveholding family.

Slaves knew more about their owners' approach to medicine than did owners and physicians about practices in the slave quarter. Doctors were only dimly aware of slave health practices, which could include conjuring (calling upon the supernatural by invocation or spell). They explained the existence of a wide range of healing customs as evidence of the slave's ignorance, superstition, and in some cases malevolence. In a letter to a Virginia medical journal, John R. Hicks, M.D., of North Carolina, derided blacks who when they did not understand the underlying cause of disease attributed it to having been poisoned. Whites, too, sometimes attributed disease to poisoning, but on these occasions doctors were more sympathetic than skeptical. Physicians attending the March 1853 meeting of the Richmond medical society spent time discussing ways of testing for arsenic and other toxins. One of the doctors present prompted the discussion by testifying that enslaved blacks had poisoned the Shelton family in Hanover County, Virginia, by putting arsenic in their ice cream. Fearful that slaves might use knowledge of roots, herbs, and conjure to harm them, whites revealed their fears about the efficacy of these measures.[49] The doctors at the Richmond meeting identified with the slaveholders' sense of slaves as a class apart—able and willing to inflict harm upon the owning class.

Despite this sense of separateness, many enslaved people accepted at least some therapies associated with the regulars. Nothing about nineteenth-century medicine precluded slaves from incorporating knowledge of orthodox treatments into their healing practices. In fact slaves more readily adopted Western ideas of medicine than Western practitioners adopted the ideas of slaves. Whereas physicians trained in medical schools held to generally prescribed standards of treatment outlined in lectures, texts, and journals, enslaved practitioners were not bound by such standards of care. A positive outcome, rather than adherence to orthodoxy, was the mark of a successful healer, who relied on the cure—the miracle of healing—to secure his or her reputation. The idea that knowledge was revealed prevented the development of an orthodox approach to healing among slaves. New revelations were continually occurring as healers encountered new conditions in their clients and as new practitioners entered the realm of healing. Anthropologists have observed that Africans from the western and central regions of the continent tended to be "relatively permeable to foreign influences" in religious matters, and their practices "tended to be 'additive' rather than 'exclusive' in their orientation to other cultures."[50] The same could be said for African Americans and healing. They willingly adopted Western medical practices when more traditional measures failed and when Western therapies proved efficacious.

When they accepted aspects of the slaveholders' medicine, slaves did not necessarily forfeit their belief in folk remedies, including the power of the supernatural to harm or heal. Indeed, most slaves relied first on home remedies. If necessary, they consulted a folk practitioner, but followed up with a visit to the conjurer or trained physician or both if the problem did not yield to traditional measures. Former slave Henry F. Pyles, for one, found nothing peculiar in consulting a physician and a conjurer simultaneously. In Virginia, former slave Duncan Gaines acknowledged, "there was much talk of 'hoodooism'" when someone was "ill for a long time without getting relief from herb medicines." Conjurer Charles Williams, once brought to court for practicing medicine illegally, defended himself by pointing out that he accepted only cases that others had been unable to cure.[51]

Conjuring was spiritual in its approach, but it differed from praying in important ways. One could learn to pray or be moved to prayer no matter what the person's identity. Conjurers were born with the gift. Generally one did not pray for harm to come to another, but conjuring could result in harm or prevent harm. One could not counter a prayer, but one could ward off a conjured spell through particular action. Simply believing in signs and omens did not mean believing in conjuring. Nor did the acceptance of herbal and root medicine mark one as accepting or rejecting conjuring as a potent life force. And in the same vein, simply knowing the steps a conjurer took to invoke a spell or tell a fortune did not mean that one could imitate the process. As former slave Herndon Bogan observed, it took a special kind of knowing to "witch somebody." Conjurers and the people who sought their help believed that illness was sometimes rooted in social causes. One worked backward from the illness to discern its origins.[52]

Former slave Sarah Felder was too young under slavery to understand exactly how conjuring worked, but she had general knowledge of it from her mother. Circumstances of birth created conjurers: anyone born during a certain phase of the moon could cast a spell on another person. A tea brewed from a particular weed in the field could keep off a spell, however. For Felder, conjuring and Christianity could not coexist. One had to choose one or the other belief system. She was a "good Baptist," she offered by way of explaining where she stood. Although she rejected conjuring as a belief system, it is clear from testimony she gave in the 1930s that she accepted other folklore. She always planted her garden in moonlight to ensure its flourishing, and she knew more than one means of bringing good luck.[53]

Their varied explanations for the cause of illness encouraged slaves to contemplate the conditions of slavery, including the human relationships, contributing to sickness. In contrast, Western medicine tended to characterize illness as a physiological phenomenon divorced from sociocultural forces. Whereas many orthodox doctors readily admitted the influence of climate on the course of disease and on the availability of particular botanical substances for treating specific medical problems, slaves went a step further to name the human environment as an important influence on health and well-being. Slaves believed that they could not entrust their entire well-being to physicians because slaves were subject to conjuring, and no white physician could counter a spell.[54] But more important, white physicians refused to contemplate the social relationships that led to many health problems in the quarter.

Physicians bore witness to the insults and indignities inflicted on slaves in the name of plantation discipline, but they generally avoided discussing health issues related to abuse. At times the practices they saw angered them. Annie Griegg's Louisiana owner once seriously injured her hand. The owner's cousin—a doctor—treated her broken bones and let his ire show. But this apparently was as far as he went. Indeed, a doctor was as likely to be a hard taskmaster as any other slaveholder. Former slave Adeline White described her physician owner as mean to his slaves, young and old alike. He beat and deprived them of food even while keeping track of their health and doling out medications as he saw fit. A. G. Grinnan of Madison County, Virginia, tentatively remarked that slave cabins in his area were crowded and uncomfortable, but he stopped short of assigning any blame for poor health. Slaves, he observed, were "generally well fed and clothed."[55]

Unable to convince the slaveholder's physician of the underlying cause of health problems in the quarter, slaves blended traditional home remedies with cures learned from others in an attempt to ward off disease and other disasters. Some of these were remembered and used by freed people after the Civil War. Former Texas slave Vinnie Brunson's description of cures "handed down to us from de folks way back befo' we wuz born" demonstrates the possible blending of several approaches to care. Ideas about the need to employ hot agents, including pepper, might have been derived from or helped to inspire Thomsonian and other forms of homeopathic medicine. Hot sassafras tea cooled the blood, and red-pepper tea cured severe colds, according to the informant. Teas made from roots and herbs might have originated in African or Native American communities. An element of magic can be seen in the advice that "two buck eyes carried in de pockets will cure de misery in old joints." And the time-honored means of dulling pain used by southern lay and medical people alike—whiskey—became more potent in Brunson's estimation when two lightning bugs (fireflies) were immersed in the bottle of alcohol. Homogeneous substances (those that bore some resemblance to the affected body part) also cured, a folk belief associated with southern slaves and other people around the world. Cures came from what was at hand, including the lining of a chicken gizzard. Slaveholders might grow medicinal plants in elaborate gardens, and physicians might import exotic substances from afar; but slaves, who had limited time and resources, generally made do with whatever they had. One woman who suffered from a general decline that lasted for more than a year found a cure in a potion made from molasses, vinegar, water, and rusty nails. A friend shared the recipe intended to cure a condition with origins in supernatural forces.[56]

Roots and herbs were important to all kinds of healing in the quarter. Ellen Butler said that slaves gathered a number of medicinal roots and herbs in her Louisiana parish: black haw root, cherry bark, dogwood bark, chinquapin bark, black snakeroot, and swamp root. Conjurers used roots and herbs in curing, as did other folk healers. When one Arkansas woman planned to marry, a conjurer had her drink a cup of herbal tea, which caused her to abandon her sweetheart and marry another man.[57] Presumably the man she ended up with had engaged the services of the conjurer to bring about this change of heart.

Most slaves relied to some extent on spells and charms. They wore coins with holes around their necks "to keep off evil spirits." Red flannel bands wrapped around the wrist instilled bravery when it was needed. Elias Thomas, a former slave from North Carolina, said that slaves wore rabbits' feet and carried buckeyes to ward off disease, even those attended in illness by regular physicians. Many slave children wore bags of asafetida (a foul-smelling resin) around their necks to prevent illness.[58]

Slaves put faith in preventive care; hence the best practitioners were those who could foretell the course of events or interpret signs of impending danger, especially death. Like physicians and owners, slaves believed that the healing art required more than knowledge of anatomy and physiology. But for slaves, the best healers could see into the future to understand the effect of a particular course of treatment. Seventh children were said by some to have this ability. Former slave Lucretia Alexander, who denied any faith in "hoodoo," did not question the psychic powers of a seventh-born child. One conjurer who began his practice at the age of twelve described his mother as "a Doctor woman." He might have inherited his skills from her, or maybe he was a seventh son or a seventh child or a child born with a caul (the inner fetal membrane) over his face—a fact of birth said to impart special powers.[59]

Ordinary people learned to interpret signs for guidance in daily living, although not everyone agreed on what the signs were or how they should be interpreted. Turtledoves might be a sign of impending death or an indication that someone in the community would move. Owls or cranes also could suggest an impending death. Almost all the slaves believed that every crook and turn in the landscape, every rooster's crow or blowing wind meant something, former slave Albert Cox observed. Lucy Donald also remembered that slaves put their store in signs, always expecting something to happen.[60]

Certain people could read signs better than others. The enslaved woman Sally was described as "a foreknower" who explained the future by observing the behavior of a rooster. Former slave Marie E. Harvey maintained into old age that she had a sixth sense for upcoming events. Nothing slipped up on her, she boasted. Spiritual interpretations of occurrences represented a form of augury, in which events in this world are examined in an effort to divine or predict an outcome. John Henry Kemp, known as a prophet in Mississippi, used his power to see into the future to discern the course of sickness, according to the former slave's testimony. Matilda Shepard, who was enslaved in Georgia, maintained that giving certain people the ability to anticipate events was God's way of revealing "things to people when we cant read or write so we can understand."[61] Orthodox doctors might do for literate people, but members of an oral culture required other types of healers.

Just as they incorporated certain Western ways of healing into their own store of knowledge, slaves shunned those they deemed ineffective or inappropriate. Skepticism concerning the ability of the owner's doctor to heal reflected the slave's understanding of whose purposes were being served. Slaveholders brought doctors in to treat sick slaves, one former bondwoman observed, to keep slaves well so that they could work. But slaves also had doubts about particular cures. Consequently, they sometimes withheld from owners information about illness. The young house servant Tilla had been unwell for some time before her mistress became aware of her dizziness and other symptoms of disease. Tilla deliberately kept her condition secret. The enslaved Laura hid her condition from Virginia planter John Walker. She apparently suffered from gonorrhea, for which neither his favored Thomsonians nor orthodox physicians had an effective cure. Mothers and fathers kept information about their children's illnesses from Louisiana cotton planter Bennet H. Barrow, even though he was known to punish the act. Luce never said a word about her son's injury for eight days; Maria did not tell him her child was ill until after the child died; no one informed him that Candis' child lay dying until the infant was "pulseless." When Robert, the child of Hetty and Demp, became ill, no one said anything for two days. Patience habitually withheld information about her health problems from Barrow, even though she was whipped for it. South Carolina physician Phillip Tidyman lamented that too many enslaved people hid their symptoms in order to consult "quacks of their own colour."[62]

Women's health problems in particular were shrouded in secrecy. Individual slave healers were innovative, so that there was considerable variation in how matters were handled; but certain traditions prevailed. Physiology and spirituality were not treated as separate. And women—not men—assumed responsibility for reproductive health.

Practices related to reproduction—from ensuring fertility to the treatment of gynecological disorders—took a particular form in the slave quarter, however, as slaveholders began exploring how the obstetric and gynecologic services of male physicians might advance their interests. Because neither obstetrics nor gynecology existed as separate fields in the modern sense, general practitioners treated any cases that came their way. They acknowledged that their interest in particular medical problems stemmed at least in part from "the pecuniary interest of the master." This state of affairs helped explain why doctors expressed concern about the ability of enslaved women to conceive and carry a baby to term and whether they knew a means of preventing pregnancy. Doctor E. M. Pendleton of Sparta, Georgia, acknowledged that "the moral and physical well-being of the slave" was another factor, but a planter's financial interest helped to focus doctors on reproductive health matters.[63]

A wide array of healers practiced in the slave quarter, ranging from regulars with medical school training to lay-taught herbalists and conjurers. At times their approaches proved compatible, but medical men and midwives, slave owners and slaves sometimes competed for the management of enslaved women's health. For the majority of slaveholders and slaves alike, the most important consideration in assessing the worth of a particular provider was not his or her education, commitment to a particular school of medicine, or even efficacy with regard to particular regimens. Rather, it was the empathy and understanding with which the provider practiced. Slave owners and slaves each hoped for attendants who would respect their needs and be sensitive to their values. Owners were most comfortable with attendants who did not challenge the existing power relations of southern society. Regulars who were of or who aspired to slaveholding status were welcome on the plantation, but so were homeopaths and folk healers—including enslaved practitioners—so long as they did not challenge the prerogatives of the slaveholders. Slaves also welcomed a variety of practitioners to the slave quarter and looked for healers who understood and respected the beliefs and customs of patients. They were skeptical of those who came too close to the slaveholders' ideal. Some practitioners (particularly those of slave status) were skilled in moving between the two worlds of the slave and slaveholder, and these gained the respect of both. Most never transcended the boundary that separated the two classes, however. Their inability or unwillingness to bridge the boundary shaped healing practices in the slave quarter.

3

Fertility

IN DECEMBER 1841 PHYSICIAN WILLIAM N. MORGAN ATTENDED the childbed of Caroline, an enslaved woman who had been in labor about twenty-six hours. He had been summoned because the infant's position was not favorable for an unassisted birth. After the baby's birth, Morgan followed Caroline's recovery for thirty days, subjecting her to enemas, tonics, blister plasters, cathartics, purgatives, opium, and morphine. Astringents, injected *"per vaginam,"* were also tried. The doctor kept note of Caroline's progress for at least three more years. Her health was "tolerable," he observed, but she experienced occasional abdominal pain, irregular menstruation, and slight diarrhea. Perhaps more important (at least to the doctor and his slaveholding client), she had not conceived, despite "frequent communications with her husband."[1]

Owners unabashedly acknowledged that the "natural increase" of slaves was a source of great profit. Slaveholders should do everything possible to ensure the health of enslaved women "and render them prolific," advised one planter in the pages of the *American Cotton Planter and Soil of the South,* a publication devoted to promoting improvements in southern farming practices. "Get as many young negro women as you can," one Texan advised a nephew, and "in ten or fifteen or twenty years you will do as well as any other man." On his own plantation, 15 children had been born in six years. Some of the mothers were young women who had just "commenced breeding," a situation that held out hope of further increase. Another

planter, this one in Virginia, boasted of his monetary gain from having purchased a young man and woman to work a small plantation.
The couple, for which he had paid $800 in 1818, had in thirteen
years produced 9 children worth in his estimation between $3,000
and $4,000. This gain was in addition to any crop they produced.
Another planter who purchased Meridie and Juda ended up with
more than 50 slaves as the result of births through several generations. Virginia planter Thomas Jefferson considered "a woman who
brings a child every two years more profitable than the best man" in
the labor force. Jefferson was not the only U.S. president to profit
from the birth of slaves. George Washington claimed 123 slaves at
the time of his death in 1799. He had started out with 10. For their
part, slaves were keenly aware of the premium placed by slaveholders
upon a fast breeder. "If a slave woman had children fast she was considered very valuable," former North Carolina slave William Mc-
Cullough explained.[2]

Because no small part of a slaveholder's future earnings depended
on the birth of children in bondage, slaveholders became concerned
when a woman past puberty failed to produce a living child with regularity. They worried about her reproductive health generally and
took action when they feared she would be unable to bear children.
They offered inducements for marriage or threatened barren women
with sale away from family and friends. They paid attention to sex
ratios and purchased potential mates, or they allowed couples to
court across property boundaries. But during the antebellum period,
slaveholders began choosing yet another approach to resolving the
"problem" of infertility among slaves. To rewards and punishments,
they added medicine. When one slave appeared incapable of completing the simple task of sewing three days following the birth of
her child, the mistress called in a physician who concluded that poor
eyesight was the culprit rather than gynecological problems stemming from the birth. The woman was healthy and could bear more
children, the doctor reassured the owner, whose relief on hearing the

diagnosis demonstrated her belief that infertility in female slaves posed more of a problem than blindness. (The woman proved the accuracy of the doctor's prognosis by having twelve more infants over her lifetime, according to his testimony.)[3]

The South's medical men both encouraged and responded to slaveholders' desire to identify the causes of barrenness among enslaved women and to discover a cure. Obstetrics and gynecology would not emerge as separate medical specialties until after the Civil War. But orthodox physicians were taking an interest in women's health problems. Eager for slaveholding clients with the means to pay medical bills, doctors began to offer midwifery services for enslaved women.[4] Physicians who promised to reduce infertility among slaves appealed to the pecuniary interests of slaveholders. Physician fees would be recouped by the addition of young slaves to the workforce. The lure of profits also appealed to physicians who wanted slaveholders' patronage. Although initially the reward for attending enslaved women might prove small, the return would come in the form of increased business all around as slaveholders called in doctors to treat slaves and recommended their services to friends and relatives in the neighborhood.

Securing medical attention for slaves offered more to owners than the promise of an expanding labor force and increased profits. Owners bragged of their willingness to obtain medical care for slaves, sometimes in contrast to manufacturers in the North and Europe, who assumed no such responsibility on behalf of wage workers. Often the same doctor who treated members of the white family attended slaves in the quarter, allowing owners to sing their own praises about their paternalistic concern for family, black and white. As the concept of the "good master" expanded in the antebellum era to include the provision of medical care, slaves benefited more or less, depending on the state of medical knowledge, the efficacy of the physician's remedies, and the compatibility of the slaveholder's medicine with the practices and understanding of slaves about the nature of illness and healing. Treatment for infertility was at best of doubt-ful benefit, and in some cases painful or harmful. Much of it was ex-perimental. Some doctors combined a reliance on experience and observation without reference to scientific theory or method to de-vise new treatments. They combined elements of the intrusive ap-proach to medicine involving purging, puking, bleeding, blistering, and boldly drugging patients. While antebellum practitioners had begun to question the efficacy of older therapies, they had not yet developed treatments that were clearly superior.

Enslaved women wanted children, but they preferred indigenous methods of enhancing fertility that were less drastic than so-called heroic measures. Their assumptions about fertility were either unfa-miliar to, misunderstood by, or ignored by medical practitioners and their slaveholder clients. Enslaved women did not so much try to en-hance fertility (which is what slaveholders wanted) as to space their children. Whereas medical men sought therapies aimed at increas-ing the number of children born to enslaved women, the women wanted intervals between pregnancies sufficient for ensuring that mother and infant were both healthy. Their different goals and ap-proaches created tension between medical men and enslaved women, each of whom thought they knew what was best for women's bodies.

Enslaved women and physicians confronted one another on un-even terrain. The women found themselves in a precarious position, needing to negotiate a means whereby they retained the right to control their own bodies while appearing cooperative before owners. But control of one's body was not a fundamental right extended to enslaved women. With the power of the slaveholders behind them, southern doctors could compel compliance, at least when they or other members of the slaveholding class were present. But neither slaveholders nor their physicians were willing to stay long in the slave quarter, a fact that left women, who found strength in one an-other, considerable discretion in managing childbearing. Generations of women shared information about how best to control fertility based on assumptions about the timing of motherhood that differed fundamentally from those of owners and doctors. A community of women thus resisted efforts by men to exert control over this most important aspect of life.

————

Among European and American doctors, infertility was in the late antebellum era beginning to gain recognition as a medical problem requiring professional intervention. There was no universal agreement, however, even about how to determine whether a woman could conceive, let alone about how to cure infertility. Eminent British physician W. Tyler Smith in 1856 claimed to find evidence of sterility in pubic hair. For some doctors, firm breasts held promise of fecundity. American doctors—both North and South—sometimes argued that people of mixed race were more likely to be infertile than others, but critics argued just the opposite. Conditions believed to prevent conception included menstrual disorders, occlusion (closing) of the vagina, sexually transmitted disease, uterine infection, "polypi in the uterus," and fibrous tumors. The last prevented the gradual enlargement of the uterus during pregnancy, making it impossible for the woman to bring a baby to term.[5] Physicians who advanced these theories had no scientific data with which to back their assertions. Yet so great was the fear of infertility that planters employed doctors to examine women whom they hoped to purchase to learn whether they were capable of bearing children.

Many owners believed that a woman's outward appearance provided clues to her fecundity, and they employed this "knowledge" in deciding whom to purchase and how much to pay. The ability to make shrewd decisions about buying healthy, obedient, productive, and prolific women factored into a slaveholder's reputation for plantation management and became a source of pride. Those slaveholders who did not trust their own judgment could consult a physician for advice. When Virginia planter Robert Conrad authorized his

wife to purchase at auction a female slave for the house (an uncommon occurrence, because most women shied away from the slave
mart), he cautioned her to have any potential candidate examined by
the family doctor to ensure that she was in good health.[6]

Would-be purchasers could insist on a thorough physical by a
physician. Doctors not only made the rounds of the slave pens in
such notorious slave marts as New Orleans; they also visited individual plantations with professional buyers looking to put together a
coffle (squad) of slaves for sale in distant localities. A woman might
be led to a private room and her body examined in intimate detail,
but she also might be made to strip in public. Auctioneers sometimes tried to head off doubts about fertility by proclaiming the
merits of a particular woman's capacity for childbearing and exposing her body in public. One purveyor of human flesh ordered the enslaved Betsy to strip above the waist so that buyers might view her
ample bosom, frequently associated with fecundity. "There's a breast
for you," he proclaimed, "good for a round dozen before she's done
child-bearing." A similar incident was seared into the memory of
Rose Williams, who was put up for auction in Texas as a "strong
young wench" capable of becoming "a good breedah." The practice of
having enslaved women strip for would-be purchasers, whether to
reassure them about a woman's childbearing capacity or as evidence
of good health and character (revealed by an absence of scars indicating punishment), contributed to the stereotyping of black women
as sexually promiscuous.[7] Proper women did not reveal body parts in
public.

Although physicians offered their services in assessing the fertility of enslaved women, there was no universal agreement among
them about how to determine whether a woman could conceive and
bring a fetus to term. Indeed, the topic of "what constitutes unsoundness in the Negro" occasioned debate among doctors with regard to enslaved women and men alike. Physician Juriah Harriss,
Savannah Medical College professor, bemoaned the lack of clear

rules for warranting slaves as healthy even though the question was of legal importance. Slaves, whether female or male, represented a substantial investment. Some buyers wanted to protect themselves from possible financial loss by purchasing a life insurance policy on the slave, but before a policy could be written, doctors examined slaves to ensure they were healthy enough to perform the "usual duties" assigned them. In the case of women, "usual duties" included childbearing. Any condition that had the potential to interfere with fertility materially diminished the monetary value of a woman in the eyes of potential insurance agents and buyers.[8]

Physicians could identify evidence of fertility more easily than infertility. They could detect whether a woman had already given birth because the size and other characteristics of the uterus indicated whether a woman had carried a child to term. Noted physician W. Tyler Smith explained in the pages of a New Orleans medical journal how to make the determination through a gynecological exam.[9] Presumably inexperienced doctors could learn how to conduct the exam by reading about it.

Like slaveholders, doctors called upon to warrant the medical condition of a slave prided themselves on their ability to "read" slave bodies and judge whether one represented a good financial investment. The skill brought monetary reward as well as professional pride to those who performed the service. One physicians' group in Texas recommended that members charge ten dollars for "giving a medical opinion on a negro for sale," and in fact B. H. Baker paid that sum in February 1860 to physician John Norwood for performing a vaginal examination.[10]

Doctors did not limit their involvement to warranting a slave's health before sale. Slaveholders who believed that they had been duped as to a slave's "soundness" sometimes brought suit to recover all or part of the purchase price, the cost of lost labor, or bills incurred in treating a particular medical condition. Generally doctors provided remarkably detailed accounts of how particular health conditions affected a slave's worth. Court appearances were public events and thus important in establishing or maintaining the professional status of an individual physician. The ability to "read" a slave's body accurately demonstrated the skills of a particular doctor and helped to establish the value of medicine and medical practitioners in the management of a labor force.[11] Consequently, doctors took court appearances seriously.

Cases charging a slaveholder with selling a woman who could not give birth were uncommon, but the fact that they existed at all suggests the importance purchasers placed on a woman's ability to conceive. The difficulty of prevailing in such cases encouraged dissatisfied buyers first to try negotiating a settlement outside of court. The "defect" of infertility might not become apparent for years, and the fact that an enslaved woman retained some value as a productive laborer further inhibited lawsuits.[12] Any perceived monetary loss might be recouped simply by reselling the woman to an unsuspecting buyer, a strategy that had the advantage of avoiding court expenses. Nevertheless, some suits went to trial.

The most likely cases to be brought in court were those in which menstrual or other gynecological problems became evident soon after purchase. In defense, sellers tended to argue that particular disorders were not disabling. When Didry's new owner cited gynecological defects as grounds for returning the enslaved woman, for example, itinerant slave trader A. J. McElveen counseled his employer not to accept her return unless she was "examined by a Doctor" who could attest to a disability. McElveen argued that she was "no more sick than women are generally."[13]

As witnesses in cases brought to rescind the sale of an enslaved woman, doctors testified to a woman's pregnancy, abortion, monthly menses, and diseases of the womb. The last were of particular concern, since they might turn out to be fatal. Three days after an eighteen-year-old woman was sold, she lay dead, possibly from puerperal fever. She was pregnant at the time of her sale and gave birth soon afterward. An autopsy revealed a tumor of the throat, which also might have accounted for her untimely death. In this case the Mississippi purchaser was a practicing physician, and both he and her previous owner had warranted her as sound.[14]

Judges and juries tended to side with slaveholders who had been deliberately misled about a woman's fertility. A Georgian who purchased a woman only to discover that she suffered from a uterine infection rendering her infertile had his money returned. An Alabama master received a refund for three women who were found to be suffering from syphilis, gonorrhea, and an umbilical hernia respectively, all because they could not bear children. Not everyone succeeded in such suits, but the fact that some secured judgments against sellers indicates that planters considered a woman's reproductive capacity important to her worth.[15]

Doctors not only identified infertility among slaves; they also attempted to rectify it. Regularity in menstrual cycles was deemed necessary not only for conception but also for performing productive labor. A planter who ignored menstrual problems would be doubly at risk. Any medical man who treated menstrual disorders successfully would be held in esteem by colleagues and slaveholders, as well as assured of a lucrative practice. The twin problems of missed work and barrenness commanded focused attention from doctors, and by the late antebellum era they were experimenting with therapies for regulating "disordered" menstruation. A Tennessee doctor identified in the record as Baskette warned other physicians of the dangers of treating menstrual disturbances "with indifference." Many believed "that nature was capable of righting herself," but this was not true. Lack of attention to menstrual problems was the greatest cause of barrenness and needed to be approached as a medical problem, Baskette argued.[16]

Physicians viewed regularity in menstruation as a sign of general health and noted a patient's menstrual history in diagnosing and in evaluating her condition. When Alabama physician H. W. Caffey diagnosed a case of catalepsy, a condition in which the patient experiences diminished responsiveness (the patient had entered into a trance), he observed that each episode (there were many) seemed to occur at the time of her monthly period. A "sub-acute inflammation of the uterus" excited a nervous reaction with menstruation, he concluded. A Virginia slaveholder thought it advisable to inform physician James Carmichael that his fifteen-year-old enslaved patient who was said to be suffering from rheumatism had not yet begun to menstruate. Physician and planter Samuel Sexton monitored the menstrual periods of one of his slaves, and when she developed pain about her abdomen that seemed related to the menstrual cycle, he performed a vaginal examination to determine the cause. Still uncertain about the diagnosis, he called in his neighbor—another planter physician—to do the same. When a slaveholder sought a return of the purchase price for the enslaved women Carolina on the ground that she was of unsound health, no fewer than six local doctors testified about her monthly menstrual cycles.[17]

Such thinking harkened back to the early part of the century, when physicians believed that the body was in a constant state of change as constitutional and environmental factors interacted with one another. Physicians, it was thought, should maintain or restore equilibrium by regulating the body's secretions: blood, urine, feces, and perspiration. Healthy performance of the menstrual cycle was considered crucial. Efforts to control "disordered menstruation" reflected this general understanding that a woman's physical and mental well-being depended on regularity. John Overton, a Nashville doctor who treated a slave woman named Mary at the request of her owner, admitted that she had not become pregnant afterward. But she was menstruating, he noted, as if to say that his attendance could not be at fault.[18]

So many afflictions seemed to stem from "unnatural" or "disordered" menstruation that a call for "the study of menstruation in our climate" by a southern practitioner appeared in the pages of the *At-*

lanta Medical and Surgical Journal. Alabama physician Robert E. Campbell considered the study important because in his estimation problems related to menstruation accounted for much of the illnesses he and other doctors observed in their female patients. Some medical students explored the subject in the dissertations they wrote in partial fulfillment for a degree in medicine. Of twenty-five graduates of the Medical Department of Hampden-Sidney College (Virginia) in 1853, three wrote dissertations on the topic. Medical students at the Atlanta Medical College in 1856 also addressed the subject in dissertations, one on healthy menstruation and another on menstrual disorders. As concern about menstrual health mounted, the physiology and function of menstruation became a subject of debate in southern medical journals and in medicine more generally.[19]

The majority of doctors interested in treating infertility focused on regulating the menstrual cycle. E. M. Pendleton published a chart derived from his eight years of medical practice in Georgia in which he listed the causes of sterility as dysmenorrhea (painful menstruation), menorrhagia (excessive menstrual flow), amenorrhea (scanty menstrual flow), leukorrhea (a whitish vaginal discharge), prolapsed uterus (displacement of the uterus), and abortion (the interruption of pregnancy). "Here," he wrote, "we have in a nut-shell, an exhibit of all the uterine affections, which might prevent conception occurring among blacks and whites." Sixty-one of the 144 cases involved menstrual disorders. The others in order of importance (according to the doctor) were "abortion, etc." (55 cases), prolapsed uterus (18 cases), and leukorrhea (10 cases).[20]

Despite the linking of menstrual health and women's general well-being and the increasing investigations of the topic, physicians had little understanding of menstruation, even the age of onset. Doctors in North America and Europe (along with the general population) commonly held that different social groups began menstruating at different ages. Some cited climate and class as causes. Other doctors characterized such thinking as old-fashioned. Physician

J. Henry Bennett wrote in 1852 that hygiene appeared to be more influential than climate. British physician W. Tyler Smith, whose lecture on menstruation appeared in the *New Orleans Medical News and Hospital Gazette*, postulated a link between climate and the age of puberty, but he believed it to be only one of several factors influencing the age of onset. Class, hygiene, race, and temperament also made a difference.[21]

Bennett put the age of onset at between eleven and nineteen. The average age of onset among enslaved women in Robert E. Campbell's practice was fifteen, which he considered the norm. Anglo-Saxons began menstruating at about age sixteen, and Amerindian women at age sixteen or seventeen, Campbell claimed, and women of mixed race began between the ages of fifteen and seventeen. Campbell based his estimates on the "good deal of research" he had conducted over a four-year period. He accounted for the difference in age of onset among the races by the order in which he supposed they became sexually active; if white women were to begin "to gratify their animal passions" as early as blacks allegedly did (especially field hands), they would start menstruating at earlier ages. House servants, according to Campbell, had their first periods at later ages than did field hands, reflecting their later entry into sexual relationships.[22]

The physiology of menstruation perplexed doctors as much as the age of onset. Campbell, who practiced medicine in Alabama, explained the process and purpose of menstruation as the elimination of an excess of blood. At puberty women underwent a number of changes, including the production of greater quantities of blood than needed. This blood went to support the fetus if a woman became pregnant, but it was thrown off about every twenty-eight days if she did not. D. Warren Brickell disagreed. He explained menstruation as the "exfoliation of the mucus membrane of the body of the uterus." The New Orleans doctor reached his conclusion after performing an autopsy on a young woman whose body lay in the "dead house" of

Charity Hospital in New Orleans. Although his ideas about menstruation were closer to actuality than those of Campbell, he mistakenly believed that menstruation occurred simultaneously with ovulation. F. H. Ramsbotham weighed in on the matter in the pages of *The Stethoscope and Virginia Medical Gazette:* at each menstrual period, one or both ovaries "burst and shed its contents." The menstrual fluid represented the "deciduous membrane" that would have formed had conception occurred.[23]

Masters and mistresses, who embraced the idea that menstrual health was crucial to the enslaved woman's performance of reproductive and productive labor, monitored their slaves' monthly cycles. Virginia planter William Bernard knew that a slave woman who had become debilitated by what he presumed to be a cold had not menstruated since coming down with ague and fever the previous fall. When the enslaved "Jenny was taken yesterday with a fluding [flooding—excessive bleeding] & [became] very much indisposed," M. Strachan sought assistance from the family doctor: "what ever you think necessary please to send." When an enslaved woman who had been treated for "an obstruction" once again became "very unwell," her owner J. A. Banks wrote to family doctor James Carmichael "to send her another Box of Pills." Yet despite such concern, not many planters granted concessions to menstruating women. One Virginia woman ran for hours chasing several hogs in a cornfield while she had her period, even though she complained of back and bowel pain, "a dragging sensation in the pelvis, and a difficulty in voiding urine and feces." Those owners who made concessions generally based them on their own (mis)understanding of menstruation or their individual judgment of the severity of a woman's complaint. Thomas Jefferson made sure his overseer knew not to force menstruating women to work in wet conditions, a practice that was believed to destroy their health. Another Virginia planter, John Fitzgerald, excused his slave Mobrina from work because she "was sick a day or two . . . from too great a flow of Her menses."[24] Generally owners formulated rules for the conduct of menstruating women that were intended to have them carry out work assignments while maintaining the degree of health necessary for bearing children.

Slaveholders sought to control customs associated with menstruation and kept abreast of a woman's monthly cycles through the distribution and storage of rags used to absorb the monthly flow. Masters, mistresses, and overseers came to know whose period was late, scanty, suppressed, painful, irregular, or characterized by excessive bleeding. The soiled rags created a problem in sanitation. Probably because they hoarded the rags for reuse and could not always wash them at once, or because they wanted their own source of rags so as to manage menstruation on their own, some women stored them in their cabins. An article "On the Duties of Overseers" published in the agricultural journal *Soil of the South* recommended that the plantation's overseer visit the cabins of slaves each week in part to "see that there are no filthy rags under their beds." This prompted an angry response from Peter Pie, an Alabama overseer who minced no words in begging deliverance from this chore. While he was satisfied to attend to the general cleanliness of the slaves both in their cabins and on their persons, he drew the line at hunting up menstrual rags and throwing them on the compost heap. "Do pray have me excused," he pleaded.[25]

When called by owners to treat menstrual disorders among enslaved women, southern doctors, like their northern counterparts, adopted an empirical approach. They experimented, observed the results, then shared their "findings" with colleagues, who were urged to give the "cure" a try. One doctor advocated electrical current "sent through the uterus" as a sure cure. A medical resident in Baltimore touted chloroform as a remedy after reading about its use as such in the *London Lancet*. Only one trial convinced him of its efficacy and prompted him to extol its virtues in *The Stethoscope and Virginia Medical Gazette*.[26]

One complication in treating menstruation was the understanding of doctors that menstrual cycles might vary from woman to woman and still fall within a "normal" range. What was profuse menstruation for one was normal for another, Thomas E. Massey of Mobile observed. The state of the uterus and the shape of the uterine neck could vary not only from woman to woman but also in the same woman from one examination to another. Women even experienced pain in different ways. What produced pain in one woman did not in another, he said, a fact that made the uterus "not exactly like any other organ."[27] These ideas complicated diagnosis and treatment without deterring southern doctors from attempting both.

Difficult or painful menstruation (dysmenorrhea) was of special concern because it accounted for much of the time women lost from work as well as for failure to conceive. No standard treatment existed for dysmenorrhea, nor any consensus as to cause. An article in *The Stethoscope and Virginia Medical Gazette* in 1853 attributed the pain to the formation of a membrane similar to the one that forms in pregnancy. Professor E. D. Fenner of the New Orleans School of Medicine, who put forth "A Remedy for Dysmenorrhea, and Consequent Sterility" in the pages of a New Orleans medical journal, insisted that the condition resulted from the formation of a blood clot in the cavity of the uterus. Doctor A. G. Mabry, called in to treat the condition in a young woman who had given birth twelve months earlier, upon examination discovered a complete occlusion of the vagina, which would have prevented conception. Physician William G. Smith encountered a similar situation in his Virginia practice. The enslaved Maria had suffered a miscarriage and subsequently developed severe pelvic pain, probably originating in an infection. Smith and other physicians attributed the pain associated with her menstrual cycle to an occlusion of the vagina, which they believed resulted from the infection. Despite the condition, Maria "became pregnant, greatly to her astonishment, and that of her owners," Smith wrote. He surmised that during one of a number of "violent paroxysms, a small passage" opened, allowing conception to occur.[28]

Doctors attempted to follow the recommendations for treatment included in medical texts and journals. Famed Scottish physician Jack Mackintosh recommended as a cure for dysmenorrhea the insertion of a bougie, a thin, flexible instrument used for dilating body passages. In Professor Fenner's opinion, a bougie might be called for in some cases, along with "the use of leeches," but the condition also required medication to prevent the clot from reforming. Determined to correct the problem (presumably at the request of the owner) using Mackintosh's method, Mabry made several incisions only to have them heal. He repeated the process again and again. At last a bougie was introduced and kept in place by a bandage, which the doctor reported "eventually made a perfect cure."[29]

Although medical texts included "remedies," many doctors of the day acknowledged that these did not always work, and they pursued further experimentation and refinement of treatment. For seven years Doctor C. W. Ashby of Alexandria, Virginia, used without success a remedy for dysmenorrhea recommended by William P. Dewees, professor of midwifery at the University of Pennsylvania. Insertion of a bougie failed as well. Ashby next tried a plant substance, stramonium, after consulting a published text by physician John Eberle. Eberle was vague about the plant's use, and Ashby began experimenting in 1840. After experience with fifteen or twenty cases, Ashby recommended his approach to colleagues. Although most of Ashby's cases involved white women, he specifically pointed to the treatment of one slave who had been married for several years without bearing a child. According to Ashby, after treatment with stramonium (coupled with a purgative, pain killers, and "hot applications"—his "usual plan"), she was both pregnant and working satisfactorily. Like many other doctors, J. V. Withers of Kentucky took a "heroic" approach in treating a case of dysmenorrhea. Finding no physical problem to account for the pain, he prescribed opium, both in the form of a medicine and in the form of a laudanum enema. The enslaved patient's suffering grew worse, and a new doctor arrived as a consultant. At first the physicians bled the woman from the arm, and when this approach did not help, more anodynes (painkillers) and bloodletting followed. Finally the physicians introduced chloroform. Uncertain as to how much chloroform to administer, the doctors recorded the dosages and times of administration, then recounted the regimen in the pages of a medical journal. Two Louisiana doctors also reported success in treating dysmenorrhea with chloroform. Their experiences appeared in the pages of the *New Orleans Medical News and Hospital Gazette* without specifying how much of the anesthetic either had administered. Other doctors wishing to follow the example would—like the originators of the therapy—need to determine the proper dose for themselves.[30]

A turn toward empiricism generally evident in American medicine in the antebellum years encouraged experimental treatment on enslaved women. H. A. Bignon, who apparently agreed with Professor Fenner about the cause of the problem, shunned what he called the common remedies for dysmenorrhea and prescribed for Celia a hip bath with mustard, Dover's powders (an opiate), and ergot. The last, a fungus that grew on rye and that promoted uterine contractions, was intended to expel a clot. The doctor also prescribed quinine and an iron compound. After six months Bignon pronounced Celia relieved. The same treatment reportedly worked for the enslaved Maria, but Ann, also a slave, "about 20 years, well made and of large stature," received a slightly different regimen, in part because she was nursing a child and experiencing pain in her back. In addition to the hip baths and drugs, Ann was given "a blister to the sacrum" and told to wean her child. This treatment worked, according to Bignon; her discharge was normal and the pain hardly noticeable.[31]

Suppressed menstruation (amenorrhea) was of even more concern to doctors attempting to treat infertility than difficult or painful menstruation. It appeared more directly linked with infertility. If the menstrual flow could not leave the body, sperm presumably could not enter the uterus. Conception was known to occur absent menstruation, but this was not normally the case. *The Stethoscope and Virginia Medical Gazette* reported the case of Hannah, a girl of mixed race who became pregnant before she began menstruating, but her situation was described as a curiosity.[32]

T. L. Ogier treated a slave girl, age seventeen, for amenorrhea when her period failed to appear over the course of ten months. "The usual domestic medicines [presumably administered by the mistress but also perhaps by the patient] had been used to promote the uterine discharges" with no effect, and the girl's mistress asked the doctor to take charge. Ogier tried a variety of treatments, which produced diarrhea but not the menses. A friend reported success in using the water pepper plant (a treatment associated with the alternative approach to medicine known as Thomsonianism) for "a case of obstinate amenorrhea." He had been urging Ogier "to make some experiments" with it in similar cases. "I thought my patient a good subject to test the efficacy of the medicine," Ogier later stated. He ordered her to ingest three times a day a concoction derived from the plant, which in his view brought about the desired result. Her menses, which appeared on the tenth day of the treatment, "flowed rather abundantly," causing the doctor to reduce, then discontinue, the medication. The following month, Ogier "commenced with the tincture three times a day as before," four or five days prior to her expected menstrual period, which appeared normal except for a yellowish discharge that preceded it. "Since that time she has menstruated regularly, without the assistance of medicine," he reported in an essay touting the cure.[33]

Other approaches to treating amenorrhea ranged from mustard and linseed poultices, hot foot baths, externally applied laudanum (tincture of opium), mineral or vegetable tonics, a generous diet, moderate food, cold bathing either in a tub or by sponge, and rest. If the condition resulted from a genital deformity or other physical abnormality, surgery might be called for, or doctors might consider dilation or incision of the cervix. Agents that stimulated the menstrual flow (emmenagogues) such as ergot or savine could be tried, though cautiously, since they proved too harsh for some women. Other reported cures included applications of nitrate of silver and scarification of the surface of the uterine cavity. One medical text published in 1848 listed electromagnetism, aloes, and strychnine among the "medicines that are regarded as emmenagogues." A southern doctor advised a black women aged thirty or thirty-two who had never conceived to assist another woman during the delivery of her baby and to "breastfeed" the infant following its birth. In May 1839 William G. Craghead discovered an occlusion of the uterus that in his estimation had caused the retention of the menses for twenty-three months in a sixteen-year-old enslaved woman. He attempted to relieve the condition by the forced insertion of a speculum, which separated the walls of the vagina. Not all cures brought immediate results, their advocates acknowledged. The best cures would bring on the menses within one to three cycles.[34]

Of course the desired outcome was not merely the restoration of the menses but general health and the bearing of children. The doctor who advised dry breastfeeding as a cure bragged of the outcome: the woman was soon delivered of her own child. In the past the outcome might have been regarded as coincidence, the doctor admitted. But medical men now looked upon the practice with interest. The doctor theorized that the mammary glands played a crucial role in conception, as did the ovaries.[35]

Despite their interest in and aggressive treatment of suppressed menstruation, as with other menstrual disorders physicians did not understand the underlying cause. Generally any discussion of origins occurred in narrow medical terms. Doctor Craghead was an exception. He attributed the cause of the occlusion he encountered in a slave to the rape of the patient when she was but a girl of twelve. His report of the case provided no clues to the social context in which the rape took place or how he learned of it. Instead he explained his effort to release the accumulated menstrual blood by forcing his way into the girl's vagina with a speculum. What the girl thought of this he did not say. His selective silences allowed readers—presumably other medical men, since the doctor wrote for a Virginia medical journal—to avoid the difficult issue of the sexual exploitation of young slave girls as they entered puberty and the troublesome thought that the young woman (child) in question may have considered herself violated twice by white men.[36]

The mistress of the slave treated by Ogier thought that the problem had begun when the young woman got wet a few days before her menstrual period, which lasted just two days and was scanty. A Kentucky doctor reported a case of suppressed menstruation in a white woman stemming from a bad cold. J. Henry Bennett noted in the pages of *The Stethoscope and Virginia Medical Gazette* that suppressed menses might result from "exposure of the body, and especially of the feet, to the cold or to the wet; of a mental shock from fear, grief, pain or anxiety, &c, or of a sudden attack of disease." Ovarian tumors and uterine inflammation also were to blame or, in rare cases, birth defects or other genital malformation. Doctor William R. Smith stated that a case of suppressed menses in a slave had originated with "exposure and a great deal of hard labor."[37] His observation was unusual, however. Most doctors did not link menstrual irregularities to conditions of slavery.

The process of determining the origins of amenorrhea was complicated by the many symptoms associated with the condition and the various circumstances in which patients lived. The condition could come on suddenly or gradually and be accompanied by "serious general symptoms," including "obstinate vomiting" and "severe hysteria." Change could be therapeutic, but the exact modification depended on the individual's situation. Curing a young lady might involve taking her out of school—an approach hardly appropriate for enslaved females, whether adolescent or mature. A change of residence from the city to the country might benefit a white woman, while a black woman might be reassigned work that limited her exposure to wet or cold. Horseback riding was sometimes recommended for white women; black women who generally performed physical labor throughout the day hardly needed additional exercise. Leeches might be applied to the vulva of unmarried women, to the neck of the uterus in married women.[38] Thus, one principle of nineteenth-century medicine—that physicians must understand their individual patients in order to prescribe appropriately—found expression in status-based treatments that reflected stereotyping by doctors more than individualized plans of care.

Antebellum doctors worked under the assumption that medical practice had to take into account particular attributes of the patient, such as environment, age, gender, race, and habits. This "principle of specificity" rejected the idea that practitioners should learn medical therapies by rote and apply them indiscriminately to patients. There were universal rules governing the doctor's choices, but the doctor's knowledge of an individual patient's idiosyncrasies would allow him to alter treatment to enhance well-being.[39] This was the theory. Actual medical practice, as exemplified by the cures for amenorrhea discussed here, suggests that treatment regimens did not reflect the specific attributes of patients so much as the doctor's understanding of social standing. Medical treatment, at least in these cases, reflected a peculiar attribute of doctors.

Many physicians believed that when menstruation was suppressed, the discharge occurred vicariously through an outlet other than the vagina. At times the cases were merely reported as curiosities, but at others doctors tried to effect cures based on this understanding. Robert E. Campbell recounted such a case involving a slave girl. She had begun menstruating at age sixteen, had one period, but missed her second and third. At the time when she should have had her fourth period, she bled from the nose. Campbell thought that almost all doctors could report similar cases. Physician J. Boring did so. The professor of obstetrics at the Atlanta Medical College thought that excretions from "the eyes, the nose, breasts, fingers, toes, skin, etc." could be "vicarious menstruation." He cited as an example the enslaved Mary (along with cases of white women), who began menstruating at age fifteen and whose periods were regular for some three years. Gradually her periods diminished and eventually ceased. Each month blood oozed instead from a wound on her leg. To cure the condition, Boring eventually amputated the leg, but thereafter the stump reportedly bled each month for about as long as a normal menstrual period.[40] Mary's situation may have been extreme, but she was far from being the only woman to suffer misguided treatment that left her no better—and in some cases worse—than before doctoring began.

Excessive menstruation (menorrhagia) could be as much cause for concern as painful or difficult or absent menses, and doctors tried various treatments recommended by colleagues or experimented with new remedies of their own making. One Virginia doctor waited some time to try a treatment he had read about in the *American Journal of the Medical Sciences,* oxide of silver, before a case presented itself in the form of a young lady, age seventeen. As this story suggests, doctors treated white women for the condition as well as black. White women could welcome or refuse treatment as they wished; black women's choices were more circumscribed by virtue of their status. Although some may have welcomed the attention of white physicians, others acquiesced in or were coerced into accepting treatment. The mistress of seventeen-year-old Dicey thought her health precarious enough that she called in a physician and declined a journey abroad so that she could stay home to tend her.[41] What Dicey thought about the matter was not recorded, perhaps not even noticed.

Twenty-five-year-old Amanda, a field hand and mother of one child born eight years earlier, suffered from "menorrhagia of seven

years standing—at times so profuse as to excite alarm for her safety."
Her periods were not only heavy but also irregular, and sometimes
did not appear at all in a month. A doctor called by her owner examined her internally using a finger and a speculum, but neither
method revealed a cause. He directed her "to wear short drawers of
red flannel" and to "use the cold hip bath daily," after which she was
to rub herself briskly with a coarse towel. He also prescribed a formula for keeping her bowel movements regular, and he provided a
tonic that included cinchona, also called Peruvian bark. (The bark,
from which quinine is derived, was an important part of the materia
medica in the United States and in Europe in the eighteenth and
nineteenth centuries.) Two weeks later he reported her "greatly improved," but the treatments continued for another four weeks. When
"some hemorrhage" returned the following month, she reportedly
resumed taking the cinchona for four or six weeks, and then stayed
well for two years afterward. Attending physician Robert Battey of
Georgia described the case in the pages of an Atlanta medical journal and recommended that his colleagues use cinchona to cure
chronic uterine ailments involving all forms of "disordered menstruation." Perhaps Amanda welcomed Battey's attention. She reportedly complained of debilitating pain, for which she must have sought
relief, although the decision to call the doctor was not Amanda's but
that of her owner. At any rate, Battey's was not the first treatment
tried. The previous fall, Amanda had taken iodide of iron, which reportedly improved her general health but did not alleviate her menstrual problems. Who prescribed it for her is unknown.[42]

Doctors were concerned about all vaginal discharges—not just
menstruation. They were unsure what caused leukorrhea, commonly
called "the whites," but they linked the condition, manifested by a
whitish discharge (mucus mingled with pus), to infertility. Napoleon
B. Anderson, M.D., of Louisville, observing that the condition
existed "in almost every case where a female does not bear children," concluded: "Unquestionably this disease is a frequent cause of

sterility." Other doctors were less certain of the cause, and the cure remained even more elusive. Anderson considered the condition to result from "the ulceration of the [uterine] neck and cavity," which interfered "with the intromission of the semen, which passes away with the profuse discharge."[43] In other words, ejaculation did not serve as a sufficient force to counteract the flow of the discharge, which meant the semen was washed away before it reached the egg.

Unable to pinpoint the cause, other doctors who treated cases of "the whites" experimented with remedies as they saw fit. Grace, a favorite house slave of mixed race, suffered from leukorrhea for twelve years during which a number of doctors attempted a variety of unsuccessful cures. The vaginal discharge was at times so copious and other symptoms so debilitating that she was confined to bed. Finally, a physician identified in the record as Russell tried injecting iodine directly into the vagina. Within three months following the initial treatment, Grace was up and about, able to "resume her occupation as cook to the family." The doctor could offer no theory about how the douche worked, but he believed the cure had something to do with the iodine's absorption into the body, citing a brown secretion from Grace's breasts as evidence. He described Grace's breasts "as full and enlarged while under the influence of this medicine," as opposed to "very small and flaccid" before treatment began; clearly, he intended to suggest a linkage between breast size or shape and fecundity. Russell then described two other cases in which he used iodine, both involving white women. Because doctors usually discussed their cases chronologically, his presentation of Grace's case first suggests that he tried the treatment upon the enslaved black woman before offering it to the free whites. Russell concluded his article by stating that he had treated other patients with similar problems, presumably of both races, and that all responded similarly to the treatment.[44]

When confronted with a case of leukorrhea in the late 1850s,

Bedford Brown, M.D., of Caswell County, North Carolina, "determined to experiment" upon the patient, a thirty-year-old slave woman who had never borne a child but had exhibited symptoms of uterine disease from an early age. Observing with the help of a speculum inflammation of her entire vaginal canal, he prescribed a solution of chlorate dissolved in rainwater—"as much of this as an ordinary female syringe contains . . . twice daily." Within two weeks the patient was cured, according to the doctor. Encouraged by this success, Brown extended the experiment to other women, first to another slave suffering from gonorrhea, and then to several other cases in which a whitish discharge appeared to originate in ulcers of the cervix. The doctor's silence on the status of the latter patients suggests that they may have been white.[45] Doctors tended in their records to ascribe race or servile status to black women while omitting references to race or status for white women, apparently on the presumption that black women represented some type of variation of the "normal" white female.

It is impossible to know how many or what types of medical treatments were formulated—perhaps on the spot—to cure problems with menstrual or other vaginal discharges. John P. Little of Richmond questioned the wisdom of an approach to medicine that stressed only the more positive or promising outcomes. Doctors who wrote about their experiences in medical journals rarely followed up with patients to investigate the long-term effects of medical treatment, although they sometimes mentioned anecdotal evidence that a particular regimen had produced desired results. This approach was wrong, Little argued. Doctors ought to make available records of failed therapies as well as successful ones. He listed some of his own botched treatments in a Virginia medical journal, challenging other physicians to do the same. Among those that did not work for menstrual disorders was guiacum (an evergreen tree resin).[46] How many experimental treatments enslaved women (or other women for that

matter) endured before he reached this conclusion can never be as-
certained. Doctors attempted cures that proved at times helpful,
harmful, or benign.

One obstacle to determining effective treatment was that articles
in the medical journals were not refereed by knowledgeable doctors.
The editor exercised some judgment but usually published what he
received and left assessment of it to others. The editor of *The Stethoscope and Virginia Medical Gazette* admitted, "We *have* published bad
articles and we expect *to do it again.*" This outcome, he maintained,
was simply the price paid for including a large amount of material
from physicians who had never before contributed to a journal.[47]
Certainly, there was an element of truth to the editor's comment, but
a bigger problem was that clients demanded action and physicians
could hardly expect to maintain a practice by acknowledging the
very real limits of medical knowledge. Doctors competed for clients
not only with one another but also with advocates of alternative approaches to healing, including promoters of home remedies, many of
which appeared to work as well as the remedies of the regulars.

By far, home remedies represented the most common alternative
to treatment of menstrual disorders by physicians. James A. Tait in
Alabama recorded in his plantation records a prescription for a tea
intended to "promote or produce the regular monthly discharge in a
woman." The concoction, made of certain berries and taken three
times a day, was readily available at no cost to anyone who hoped for
a cure.[48] Apparently Tait expected or at least hoped the tea would
work. If it did, there would be no need to employ medical assistance
for the promotion of menstrual regularity. Doctors were careful to
distinguish between professional medicine and folkways, some of
which originated in the slave quarter. Only in this way could they
hope to present themselves as professionals.

Enslaved women took measures of their own to regulate the
menstrual cycle, which they viewed as important to motherhood.

They did not consider conception to require medical attention, but they, too, were concerned about a woman's fertility and general wellbeing. The women were pressured by members of both the enslaved and slaveholding communities to bear as many children as their bodies would allow because slaves and slaveholders alike placed a high value on motherhood. Slaveholders encouraged the birth of children because it enhanced their financial position and helped them cultivate an image of themselves as stewards of slaves whose "benevolent" rule allowed bondwomen and men the privilege of a family life. Slaves valued children for their universal ability to charm, entertain, love, and be loved and because the birth of a child strengthened families and communities while contributing in important ways to the family economy. The presence of children allowed mothers and fathers alike to experience life beyond the role of slave. The survival of their people depended on the birth of infants.[49]

Societies that place a high value on motherhood consider barrenness a tragedy. Enslaved women who did not bear children early and regularly had to contend with the disappointment of husbands as well as owners. When a Georgia woman failed to bear a child within what her husband and owner considered a reasonable period of time, both showed displeasure. Her husband left, and her owner stopped showing her much attention. When her master sent her to work for a doctor in the hope that medical treatment might help her conceive, she was happy to go. She avoided for a time both her master and her husband, whom she described as "cross." Occasionally a woman rejected motherhood completely in retaliation for the wrongs inherent in the slave system. Mary Gaffney of Texas maintained that she deliberately "cheated Master" by having no children while she was enslaved.[50] Such situations were rare, however. Most women wanted children.

Because they valued children, enslaved women were more concerned with regulating fertility than with preventing conception.

The women worked hard from sunup to sundown to complete tasks for owners. After finishing this work, they faced family responsibilities in the quarter, which ranged from breastfeeding infants to cooking for and clothing families. Because repeated pregnancies took a toll on a woman's body, most mothers tried to space children to avoid taxing their health beyond the point of recovery and to allow time to breastfeed their children and care for other family members according to their own ideas about what was possible and proper.

Given the emphasis on motherhood by both the enslaved and slaveholding communities, women were left on their own to ensure that repeated pregnancies did not exhaust their strength or interfere with their ability to care for older children. They relied on secret, indigenous means of doing so, as have other women who have found themselves living in societies unwilling to grant them power to manage pregnancy and childbirth on their own.[51] Their behavior suggests that they welcomed pregnancy as long as children were spaced appropriately. They worried if they bore children too frequently, but they were equally anxious if they did not become pregnant often enough. Instead of promoting or inhibiting a particular pregnancy, most women tried to prolong the period between childbearing through extended breastfeeding.

Slaveholders preferred that infants be weaned as early as practical, usually between eight and twelve months. Mothers wanted to breastfeed for two or more years, a practice that helped to ensure not only the health of the child but also that of the mother. Although the role of breastfeeding in suppressing ovulation was not clearly understood, women knew that they diminished the chance of becoming pregnant by breastfeeding. Slaveholders who arranged for mothers to leave their babies under the charge of a caretaker while they worked elsewhere encouraged early weaning by feeding babies supplementary foods during the day. They let mothers leave worksites periodically to nurse infants but gradually stretched the time between feedings as the children aged. By the time infants were a year old, mothers were prohibited from breastfeeding at all during day-light hours. But after mothers retired to their cabins for the night beyond the sight of owners and overseers, they did as they pleased. Many continued to breastfeed children at night to the age of two or even older. "It was a common occurrence," former slave Amanda McCray testified, "to see a child of two or three years still nursing at the mother's breast." Perhaps in the realization that rules against the practice would be impossible to enforce, one planter expressed an ex-pectation that a mother would probably be "up with her child" at night.[52]

Despite widespread knowledge that breastfeeding was best for the baby, a few physicians weighed in on the matter in line with the slaveholders' desire to limit its duration. Tennessean T. Lipscomb went so far as to argue that overlong breastfeeding produced false pregnancies, the development in utero of all or part of a malformed embryo or placenta and membranes. Lipscomb, whose practice con-sisted of "many cases peculiar to females," styled himself something of an expert on false conceptions. In 1855 he cited the case of an en-slaved woman who developed a mass in her uterus (known as a mole) because she continued to breastfeed her child for fifteen months fol-lowing its birth. Although the doctor admitted that false concep-tions did not occur in every case of extended nursing, he thought that at least four-fifths of them could be traced to this cause. Pro-longed nursing supposedly blighted the development of the fetus. Lipscomb's linkage between prolonged breastfeeding and moles lent a certain scientific credibility, however spurious, to the wishes of planters that enslaved women would wean children early and be-come pregnant quickly following a birth. So did the position taken by other southern doctors that weaning should occur between the ages of six and twelve months.[53]

Women found ways other than through breastfeeding to regu-late fertility. They could track regularity in menstruation by mark-ing lunar phases. When menstruation ceased or became irregular, enslaved women employed agents (emmenagogues) to achieve the regularity in menstruation they desired. Sage tea was "good for painful menstruation or slackened flow," for example.[54] They did not think of themselves as inducing abortion, because (like white women) they believed that pregnancy was not the only cause of suppressed menstruation, nor did they believe that a fetus was formed from the moment of conception. Ambiguity about why the menses had ceased and when life began allowed women a degree of flexibility in controlling fertility without encountering resistance within the slave community, where motherhood and children were highly valued. The fact that the same substances that brought on the menses might also enable women to detect a pregnancy removed any stigma attached to their use. If a woman used an agent believed to stimulate the menses without achieving this effect, she understood herself to be pregnant and acted accordingly.

The most popular emmenagogue used by enslaved women was the root of the cotton plant, which was both effective and widely available.[55] Cotton was the cash crop most commonly cultivated in the antebellum South, and indeed it was the expanding cotton belt that fueled the slaveholders' desire for increased numbers of slave births. As the United States expanded its borders westward first into areas purchased from France and later into areas wrested from Mexico, slaveholders followed. Expanded territory called for more laborers, who could be purchased from older slaveholding states or raised from infancy. Slaveholders sought a means of ensuring that children were born in bondage to cultivate the cotton plant, even as a female network of enslaved women shared knowledge of the plant to ensure that the number of children born met their judgment about the appropriate timing of motherhood. The fortunes of slaveholders rested on the portion of the plant that grew above ground, the destiny of women on the part below.

The ubiquitous cotton plant proved advantageous to women who wished to use it without arousing undue suspicion among owners, husbands, or others. It could be brewed into a tea or chewed. And consumption could be stopped as easily as started when a woman wished to become pregnant.

Both husbands and owners knew of its general use among enslaved women, and worried that women were deliberately avoiding pregnancy. Former slave Dave L. Byrd believed that deliberate abortion was so widespread among enslaved women in Texas that the entire black race "would have been depopulated" had not emancipation changed attitudes toward childrearing among black women, who presumably were more eager to bear children in freedom than in slavery. All the women used cotton root for this purpose, Byrd said. Slaveholders watched them carefully in an effort to put an end to the practice, but with little success. The women "would slip out at night and get them a lot of cotton roots and bury them under their quarters."[56]

Former slave William Coleman described the use of cotton root as ubiquitous in Tennessee. It was a wonder the entire race was not wiped out, he said, given the tendency of women to chew it. When his master finally realized what was going on, he tried to prevent the practice by severely punishing—Coleman said almost killing—any woman engaging in it. His actions had little effect, however; the women "would slip [out] and chew it in spite of all he could do about it."[57]

Southern doctors knew of the root's use by enslaved women; some even incorporated it into their medical practice. Physician Thomas J. Shaw urged his colleagues to give the cotton plant "a trial" in regulating menstruation among white clients. In the pages of the *Nashville Journal of Medicine and Surgery*, he listed its desirable attributes as "handy to all, and free of expense." Shaw recommended a decoction of four ounces of cotton root to two pounds of water, boiled down to one pint and taken (a wineglass full) every hour. He noted the root's "most salutary effect . . . in aiding or augmenting menstruation; its action is very speedy." Doctor Bouchelle of Mississippi also readily acknowledged its habitual and effective use by slaves. He thought it as efficient as and safer than ergot, a treatment favored by physicians. It had no other effect than "the excitation of the menstrual secretion, excepting, perhaps," pain relief. John Travis, M.D., of Tennessee openly sought a cure for obstructed menses in a white woman from the materia medica known to slaves. In 1852 he reported to readers of the *Nashville Journal of Medicine and Surgery* that the cotton root "worked like a charm" in inducing menstruation. He had learned of the method ten years earlier when reading another medical journal, the *Western Journal of Medicine and Surgery*, which attributed the source to "a negro woman" living on a Mississippi plantation.[58] Physicians turned to the remedial substances used by slaves because many of their own medicines and therapies did not prove efficacious.

Skeptics existed. E. M. Pendleton, who practiced medicine in Sparta, Georgia, found absurd the theory "prevalent among planters and some physicians" that enslaved women could control their own fertility. It was not possible, he opined, for the "stupid negro" to have discovered a reliable means of doing so, when "sober, thinking men have failed for ages" to find a means of regulating the menses. The fact that masters, mistresses, and physicians kept a watchful eye over the reproductive lives of enslaved women made the possibility even more remote.[59]

To admit that enslaved women could control their own reproductive destiny was to acknowledge the limits of the slaveholder's power. If black women could not be made to bear children in sufficient numbers to expand or at least maintain the size of the labor force, southern slave society would soon cease. Future generations of planter children would have no source of bonded labor. Many men like Pendleton were unwilling to entertain this sobering thought; others took no chances and joined in a quest to obstruct the ability of enslaved women to abort children.

Meanwhile enslaved women tended or gathered other medicinal

plants that aided in fertility regulation. Most of these treatments, like the tea made of the cotton root, were favored because their preparation was easy and could be undertaken by anyone—not solely by a person with special knowledge or powers. They were readily available and entailed no expense. Like the cotton root, they could be used in secret. Neither owners nor husbands nor anyone else had to know.[60]

An early twentieth-century survey of African Americans living in the South identified the joint use of dogwood root and dog-fennel root as a traditional means of preventing conception or producing miscarriage in women who had already conceived. The dogwood was made into a tea; the dog-fennel root was chewed and the juice swallowed. Jimsonweed (stramonium), highly toxic if not used correctly, was also said to have been brewed into a tea and used to promote regularity of menstruation. The "ground mole," according to a former slave, had also been used "to bring the women right"—that is, to treat dysmenorrhea or obstructed menstruation.[61]

The substances favored by black women for regulating menstruation were not the same as those employed by white women to effect an abortion. John H. Morgan, who practiced medicine in Tennessee, did not question the habitual use of the cotton plant by enslaved women, but he doubted that black women could obtain ergot and other means of abortion available to white women. Rue, widely considered an effective emmenagogue, was not commonly cultivated. Tansy, a dangerous substance, was widely grown in gardens, but enslaved women—with little time on their hands—preferred to gather rather than grow medicinal herbs and roots. Morgan maintained that both black and white women inquired about the abortive properties of camphor, but it needed to be taken before and after menstruation. This fact, together with the difficulty of obtaining it, meant that it would have been used more often by white than black women.[62]

Morgan's myopic view failed to consider the different purpose black women had for employing emmenagogues and other agents affecting vaginal discharges. Enslaved women attended to their menstrual cycles to ensure their own well-being, not merely to regulate fertility. The leaves of the squaw weed, or golden ragwort, which grew wild in the Georgia piedmont, were brewed into a tea and drunk at bedtime to relieve the discomfort associated with menstruation. Tansy, when obtained on rare occasions by black women, could be used to alleviate the pain associated with the menstrual cycle—not solely to induce an abortion. Slave women probably treated vaginal infections by ingesting herbs or inserting substances into the vagina to stop the discharge. Southern folklore recognized a number of simple cures for the whites, including alum, dragon's blood, motherwort (for women's disorders generally), that were probably used by black and white women alike.[63]

Sometimes plant substances that were chewed or ingested as teas required elaborate, ritualistic preparation. For example, "black haw" root—a means of preventing conception mentioned by African American informants early in the twentieth century—had to be dug from the north and south sides of the plant to be effective. It needed to be boiled with "bluestone" and the liquid strained carefully before being bottled. Even then the preparation was not complete: the black-haw potion had to be used in conjunction with another tea made from "red shanks" roots, red pepper, and gunpowder. Finally, the woman had to wait for a new phase of the moon before drinking a little from each bottle.[64] Such substances were less favored by enslaved women than the cotton root precisely because they took time and frequently involved another person—usually a healer, who might be identified and pressed by an owner to tell what she knew.

Chemical, mineral, and animal substances were all used to regulate fertility, sometimes alone or alongside botanicals. African Americans also recalled regulating fertility by manipulating the mechanics of lovemaking. Although modern people would consider the practices a manifestation of superstition, folk belief held that such practices worked. Holding a brass pin or copper coin under the tongue during coitus prevented pregnancy. If a woman lay perfectly motionless during intercourse or if she turned on her left side immediately after the act, she would not become pregnant. Gunpowder mixed with milk could prevent conception, as could swallowing nine pellets of birdshot. A teaspoon of turpentine ingested each morning for nine days did the same. A woman could produce the menses with a douche made of a tea concocted from the roots of the cocklebur mixed with bluestone. This method was dangerous, however, and required the woman to take special precautions.[65]

Slaves did not limit their efforts at regulating fertility to preventing conception. They also attempted to promote it when the timing was right. They identified substances that men might use as aphrodisiacs, for example. Some—but certainly not all—believed that union with a man who had a large sex organ would ensure fertility. Anna Humphrey for one assumed this in her youth. Couples who made love during cotton-picking season were said to have a greater chance of conception than those who made love at other times.[66]

Some of the ideas of slaves about why certain women were barren were similar to those held by members of the dominant class, and they may have originated with that group. Former slave Sophie D. Belle married twice following slavery, but she never had any children. Her friends advised her that she might have given birth to a child if she had married a darker-skinned man. Belle married "very light men both times." She described herself as eight-ninths white. Her mother had been of mixed race, and her father was a local (white) physician. These ideas echoed those of physician Josiah C. Nott and certain other doctors, as well as the broader society, who believed that people of mixed race could not mate successfully.[67] However, these ideas were not widespread among blacks, especially before the Civil War.

Fertility regulation generally was not practiced by unmarried women, only by those who had already born a child; slaves considered any discussion of the topic among children or unmarried women taboo. They restricted information about sexuality and menstruation to mature women in the hope that young women would remain naive or modest and not grow up too fast. By remaining silent about sexual matters, adults tried to shield girls from entering into marriage too soon and from the sexual abuse that sometimes followed a young woman's entry into puberty.

Modesty about sexual matters inhibited young women from broaching the subject before marriage. Frances Fluker started menstruating before she understood what it meant. She had older sisters, but even they did not tell her about puberty. They must have sympathized with the situation of their younger sibling, but they followed the custom of not discussing bodily changes associated with maturation in the presence of children. Minnie Folkes married at the age of fourteen without understanding that her husband expected more of her than cooking, cleaning, washing, and ironing. One older girl believed her siblings when they told her that their mother's new baby had come from the chimney. Henri Necaise, who grew up a slave in Mississippi, recalled adults telling children, whenever they asked where they came from, that babies were found in hollow logs or in the canebrake. On the Florida plantation where former slave Duncan Gaines grew up, adults told children that babies came from tree stumps or simply to "shut up."[68] Childhood could be prolonged only so long in a society in which owners pressed youths to marry and in which children were highly valued, however. Many slaves became mothers at early ages.

Once a woman had a child, the restriction on information about sex and the regulation of fertility was lifted. Following the birth of a child, the new mother could ask almost any older woman for advice, because knowledge about controlling fertility was widespread. Part of the older woman's job was to dispel the superstitions or folklore that sometimes circulated among younger women. An older woman set Anna Humphrey straight about the relationship between the size of a man's penis and his ability to father children, for example.[69] The need for younger married women to consult older women for advice fostered a sense of female community across generations.

Women seeking information about regulating fertility at first followed popular advice, which tended to be secular in nature and readily available from kin and acquaintances. If that did not produce the desired result, a woman might consult a traditional healer, a midwife who provided a mixture of secular and spiritual advice intended to enhance or inhibit fertility. Some women who wished for children but who did not bear them also turned to medical men for advice if they had access to them or to a conjurer if the problem originated in a social relationship and if the women believed in supernatural healers.[70]

Certain indigenous methods may have proven effective, although the concept of efficacy in its modern sense had not developed within either the enslaved or the slaveholding community. Belief in effectiveness for enslaved women would have followed empirical use of particular substances or methods or stemmed from the doctrine of signatures, in which characteristics corresponding in structure or relative position suggested efficacy. (For example, the whorl of lavender flowers set in the axils of the motherwort's leaves was suggestive of a woman's sexual organs, which in turn recommended the plant's use in treating women's problems—an idea embraced by blacks and whites.) The efficacy of the method may not have been as important as female solidarity in the transmission of folk knowledge.[71]

For enslaved women, the sharing of knowledge about how to regulate fertility helped create the concept of community among women who offered advice not only about spacing pregnancies but also about caring for infants. When efforts to space children failed and a woman became pregnant sooner than she had hoped, her female friends and relatives offered practical advice and assistance on

bearing and caring for the child. The woman did not consider her
child unwanted; she did not think of herself as avoiding pregnancy.
Rather than rejecting motherhood she was ensuring its success. The
women who used emmenagogues or other methods of regulating reproduction hoped to space children more than two years apart so as
to ensure their ability to care for those already born and to preserve
the strength necessary for bearing other babies in future years.[72]

Enslaved women who used indigenous methods of spacing children appear to have succeeded to some extent. In Loudoun County,
Virginia, enslaved black women on average began having children at
an earlier age than did free white women. They nevertheless had
fewer children over the course of a lifetime. Although it is possible
that more black than white women became temporarily or permanently infertile because of poor health due perhaps to hard labor
or to a less-than-nutritious diet, enslaved women tended to space
their children farther apart, a fact that suggests a deliberate effort to
regulate fertility. Black women in Loudoun began having children
around the age of twenty, and they gave birth on average every two
and a half years. Local white women, in contrast, married between
the ages of twenty and twenty-two. They bore their first child within
the first twenty-four months of marriage, and they gave birth ap-
proximately every two years. It seems likely that enslaved women in
other parts of the South gave birth at a similar age and at similar intervals to those of Loudoun County. One historian who has studied
enslaved women throughout the South believes they had their first
child around the age of nineteen and subsequent children at two-
and-a-half-year intervals.[73] Perhaps this trend in spacing children
was not lost on the slaveholders, who hoped through medicine to
enhance fertility by bringing the experience of enslaved women in
spacing children closer to that of their wives and daughters.

Census data and slave registries from Virginia suggest that enslaved mothers became pregnant more often in 1860 than in 1800,

both because they gave birth at earlier ages and because the spacing between children grew shorter. The change was nothing short of remarkable on Samuel Vance Gatewood's plantation. The average spacing between live births fell from nearly thirty-two months in the period 1794–1813 to less than twenty in 1835–1854. Yet no evidence exists that greater attention to fertility by doctors had any bearing on the outcome. Increasing pressure by slaveholders or factors internal to the slave community probably account for this trend. And even though the birth rate among slaves was increasing, slaveholders failed to achieve their overall goal of increasing the number of children who grew to adulthood, because infant mortality increased proportionately to the increase in births.[74]

Gynecology emerged in a peculiar fashion in the Old South. By the late antebellum years, slaveholders were soliciting the assistance of physicians in treating slave women's infertility. Many of the physicians' therapies were experimental, ineffective, painful, even dangerous, and implemented with the slaveholders' needs in mind. Enslaved women thus found themselves subject to invasive procedures that benefited physicians and slaveholders more than the women they were supposed to assist. The women (who had their own reasons for cherishing children) preferred indigenous methods of regulating fertility to those offered by physicians and their slaveholder clients. Even those methods that in hindsight appear incompetent no doubt imparted to the women a sense that they could control this important aspect of life—not an inconsequential achievement in a society that granted slaveholders an unbridled right to control life in the slave quarter. The therapies of the slaveholders' physicians were not effective so far as the women were concerned. In addition, they represented an expansion of the slaveholders' intrusion into the lives of enslaved women. The physical dominion of slaveholders expanded as their doctors probed and prodded enslaved women's most intimate bodily secrets. However much the new procedures unsettled the women, they eased the minds of the slaveholders, who believed that something was being done to ensure the continuation of slavery into future generations through the birth of bonded children. In addition, they reassured members of the dominant class (even those who opposed the institution) that the worst conditions of slavery were mitigated by the benevolence of owners who sought medical care for the women under their charge. Doctors and slaveholders joined in an alliance that focused on issues related not only to fertility but also to bringing a baby to term.

4

Pregnancy

IN 1848 KENTUCKY PHYSICIAN W. W. HARBERT WATCHED A SLAVE woman die of internal hemorrhage, which he discovered only through the autopsy that followed her death. Jane was six months pregnant. Called because of complications that seemed connected to her pregnancy, Harbert was unalarmed at first because he felt the baby move. He prescribed pain relievers, bed rest, a bland diet. When her condition deteriorated, he escalated treatment to include bleeding, a laxative, and other medications typically associated with antebellum medical practitioners. Eventually Harbert attempted an abortion. After nine days of treatment, which now included cotton oil and enemas intended to end the pregnancy, the patient died.[1]

Harbert's actions—despite the unfortunate outcome—reflected the prevailing attitude among physicians and planters in the South that if forced to choose, one should save an enslaved mother at the expense of her infant. Physician J. W. H. Spann of Missouri had this goal in mind when he manually delivered an enslaved woman who was five months pregnant. In reporting the case to colleagues, Spann deemed it unnecessary to justify his decision other than to emphasize the positive outcome for the mother. Joseph P. Logan, M.D., of Atlanta also affirmed the established medical principle that the life of the mother was more important than the continuation of a pregnancy. Called in March 1855 to treat Lavinia, a thirty-eight-year-old mother of nine living children, he determined that she was about six weeks pregnant and possibly suffering from typhoid. Various remedies yielded only temporary relief. When she appeared near death, Logan—in consultation with two other doctors and with the assistance of one of them—performed an abortion to save the mother's life.[2]

Abortions were not without controversy, but southerners generally accepted them to save the mother's life whether she was black or white. When it came to enslaved women, physicians followed the wishes of owners, who favored the mother over the infant. The fact that premature infants did not tend to thrive encouraged everyone to focus on the mother's health. But slaveholders were concerned that enslaved women bring infants to term, especially after Congress ended the importation of slaves. As the perceived value of enslaved children increased, medical men grew more sensitive to debate surrounding abortion. Some doctors gave increased attention to medical means of preventing spontaneous and deliberate miscarriage in the slave quarter; others scrutinized more closely the indigenous practices employed by enslaved women to regulate fertility.

The concern of antebellum slaveholders for infants in utero corresponded with changed attitudes more generally in the United States. *The Stethoscope*, a medical journal published in Virginia, carried in 1855 a favorable notice of a book by a New York medical school professor that urged doctors to exercise caution in the treatment of pregnant women lest they induce abortion. Doctors "have no more right to trifle with the life of the child than . . . with the life of the mother," the commentator intoned. That having been said, however, when the mother's life was endangered, every measure might be taken to save her whatever the "consequence that may result to the child."[3] Whereas doctors once had referred to all cases of failed pregnancy interchangeably as abortion or miscarriage, they began to discriminate in their terminology to assign blame for why an infant had not been carried to term. By the late antebellum era there were deliberate abortions by women to regulate pregnancy, deliberate and inadvertent abortions instituted by the practices of physicians, and unexpected miscarriages, all of which appeared to occur with some regularity within the slave quarter. Still, considerable variation characterized the use of the terms.

Part of the imprecision surrounding the discussion of abortion and miscarriage stemmed from a failure among physicians and laypersons to agree on when life began. J. Boring, professor of obstetrics at the Atlanta Medical College, disputed two popularly held ideas: that life began at birth and that life began at quickening (the time when a pregnant woman first feels fetal movement). Boring contended that life began at conception. The distinction had the potential to alter medical practice. Under Boring's definition the introduction of a bougie (a slender cylindrical instrument used for dilating) into the uterus or the administration of ergot to expel the contents of the womb constituted taking a life no matter how early the procedure occurred in a pregnancy. Only God could give or take a life, Boring argued. Yet doctors willingly did so for money. Some of the women who sought an abortion did so to escape the chastisement meted out to single mothers who gave birth illegally, he charged, but it was not just the unmarried who sought an abortion. Wives sometimes wished "to escape the pangs of parturition, and the seclusion of the season of nursing."[4]

An editor of the *Atlanta Medical and Surgical Journal* agreed that the destruction of "the product of conception" should be regarded as murder. Although the editorialist contended that criminal abortion occurred less often in the South than in the North, he nevertheless thought that it was performed often enough among southerners to alarm people interested in "the welfare of the [white] race." Eminent Philadelphia physician Charles D. Meigs sounded a similar alarm in his obstetrical manual. Noting that it was a felony to take the life of a fetus at four or four and a half months (quickening generally occurs between the fourth and fifth months of a pregnancy), he argued that the distinction was "without a difference, for the child of six weeks or of two months is as essentially quick with life as one of five or seven, or even nine months. The only difference," he went on, was that one was "strong enough to make itself felt, while" the other was "so feeble as not to be perceptible by the mother." Doctors who performed abortions, even before quickening, should be punished for the crime of murder, Meigs maintained.[5]

Discussions of deliberate abortion among black and white women differed in important ways. Black women—already degraded in the eyes of whites by class and race—could hardly be accused of debasing themselves morally in performing abortion. And so moral repugnance was reserved for the white women who avoided childbirth for selfish reasons: "to escape the pangs of parturition, and the seclusion of the season of nursing." Yet abortion among black women remained a source of worry. An enslaved woman who aborted a child without the approval of an owner challenged the slaveholder's authority.

The ability of enslaved women to regulate their own fertility undermined the ideal that owners could and should exercise mastery over their slaves. The herbal wisdom of black women represented an alternative approach to orthodox medical care—one that challenged the "scientific" knowledge of white physicians. It also posed a threat to southern society. Slavery could not continue if black women ceased bearing children. No demographic evidence suggested that black women would stop having babies. The evidence, in fact, suggested that enslaved people, male and female, revered motherhood. But in the political climate of the late antebellum years, slaveholders worried about the future of slavery and countered any challenge to its continuation whether real or imagined. Doctors joined slaveholders in attempting to prevent abortion in the slave quarter, but even as they castigated black women for reportedly aborting infants, they reserved for themselves the right to go forward with an abortion when the life or health of the mother was in jeopardy.

Southern physicians and their slaveholding clients were well aware that enslaved women used cotton root and other means to regulate fertility. Eager for a growing population of slaves, slaveholders began by the late antebellum era to label any effort by enslaved women to space children as "abortion" and to speak contemptuously of the practice. When one Natchez planter sued another on the ground that the woman he had purchased was falsely warranted as sound, he produced a witness testifying that a short time before her purchase she had "taken some medicine to clear herself" (induce an abortion). After a twenty-year-old woman miscarried while working in the field, her owner brought in a doctor specifically to determine the cause. The owner suspected that the miscarriage had been the result of what he termed self-inflicted violence intended to abort the child. Doctor J. S. Dixon, who arrived fifteen minutes after the delivery, confirmed his supposition that the woman had aborted the child using a blunt object.[6]

Doctors helped fuel suspicion among the slaveholding class that enslaved women commonly aborted their children. One country doctor maintained in the pages of a New Orleans medical journal that barrenness occurred more often among black than white women, an observation that in the minds of many slaveholders suggested deliberate abortion by enslaved women. Another doctor charged a black woman with assisting in the abortion of nearly all the infants on a Tennessee plantation. Only two infants had been born at full term on the place in the preceding twenty-five years, according to the doctor's testimony. He apparently thought the woman was administering an abortive weed to all the pregnant women (with their consent). No less than two medical journals reported that the low fertility rates on a Mississippi plantation were no accident but rather the consequence of slave women's deliberate use of a tea brewed from the cotton plant. Physician E. M. Pendleton, of Sparta, Georgia, philosophized in 1849 about what he termed "an unnatural tendency in the African American female to destroy her offspring." Noting a compilation of statistics from Georgia purporting to show that black women were four times more likely than white women to experience abortion or miscarriage, he speculated that either slave labor was "inimical to the procreation of the species" or the women knew "a secret by which they destroy the fetus at an early stage of gestation."[7] Most white southerners considered only the latter explanation plausible.

Despite the frequent circulation of stories about abortion among black women, a few members of the medical profession harbored doubts about their accuracy. The "country doctor" cited above allowed that in his twenty years of practice he had never observed a case of deliberately induced abortion in the slave quarter. Instead, slave women appeared eager to bear children. As evidence, he cited women who had beseeched him to help them conceive. A physician identified in the record as Avent posited that no one—white or black, professional or lay—knew of a sure method of deliberately ending a pregnancy. It was difficult to induce an abortion in a healthy woman. Even Pendleton entertained doubts about the prevalence of abortion. Although several means of producing miscarriage were available, he was uncertain whether enslaved women were acquainted with them. Pendleton charged planters with being too quick to accuse black women of aborting children as well as of avoiding pregnancy. When the planter asked a doctor whether the patient "has been taking something to keep her from having children," he responded affirmatively "just to please the prejudices of the inquirer." Statistics collected for Hancock County, Georgia, suggested that blacks were "much better breeders than the whites." It would be a mistake, Pendleton insisted, to believe that only white women wanted children. The "general laws of nature" ensured that all women (indeed all female mammals) wanted to bear and nurture offspring.[8] Despite such protestations, slaveholders held to the belief that black women were deliberately aborting infants in large numbers.

Blacks appeared less likely to bring a baby to term than whites. Pendleton thought that some of this difference reflected "overexertion at the wash-tub, scouring mop and plough" and other work assignments. If the different labors of black and white woman were switched, white women would have more abortions than blacks, he maintained. Only the black woman performed "the severe labor of the sterner sex" while pregnant.[9] This was a message that the majority of slaveholders did not want to hear and that few physicians dared to deliver. If not couched carefully, it could lead not only to calls for a reduced workload for pregnant slaves but also to criticism of slavery in general. Slavery's foes looked for ways to discredit the system. Punishing work regimes said to promote spontaneous abortion could be cited in support of the abolitionist cause; consequently, doctors and slave owners tended to refrain from discussing the issue openly.

Pendleton, who maintained he was no "Negrophile" (a derogatory term used by contemporaries to identify people who sympathized or fraternized with blacks), promoted his ideas as scientific observation, not as a moral indictment of the slave system. Lower fertility rates in the slave quarter were a fact of life intrinsic to a system of labor in which women performed the physical chores necessary to getting a crop in and out of the ground, it was true. This was not the whole story, however. "Intemperate sexual indulgence," he claimed, contributed to low fertility rates among slave women. Frequent and indiscriminate sex was not only immoral but also supposedly injured "the generative function." Black women who married and lived "respectably like white people" would encounter no problem with fertility. Although he acknowledged the possibility that arduous work helped account for low fertility rates in the slave quarter, Pendleton stopped short of accusing slaveholders of creating conditions under which black women could not bring a baby to term. The women's personal choices were equally to blame for low birth rates.[10]

Pendleton's skepticism about deliberate abortion in the slave quarter went largely unnoticed. Racism and worries about the future of southern society fueled fear among slaveholders and doctors that black women were purposefully aborting in large numbers the children upon whom slave owners depended. Hope grew that medical men would devise a means of intervening in abortion. Meanwhile planters did little to address either the problem of work assignments or the supposed "intemperate sexual indulgence" of the quarter.

Physicians who deplored the use of abortifacients among black women expressed greater sympathy for white clients, reflecting a tendency of doctors generally to accept the interpretations of their slaveholder clients when it came to medical matters. Doctors regularly and readily prescribed substances for stimulating the menstrual flow (emmenagogues) for white women to stave off pregnancy even as they deplored the actions of enslaved women to regulate the menses. The tendency to accept the word of a "lady" that she was not attempting an abortion extended to doctors outside the South. One Canadian physician went out of his way not to know that the adolescent daughter of a "lady" was pregnant—refusing to conduct an internal exam or even to ask indelicate questions. He prescribed emmenagogues throughout the pregnancy and recommended horseback riding toward the end—an activity the mother forbade on the ground that people would talk about her daughter's appearance. (Both the doctor and mother acknowledged that she looked pregnant.) Eight and a half months after the cessation of her menses, they reappeared in the form of "hemorrhaging." Now the doctor was summoned urgently to treat the young "lady." Although he found the sofa and floor covered with blood and other liquid and learned of the father's furious response to the situation, the doctor continued to write about the case as if it were a menstrual problem rather than the result of months of attempted abortion, possibly followed by infanticide. The fact that the case appeared in a Virginia medical journal suggests that the editor thought southern doctors would find it relevant to their own practices.[11]

Suppositions based on race and class clouded doctors' diagnostic ability as they strove to fit observations about bodily functions into preconceived ideas about black and white sexuality and morality. One nine-year-old slave girl suffering from an extended abdomen died when her owner, J. Haywood Jones of Alabama, and the physician he employed diagnosed the problem as pregnancy rather than illness. Not even the inability of the doctor to conduct a vaginal exam because of the small size of her vagina dissuaded him from his diagnosis. An autopsy by attending physician W. H. Gantt and four other doctors revealed a large abdominal tumor instead of a fetus. Apparently in self-defense, Gantt observed that it was "the undivided opinion of all who saw her that she was pregnant." He further rejected any responsibility for her death by noting that grapes brought to the patient by some black children triggered the convulsions that led to it.[12] The preconceived notion of black promiscuity evidently persuaded the girl's owner and doctor that no cause other than precocious sex need be considered—even in the face of evidence to the contrary (the impenetrable vagina and the child's age).

Slaveholders did not limit their investigation of interrupted pregnancy to ferreting out deliberate abortion. Rather, they insisted on investigating all cases of miscarriage and stillbirth to determine the cause. Physician and planter Joel Shelby, of Liberty, Texas, personally examined the dead fetus of his enslaved woman although she resided on a plantation located thirty miles from his home place. He evidently sent orders directing the old woman who attended the birth to save the fetus for his inspection. Fifteen days passed before Shelby got around to the task. By then its condition would have deteriorated and rendered any analysis of the remains suspect; nevertheless, the doctor exhibited no uncertainty in his conclusion that the baby had died six weeks before the miscarriage while the woman

was out gathering corn.[13] Farfetched as his deduction might have
been, this case together with the one involving the nine-year-old girl
illustrates the determination of slaveholders and their physicians to
control all aspects of enslaved women's reproductive health, including any interpretation of negative outcomes.

Of course, determining the cause was only one reason slaveholders paid physicians to examine women whose pregnancy had ended
in miscarriage or stillbirth. Dreading the loss of valuable property
and accustomed to taking command of a situation, they called in
doctors in the hope that something could be done. Unfortunately,
given the limits of obstetrical knowledge, physicians could achieve
little. Dixon, called to treat the twenty-year-old described above,
bled the woman and gave her calomel (mercurous chloride used as a
cathartic and diuretic), morphine, and oil to aid her recovery. Some
doctors prescribed the botanical substance black haw to prevent miscarriage or abortion already in progress. Physician W. W. Durham
claimed to have discovered another means of interrupting abortion
when his supply of black haw ran short. "At one period of my practice the Negroes used the cotton root so frequently to produce abortion that my supply of black-haw became exhausted," the doctor
wrote in 1867, "and having heard of the power of the hazel to effect
the purpose . . . I resorted to it with perfect succes." Durham's intended readers were medical men, and he included a recipe with his
comments: "Steep one ounce of the leaves in one pint of water, and
drink freely."[14]

As Durham's statement suggests, slaveholders called physicians
to attend enslaved women when miscarriage threatened. Planter
Bezaleel Brown summoned a doctor on 4 July 1816 because Jane, the
house servant, who was several months pregnant, "threatens a loss."
Miscarriage represented a lost opportunity to expand the labor force.
In addition, it usually entailed some cost to the planter who owned
the slave. In some cases, concessions had already been made to the
expectant mother to ensure her successful delivery—often in the

form of a reduced work assignment late in the gestation period. More of the woman's work might be lost or reduced while she recovered.[15] The doctor's fee represented a cost, but it had to be weighed against the possible loss of the mother's labor and the child. Of course, women did not work at full capacity when they were recovering from childbirth, but the planter in this case gained an additional asset—the newborn slave.

When a woman suffered a miscarriage, the financial cost was not offset by the birth of a child. One study of pregnancy among slaves on a Georgia cotton plantation found that mothers tended to avoid field work for twenty-five days whether their infants lived or died. Medical expenses for complications of pregnancy could be high, especially if the mother required ongoing care. In May 1817 South Carolina physician Henry Ravenel charged $3.50 for visiting, prescribing, and furnishing medicine for Charlotte, who "threatened miscarriage." When he returned the following day, he assessed a fee of $2.50. Later in the month Ravenel charged $7.50 for attending "Judy at labour" on the same plantation. The size of the fee indicates that this birth went smoothly. The previous year, Ravenel had been called to see Bess, who miscarried in the night. For this visit, Ravenel charged $13.00. A follow-up call two days later added $7.00 to the bill. A Virginia planter paid $10.00 to Doctor J. Lyle for visiting and furnishing medicine after a woman miscarried.[16] In this case the mother lived. The financial cost to the planter from miscarriage rose dramatically, of course, if the woman died, as sometimes happened.

Frequent miscarriages challenged the planter's ideal of slaveholding. Owners maintained that slaves were better off under their stewardship than if they fended for themselves, but women who could not bring a baby to term hardly supported this claim. By calling in a physician when miscarriage threatened, the slaveholder demonstrated a concern for the mother and child's welfare. This was one reason owners eagerly summoned medical men in the face of miscarriage despite the medical profession's poor record of success in such situations. One master was so sure that his slave would die after a miscarriage that he refused to bury the fetus "until he saw there was no probability of putting the mother with it." Nonetheless, he sent for a physician.[17]

Incidents of miscarriage were said to be high among slaves and may have been increasing during the cotton boom years, when planters pushed slaves to work hard at planting and harvesting the lucrative crop. James Henry Hammond in South Carolina described the enslaved women on his Silver Bluff plantation as acquiring "habits of miscarriage." Alabama planter John Horry Dent made numerous entries about failed pregnancies in his plantation journals. In 1841 he wrote: "Tenah very sick this morning . . . miscarried at 11 O clock AM." In 1853, "Phillis threatened Abortion." Tyrah miscarried in 1858. In January 1860, "Helen abortioned last night."[18]

Sensitive to slaveholders' concerns, doctors sought ways of improving a woman's ability to bring a child to term. In 1853 the *Nashville Journal of Medicine and Surgery* carried an article by a physician with "a pretty extensive practice in midwifery" who had developed a pill that he claimed worked even for women with histories of repeated miscarriage. He cited success with one thirty-five-year-old enslaved woman who had miscarried a child "nearly every year" and another who had experienced five miscarriages in quick succession, as well as other cases. Made from the "extract of Hyosciamus and Oil of Sassafrass," its developer, Doctor R. Thompson, considered it valuable "in all cases of threatened abortion, when not caused by accidents or severe sickness," as well as "for all the nameless pains, aches and disquietudes attendant on conception and gestation." He prescribed it a week before the expected due date and after the delivery to calm the nerves of black and white patients alike. Thompson took care to describe his experience in developing the drug. He told how he first concluded that it would work and explained that he had tested it first on himself. The ordering of the case histories in his account suggests that the black women were the first patients to receive the medication.[19]

Thompson's testimonial to the contrary, doctors could do little to avert an imminent miscarriage. But poor outcomes did not prevent physicians from developing other plans of treatment and boasting of an ability to assist, which encouraged slaveholders to call in a physician in hopes of staving off a slave's spontaneous abortion. A Georgia physician publicly took credit for preempting a miscarriage through bleeding and the use of "opiates, astringents, &c." A Doctor Currey reported some of his cases to the East Tennessee Medical Society, including one involving the enslaved Lucy, who miscarried in her third month while spending the day washing. He indicated which medicines he had tried in the belief that other doctors in attendance would be interested in discussing the protocols.[20] Apparently it never occurred to him to suggest a lightening of a pregnant woman's workload, which might have proven more effective. Laundering in particular involved heavy physical labor. Buckets of water had to be carried, cauldrons of hot water had to be stirred, stains had to be beaten by hand from the clothes, and baskets of wet clothes had to be toted where they might be spread and dried.

There is little evidence that doctors were blamed for negative outcomes from pregnancy. Everyone recognized the very real limits of medicine, and few clients in the South filed malpractice suits. In the North, however, dissatisfied patients in the late antebellum era were increasingly seeking redress through the courts, often for obstetric cases. The disparate experiences of northern and southern doctors suggest a difference in attitude toward the doctor as authoritative figure.[21] Because many orthodox doctors came from elite families accustomed to command, some patients may have been intimidated or believed they did not have the standing necessary to challenge the doctor. Such attitudes would certainly have prevailed in the slave quarter, where no one had legal authority to file a case in court and where neither the patient nor other black witnesses could by law testify against a white man. Only the slaveholder could complain, but owners had much in common with physicians. Both equated boldness of action with manhood, and each accepted the idea that unfortunate outcomes could not be avoided. The attitude among elite men that only they could accurately judge one another helped ensure that any blame for miscarriage remained with the expectant mother or her female attendant. Moreover, the advice of physicians seemed grounded in modern science and was respected by men more than the folk wisdom associated with women. Attitudes about status and ways of knowing thus combined to discourage the filing of malpractice suits in the South.

Physicians more commonly appeared in the aftermath of miscarriage to treat complications than at the outset. A. R. Nelson of Tennessee was called to attend a woman who had lately miscarried a fetus of four and a half to five months. The afterbirth had not been expelled with the infant. The doctor tried friction on the abdomen before resorting to a hook to extract the placenta. He then turned to drugs: blue mass (a blue pill made from metallic mercury and other ingredients) and an emetic (ipecacuanha). When these failed, the doctor prescribed salts as a remedy for constipation, which produced "two passages." The doctor tried the hook once more, and an hour or two later the afterbirth was removed. Again the doctor prescribed blue mass along with Dover's powder (made from ipecac and opium). The latter would have been intended to calm the patient, who had been forced to endure quietly the excruciatingly painful process. The thirty-seven-year-old woman recovered. It was her ninth pregnancy, seven of which had ended in miscarriage.[22]

Such women were of concern to slaveholders. The physician who perfected a method of preventing multiple miscarriages or stillbirths would enjoy widespread admiration and no doubt a lucrative practice from slaveholders who regretted the loss of the mother's labor as well as the loss of the child. Medical students explored the causes and prevention of miscarriage in dissertations while doctors discussed methods of bringing a baby to term. Doctors D. Warren Brickell and E. D. Fenner, for example, concluded that a woman with a small pelvis might yet bear a healthy child if labor was induced at eight months, before the fetus was fully developed. The smaller infant might pass through the pelvis without difficulty.[23] The problem, of course, was that premature infants rarely thrived.

Most antebellum slaveholders waited for problems to develop during childbirth before summoning a physician, but some were willing to take preventive measures based on experience. A woman's previous history with childbirth could prompt a master or mistress to take the extra precaution of consulting a doctor in advance of labor, as several cases from the 1850s substantiate. Master Joseph P. Manly of Georgia engaged E. F. Knott on behalf of Jane because he expected difficulty; she had suffered a prolapsed (displaced) uterus when she had given birth previously. Brickell and Fenner reached their conclusion about the difficulty posed by a small pelvis following the examination of a pregnant woman who had conceived five times previously but who had not yet produced a living child. They were unable to save the sixth child either, this time because of the condition known as placenta previa, a life-threatening condition that occurs most often in women who have experienced multiple births. (The placenta is abnormally buried in the uterus so as to cover partly or completely the opening of the uterus.) Doctors know today not to examine vaginally a woman with the condition, because feeling with the hands can induce the bleeding that leads to death. But doctors Brickell and Fenner did not know this when they conducted the internal exam that led to their finding. M. J. Greene was summoned to see an enslaved woman in labor even though there were no signs of complications. When the doctor arrived, the woman's owner informed him that she had been bled during each of her previous four labors. Uncertain as to why, Greene waited three hours. Concluding that she was slow to dilate and possibly feeling pressure from the owner, the doctor decided to follow precedent and bleed the patient. Eventually, however, the doctor realized that the problem was more complicated than he first supposed. This was "a case of partial placenta previa, with transverse presentation—the right foot and hand," he wrote later. Despite heavy hemorrhaging, the mother convalesced, but the child was stillborn.[24]

At times other conditions than a threatened miscarriage drew medical men into a drama centered on pregnancy. Nineteen-year-old Amelia developed eclampsia, a condition occurring occasionally in the latter half of pregnancy and characterized by convulsions and sometimes coma. After finding Amelia unconscious, her mother notified the overseer. He in turn sent for the doctor, John Butts, who arrived five hours later hoping to deliver the child manually. He planned to wait until the woman was dilated sufficiently to allow the passage of the child, meanwhile controlling the convulsions. He bled Amelia in each arm and sent for chloroform to be delivered from his office. Through trial and error, Butts established that chloroform administered by handkerchief over the nose stopped the convulsions, at least temporarily. Altogether, he used half a pound of chloroform to sedate the woman over a period of three hours. Then, having grown impatient with the slow progress of labor, the doctor inserted his fingers into the uterus to break the amniotic sac by force and speed the process. He grabbed one of the baby's feet, pulled, and removed the dead child over the course of half an hour. After removing the placenta, he left the plantation to attend other duties but not before advising a black nurse about administering the chloroform as needed during his absence. For weeks the patient appeared in a stupor, unable to speak or to recognize anyone.[25]

Although the doctor eventually pronounced the patient "entirely well," he remained troubled by the case. He could not fit the episode into any previously known narrative of disease or pregnancy. His discomfiture led him to seek opinions of colleagues about what might have caused the lengthy coma. Was the cause of the prolonged stupor the original epileptic convulsions or the chloroform or a combination of the two? In other words, was the case more about the course of epileptic convulsions or about the administration of chloroform or both?[26] He used the episode to present himself as a man of science studying an abstract phenomenon. The patient's health was of course important, but so was the professional practice of medicine.

As concern over miscarriage mounted, some physicians wondered more broadly about the linkage between disease and pregnancy, for white women as well as black. They asked, for example, how pregnancy affected the course of disease. The Fisk Fund offered a prize of $100 for the best medical dissertation on the subject of whether pregnancy accelerated or retarded the development of tuberculosis in persons predisposed to the disease. The *Atlanta Medical and Surgical Journal* carried news of a conference paper read before the Association of the College of Physicians of Ireland purporting that pregnancy generally protected women from contracting diseases such as cholera, while conceding that when such a disease struck a pregnant woman, it generally did so with ferocity. The author of the paper further hypothesized that certain types of diseases such as phthisis (understood as pulmonary tuberculosis, consumption, or a general wasting away) went into remission when women became pregnant.[27] The appearance of such notices in southern medical journals indicates physician concern about the linkage between disease and pregnancy, but this concern did not produce understanding. Women who experienced pregnancy and illness simultaneously continued to confront practitioners who did not know how one affected the other and did not agree upon methods of treatment.

The uncertainty about the link between disease and pregnancy raised questions about whether physicians inadvertently induced miscarriage. A great medical debate evolved over whether certain drugs used to treat other health problems in pregnant women resulted in abortion. Through this debate doctors demonstrated their commitment to avoiding miscarriage and bringing a pregnancy to a successful conclusion.

Particular controversy centered on the use of veratrum viride, also known as hellebore, which slowed the pulse and was thought to be useful in cases of croup, bronchitis, laryngitis, asthma, pleurisy, pneumonia, and other sicknesses. One theory promoted its use as a substitute for the bleeding that was part of the standard treatment for these conditions. When an article appeared in the *Nashville Journal of Medicine and Surgery* questioning the association between veratrum viride and miscarriage, physician W. A. Brown, one of the first doctors to write about hellebore's abortive property, responded promptly. Since writing his original thesis, he had given the substance to two pregnant women. Both were slaves and the master of each had been apprised of the likely result. The owners had consented to its administration because it appeared the lesser of two evils. As expected, both women miscarried. Brown included with his rebuttal the testimony of other doctors who recommended against prescribing it for pregnant women because of the risk of abortion. "Hundreds of women are sure to . . . abort," Brown warned, if doctors persisted in its use. Doctor W. H. Robert also reported a case of miscarriage following the administration of veratrum viride. He prescribed the drug along with a blister for a woman with pneumonia. The slave, in her sixth month of pregnancy, miscarried the next morning. In a subsequent issue B. F. Newsom of Georgia disputed Brown's explanation for the cause of the miscarriage.[28]

The debate over the use of veratrum viride spilled over into the *Atlanta Medical and Surgical Journal*. There V. H. Taliaferro acknowledged that the medication could do harm if used without proper supervision. He stopped short of avoiding its use, however. If physicians gave up veratrum viride, Taliaferro protested, they might as well give up "arsenic, mercury, opium, antimony, &c." because they are dangerous, and in that case doctors might have no remedies at all. As a matter of fact, Taliaferro declared, veratrum viride had a distinct advantage over other dangerous drugs in that the stomach could not retain enough to cause death except in repeated large doses. To bolster his case, Taliaferro argued that the drug might have value in treating puerperal (childbed) fever. Having used it himself in practice, Taliaferro thought it more likely to retard uterine contractions than to encourage them, although he readily admitted that the medication sometimes produced violent nausea and vomiting, which in themselves, he admitted, could result in abortion.[29]

A belief among physicians that blacks did not react as well as whites to sedatives added to the reluctance of at least one physician to prescribe veratrum viride.[30] But for the most part, discussions concerning the use of drugs during pregnancy proceeded without reference to physiologic racial difference. Any distinction in their use for blacks and whites reflected instead the social environment in which physicians operated. For physicians reading the Atlanta journal, the warning was clear: eliminate this plant substance from your remedies in treating pregnant slaves, or at least gain the owner's informed consent before administering it. In the end, some physicians spurned the drug's use in pregnancy for fear it would cause women to abort; others continued to recommend it in cases in which the mother was otherwise at serious risk.

Questions about the safety of drugs for pregnant women extended to quinine, a crystallized substance derived from cinchona bark. Interest in this drug ran high in the late antebellum era. It was proving a successful treatment for malaria and held out hope for a variety of ailments. Doctors submitted so many articles about the drug that the editor of one southern medical journal felt compelled to suspend publishing them (if only temporarily) to make way for other subjects. "If we were to publish everything which has been sent to us on the subject of quinine, there would not be room left for anything else in the next two numbers," he explained in defense of the ban.[31]

Use of quinine engendered controversy because some doctors considered it an abortifacient. Not all agreed. Joseph J. West, adjunct professor of anatomy at Savannah Medical College, thought it was wrong to deny pregnant women this protection against malaria without proof of a harmful effect. Citing half a dozen successful outcomes in his practice, most of which involved white women, West continued to prescribe quinine without worrying about its potential to induce abortion. In fact West went so far as to assert that quinine prevented rather than promoted miscarriage in an enslaved woman whose hemorrhaging suggested the possibility of an impending miscarriage. He acknowledged that many abortions accompanied the introduction of quinine, but he thought that these would have occurred anyway as a result of the malaria for which the drug was prescribed. The *Charleston Medical Journal and Review* in 1860 carried an article by Georgia physician J. S. Rich exploring the worth of quinine in arresting hemorrhage, to be used in certain cases "where all the usual remedial agencies have proven abortive, and where the patient is rapidly sinking." Despite the controversy, doctors continued to prescribe quinine for large numbers of slaves. Doctor William Pettigrew reported at the February 1860 meeting of the South Carolina Medical Association that while in Louisiana he had advised one of his clients to administer quinine every day to each of his slaves. The major health problem on the plantation was malaria, and the doctor considered this the most effective way of handling the disease.[32]

Whereas some slaveholders sought physician assistance only in the face of a medical crisis, others looked to physicians for help in determining the fact of pregnancy. They hoped to ferret out any woman who might be feigning pregnancy to gain concessions and to project effectively their available supply of labor. One South Carolina planter expressed frustration with his inability to distinguish the truth of the matter on his own: "Very much [vexed] with *sick women*, either real or pretended, the latter in most cases." In fact some women who reported signs of pregnancy—cessation of menses, a swelling abdomen, nausea, even quickening—did not produce a child within the period normally observed in gestation. Rice planter and physician James Ritchie Sparkman may have felt twice duped by the slave woman known as Bella. Her first pregnancy lasted more than the usual nine months; her second reportedly ended in miscarriage. Of course, Bella may have miscarried twice; other women may have done the same or suffered from gynecological conditions that produced symptoms similar to the signs of pregnancy. But some may have intended to mislead owners in order to gain concessions extended to pregnant women. The situation encouraged slaveholders to call in physicians to examine women before excusing them from demanding physical labor. Another benefit of verifying pregnancy was the ability to plan ahead to meet agricultural needs with a reduced workforce. Nelson Berkeley's overseer was unsure in January 1828 how many hands he would have to work in the crop that coming season. All the hands were "well at present," but some were pregnant. He was unsure exactly how many; he guessed two or three.[33] Knowing would have allowed him and the plantation owner to arrange for additional workers at peak periods of labor.

Most planters expected to excuse pregnant women from the most arduous labor late in the gestation period. Agricultural journals of the day carried essays, letters, and other articles reflecting the latest thinking on the subject. One South Carolina overseer in 1828 suggested that pregnant women have their usual work assignments cut by half during pregnancy and that they be excused from working in wet areas. Another South Carolina overseer went even further, advocating that pregnant slaves be in "great measure exempted from labor, and certainly from exposure and undue exertion for some time before confinement." Most planters granted concessions, but few went so far as to reduce work assignments to the extent advocated by these agricultural reformers. In fact some slaveholders dealt with the

"problem" of pregnant laborers by refusing to grant reduced work assignments at all. Although planters welcomed the birth of a slave, no
one wanted to be left shorthanded in cultivating a crop. Planter
Kenyon Morps of Georgia expected pregnant women to work "right
up to the last minute" before giving birth. John Horry Dent's biogra-
pher has concluded that the Alabama planter's practices consistently placed the welfare of the crop before that of pregnant women
and their infants; generally, his women worked almost up to the time
they delivered. Dent wrote frequently about his slaves' pregnancies, indicating great concern about their effect on his agricultural
output.[34]

Those planters who made concessions to pregnant women fell
back on disciplinary measures to ensure that women did not claim
privileges of pregnancy to which they were not entitled. The enslaved Markie, described as having been pregnant "for many more
months than are generally required for the process of continuing the
human species," received a flogging for her false claim. Perhaps she
said she was pregnant to gain the increased rations her owner allowed pregnant women, as the informant who told her story believed. Or perhaps her owner unknowingly punished her for having
medical problems whose symptoms mimicked those of pregnancy.[35]

Slaveholders could turn to medical men to help determine
whether accommodations were necessary by verifying the pregnancy.
As men of science, doctors were beginning to spurn the would-be
mother's word in favor of symptoms verifiable by observation. J. Junius Newsome of Georgia, who penned a "Thesis, on the Signs of
Pregnancy" in 1855, considered unreliable symptoms to include cessation of the menses, morning sickness, changes in the breasts, enlargement of the abdomen, and quickening. More reliable diagnosis
was possible by manipulation of the uterus through an internal examination (ballottement) or listening for the fetal heartbeat. Although some doctors maintained they could ascertain a pregnancy as
early as the third month, Newsome thought five months was more

realistic in determining a pregnancy by internal examination; the fetal heartbeat could be heard at about four and a half months.[36]

Doctors could hardly discount completely the signs and symptoms women had relied on traditionally to determine if they were pregnant. Newsome himself admitted that cessation of the menses when coupled with morning sickness was a pretty good sign of pregnancy. Nevertheless, the message he hoped to convey was clear: women could not be relied upon to establish the fact of pregnancy. Only medical men trained in the latest scientific techniques could be counted upon for accuracy. This line of argument appealed especially to slaveholders, who generally believed their bondwomen prone to deceit. It also reflected a shift in medicine as doctors began to rely less on patient narratives in diagnosing disease and more on physical examination of the patient.[37]

The task of verifying pregnancy was indeed daunting. The condition could not even be verified by the appearance of a child nine months following the cessation of menses because doctors were uncertain exactly how much time separated the two events. Statistics first published in the *American Journal of the Medical Sciences* and appearing in the *Western Journal of Medicine and Surgery* noted great variety in "the relation between the time of the last menstruation and the birth of the child." The highly respected physician William P. Dewees acknowledged "many causes" that shortened gestation and "some which may procrastinate the period." Some physicians believed that gestation might be prolonged well beyond the usual term. Doctor J. S. Chisolm, who presided at the birth of a baby weighing nearly fourteen pounds, promptly proclaimed the mother to have been pregnant for eleven months. His assessment seemed to reflect his sense of the infant's size along with the owner's assessment of when the woman had stopped menstruating. Wooster Beach's medical text noted that while gestation lasted 280 days or forty weeks, the difficulty of pinpointing a date of conception together with variations produced by nature required some flexibility in predicting a

birth date. Even the well-known Philadelphia obstetrician Charles
D. Meigs acknowledged in his popular obstetrical text that pregnancies lasting longer than 280 days were not unknown.[38]

Cases of prolonged pregnancy could last for years if the fetus
died, according to medical literature of the day. A Richmond doctor
reported a case in which an elderly slave woman was believed to have
retained a dead fetus in her abdomen for forty years. She began passing bones in her stools, and more than one doctor attributed the
phenomenon to this cause. An Alabama doctor gave an account of a
similar case. The slave Mary had ceased to menstruate at the age of
twenty-eight. She experienced periodic headaches, painful urination, and a constant blood-tinged discharge from the vagina and
urethra. She also had chronic respiratory problems. Five years later
she miscarried what appeared to be a badly decomposed fetus of
about two months. Fetal bones continued to be expelled from her
body for fifteen more years, whereupon she developed pneumonia
and died. The doctor who attended her during her final illness described her as a "feeble, old woman," age forty-eight.[39]

Superfetation—the development of a second fetus after one has
already begun to grow—was also reported in medical journals,
adding to the confusion surrounding the length of gestation. North
Carolinian W. C. Sanckford described a case in the neighborhood of
Flanklinton in which a slave woman miscarried a fetus at six
months, then six weeks later miscarried a fetus determined to be
about three months. As to why both were not aborted at the same
time, Sanckford speculated that the woman had a double uterus. The
doctor did not know whether she had secreted milk or had the "usual
flow of lochia" (the uterine and vaginal discharge that follows miscarriage or childbirth). His interest in the matter led him to investigate similar cases disclosed in medical journals. Four were European,
but in New Orleans a woman reportedly delivered two fetuses at
eight and four months, one black and one white. The attending
physician said that in this and perhaps similar cases the woman had

not only a double uterus but also two vaginas.[40] A fascination with abnormalities of birth led doctors to overstate their occurrence and certainly encouraged them to share their experiences with other physicians in the pages of the nation's medical periodicals.

The argument for involving medical men in verifying pregnancy was, for some, grounded in the very real concern that certain women who exhibited signs of pregnancy were actually suffering from other conditions. Absent menses, a swelling abdomen, enlarged breasts, and darkened nipples made a fourteen-year-old Tennessee slave appear four months pregnant, but in fact she had an abdominal tumor with adhesions, which claimed her life. Another Tennessee slave woman reported "all the symptoms" associated with pregnancy. She began hemorrhaging and experiencing labor pains at four months, but her symptoms in fact reflected the presence of cysts. Doctors Sharber and Hall performed an autopsy following the death of a Tennessee woman known as Grace. Her friends thought she was three months pregnant because her breasts were enlarged and her menses had ceased. Even the doctors thought she had died following a miscarriage, but the autopsy revealed that she was not pregnant. She instead had suffered from uterine cancer.[41]

Mistakes in verifying the fact of pregnancy cut both ways, of course. Doctor William R. Smith mistakenly attributed symptoms resembling pregnancy to disease. The woman believed she was pregnant, and an old woman, probably a midwife, agreed, but the doctor discounted both women's testimony; the fact that they were black, female, and enslaved no doubt contributed to his dismissal of their statements. The patient soon went into labor and gave birth to a healthy child. Smith later ascribed his error to the presence of pregnancy and disease in the same woman, rather than to his failure to listen or observe. His confusion stemmed from the patient's having symptoms of disease (namely urinary and bowel complaints), which he described as continuing after the child's birth.[42]

A fifteen-year-old slave in Virginia complained for three days of

being sick before taking to bed. When the home remedy employed
by the mistress failed to relieve her fever and pain, a physician was finally called. The doctor, identified as Parker, could discern nothing
wrong at first. When he asked the patient about menstruation, the
girl said she had been "unwell" for some three weeks. Parker concluded that her case was "one of rheumatism from exposure," although he was not entirely certain, given the girl's "indisposition to
talk." The doctor left a prescription for calomel and opium and orders that she be given castor oil to purge her bowels. That evening
Parker returned and thought he discerned the signs of tetanus in his
patient. He immediately left to consult with another doctor. The two
returned to administer chloroform, which Parker happened to be
carrying, along with more calomel, now laced with quinine and morphine. They raised blisters over the woman's chest, abdomen, and
back; administered more chloroform; then left. Out of what he
termed curiosity, Parker returned at one o'clock to find the patient
delivering a fetus of about three or four months.[43]

While physicians and their slaveholder clients worried about
shamming and deliberate abortions by enslaved women and inadvertent miscarriages initiated by doctors, slaves held different fears
about the future of mothers and infants. Enslaved women were far
more likely to be deprived of sufficient material resources or subjected to harsh work regimens and physical chastisement during
pregnancy than to doses of veratrum viride. In the twentieth century,
long after slavery's end, former slaves and children of former slaves
expressed indignation at the everyday conditions of their lives and
the danger these posed for pregnant women and children, rather
than at the physician's drug regimen.

When it came to protecting unborn children, enslaved people
understood that their actions could affect negatively the development of the infant. The mother's experiences were said to mark an
infant in utero. Isabella Duke limped, she said, because during her
mother's pregnancy her father had sustained an injury that left him

disabled. Isabella's own son was similarly "marked at birth after his grandpa." Betty Coleman of Arkansas explained that she had "a birthmark on my thigh" in the shape of a chicken breast because her mother allowed one to spoil while she was pregnant and scratched her thigh at about the same time. Emma Foster bore a child with six fingers on each hand, which she thought was the result of having rubbed a friend's injured finger while she was pregnant.[44]

Such beliefs were not limited to the inhabitants of the slave quarter. One enterprising white woman who was charged with giving birth to a child of mixed race offered as a defense at trial that she had expressed a fear of slave insurrection during her pregnancy, which might have marked the baby. A doctor who oversaw the birth of a severely disabled child to an enslaved mother attributed the event to the mother's having seen an elephant—a part of a traveling menagerie of exotic animals—during her pregnancy. Members of both the owning class and the medical community expressed a similar understanding that events occurring during pregnancy could mark a child, often for life. North Carolina physician Edward Warren thought there was too much evidence to the contrary to deny that an impression made on the mind of a pregnant woman could physically mark a fetus. In the pages of *The Stethoscope,* he cited cases involving children of both whites and blacks. One black boy was said to resemble a fox in his habits and looks. The doctor interviewed the mother for details, which he passed along to readers. While she was pregnant, her master had obtained a live fox, and she had looked upon the chained animal every day.[45]

The matter of mother's marks was subject to controversy within the community of medical practitioners. W. P. Moore, for one, read a paper before the Tennessee Medical Society that was published in an 1857 issue of the *Nashville Journal of Medicine and Surgery,* denying the ability of the mother to mark the baby in utero. The fact that members of the medical society and editorial board of the medical journal determined a need for the dissemination of such ideas at that time indicates their persistence among medical men as well as laypeople. In fact the Nashville journal carried another article on the subject in 1860, which argued that mother's marks were real.[46] The circulation of such stories among doctors and laypeople reflected a general concern about pregnancy. Danger lurked everywhere, and only with proper management would mother and baby survive the ordeal.

In the case of slaves, limitations on their material conditions of living occasioned special anxiety because they could not easily indulge the food cravings that would have prevented the appearance of many mother's marks. Emma Foster believed she had marked one of her babies by craving beer that was unavailable to her. Her daughter was born with a mark resembling beer on the back of her neck, and she reportedly had a tendency to foam at the mouth. Fortunately, Foster was able to obtain some beer when the girl was about a week old. A teaspoon administered by mouth appeared to eliminate the infant's foaming, although the mark on her neck remained. Mandy Tucker while pregnant craved buttermilk belonging to another woman. "The milk smelled so good, but I wouldn't ask for it," she explained later. Consequently, her daughter bore a white spot on her stomach that looked just like milk.[47] Cravings for particular foods were common, and slaves thought them best indulged.

Yearning for food did not necessarily reflect a lack of proper nutrition. Yet some women no doubt suffered during pregnancy for lack of an adequate diet. Part of the problem was that any pregnant woman who was unable to work as a full hand might have her rations reduced, as was customary for other slaves whose illness, age, or disability kept them from working as a "prime" hand. James Henry Hammond of South Carolina specifically instructed his overseers not to reduce a woman's rations when pregnancy prevented her from performing a full day's labor. The fact that he felt obliged to spell out his wishes in writing suggests that at least some planters or overseers customarily reduced rations for an expectant mother unable to work at her usual capacity.[48] Through such actions, slaveholders demonstrated priority for the bottom line even as they granted concessions to pregnant women.

Pregnancy represented a time when slaves needed to exercise caution not only for fear that the child would be marked but also because the mother's health could be ruined. When pregnant women were fed an inadequate diet, slaves sometimes resorted to appropriating food without an owner's permission. They referred to the practice as "taking" rather than stealing, justifying the distinction on the grounds that slaveholders had stolen the labor—indeed the bodies—of the slaves, and thus were the bigger thieves; that everyone was entitled to a subsistence; and that as their owner's property they were incapable of stealing from him or her in the legal or moral sense of the word. Eliza Elsey, who had been born a slave, regretted the practice of "taking." Pregnant women who appropriated goods would pass on to a future generation the habit of stealing, she feared. It is not clear whether her objection reflected a sense of morality that opposed taking from owners, a concern that slaves who stole habitually would probably be caught, or a fear that slaves who stole out of habit might take from other slaves as well as from owners. At any rate, Elsey believed that taking had the potential to emerge as a type of birthmark—not visible to the eye except in the pattern of behavior.[49]

Demanding work regimens posed a problem for pregnant women. Not all owners reduced work assignments to any extent, and almost no one reduced work throughout a pregnancy. Physician Thomas J. Shaw may have pronounced the cotton plant to be "handy to all, and free of expense," but of course enslaved people paid a high price for its cultivation. The strenuous nature of its cultivation (which for women frequently involved long hours in a hot field lifting heavy hoes), along with that of rice, sugar, tobacco, and hemp (all crops cultivated by slaves in the South), represented a serious threat to the successful completion of a pregnancy. Although physician Dixon attributed miscarriage by the twenty-year-old enslaved woman to deliberate abortion, her friends and family no doubt noted that she had been compelled to labor in the field through seven months of pregnancy. Indeed, even the editor of the medical journal reporting the case scoffed at the doctor's explanation: 999 times out of 1,000 the mother was not at fault. Those rare cases in which she was were difficult to decide and could never be determined with certainty. Betty Krump complained that her enslaved mother had the same work to complete when she was pregnant as when she was not. When interviewed about slave life, Annie Coley said that her mother bore twelve children in bondage before she was excused from difficult field labor and put to weaving at the loom.[50]

It was not merely the standing, bending, and lifting in hot fields that troubled pregnant woman. When former slaves were interviewed about their experiences under slavery in the decades following the Civil War, stories emerged about deliberate abuse. Physical punishment occurred regularly and galled fellow slaves, particularly when it resulted in loss of life—the mother's or the child's. Reverend Wamble described how at age two he was left motherless: his mother died as the result of a miscarriage originating with a severe whipping. Kump also told of a pregnant woman who miscarried after an overseer's harsh punishment.[51]

Slaves understood that physical punishment posed a danger to pregnant women and their unborn children. Slaveholders and their plantation managers did, too, but their attempts to avoid miscarriages resulting from harsh punishment often consisted in digging a hole in the ground and having a woman lie face down with her swollen abdomen in the hole before a beating began. The practice afforded some protection for the fetus while allowing a pregnant woman to suffer the full measure of punishment that owners and overseers considered her due. Had she been beaten while standing, her baby might have been harmed by a blow to the abdomen. In addition, she probably would have fainted, and thus brought the beating to a halt or been rendered oblivious to the pain that accompanied

it. Marie E. Harvey, though born some years following the end of
slavery, recalled such an incident involving her grandmother, which
members of her family had continued to talk about for decades after
emancipation. Other former slaves told similar stories. Of course not
all owners took the precaution of digging the hole. When a Virginia
woman angered her mistress by burning the bread or biscuits, the
mistress ordered the pregnant slave to strip and beat her with a strap.
A Mississippi man hit Candies Richardson so hard shortly before
the birth of her daughter that she was knocked to the ground. He
faulted her for failing to pick cotton fast enough. In North Carolina
a pregnant woman died after she was partially buried, beaten, and
left in the hot sun for a time. Her overseer devised the punishment
after she fainted in the field. The punishment was for shamming.[52]

When called to attend a miscarriage or to perform an autopsy on
a woman who died as the result of a miscarriage, medical men generally did not explore the possibility of physical abuse, at least not publicly. Indeed, the only nonmedical explanation they entertained with
any regularity was the possibility that the woman had tried deliberately to abort the child. Practicing medicine at the plantation
owner's behest precluded their asserting physical abuse at the hands
of an overseer or owner as a cause of miscarriage. Medical men rarely
questioned the work regimens of enslaved women or reported cases
of physical abuse in the pages of medical journals. Corporal punishment of pregnant slaves, like that of any other slave, was deemed a
necessity. Those doctors who owned slaves evidently punished them
in the same fashion as other slaveholders. A week before his slave
Patsy gave birth, Charles A. Hentz physically chastised her for
charging items to his account at a local store.[53]

Physicians generally exerted more effort toward promoting
motherhood for black women through medicine than toward improving the terrible conditions which many endured and which in
retrospect appear to account for the low fertility rate among enslaved
women. When her mistress beat a young woman, Mary, about the

head and left her groaning in the basement, the doctor summoned to the scene "put a silver plate in her head." He also took the time to counsel her about the future. Mary might be bothered by the incident now, but her health would improve later "when she got married and had chill'un." The doctor's advice comported with slaveholder ideas about the appropriate role of women within the enslaved community.[54] Perhaps his intent was as much to reassure Mary's owner as to encourage Mary. Despite the serious injury, all would be well if only she became a mother.

John H. Morgan of Tennessee was one of the few physicians willing to admit that "hard labor and exposure in bad weather" resulted in a high incidence of aborted pregnancies among enslaved women. If the women "were kindly treated, and proper regard paid to the catamenial [menstrual] periods, we should hear of but few cases of abortion among them," the doctor assured members of the Rutherford County Medical Society in 1860. Inadequate food and clothing contributed to uterine disease, which in turn inhibited conception and the woman's ability to carry a child to term, Morgan said. His colleagues were far less certain that the blame for miscarriage lay with the conditions of slavery. A doctor identified in the record only as Smith responded to Morgan with a story about an enslaved woman who for twenty-five years had supposedly provided abortive weeds to all the women on one plantation. Doctor Baskette agreed with Morgan that enslaved women were falsely accused with some frequency of aborting fetuses, but he stopped short of indicting the conditions under which women were made to labor. Instead he blamed owners for paying insufficient attention to menstruation. With proper medical attention, problems of this nature might be eliminated, he concluded, drawing the discussion back to narrower, medical matters.[55] Acknowledging adverse conditions would have placed these doctors at odds with their patrons.

The poor outcomes associated with orthodox medical practitioners, coupled with their lack of sympathy for enslaved women and their failure to know or appreciate the importance of customs within the slave quarter, meant that some women preferred to keep pregnancies hidden from view rather than to reveal them and risk subjecting themselves to the invasive procedures of medical men. Speaking about pregnancy invited interference not only from the slaveholder and the slaveholder's physician but also from malevolent spirits or individuals in the quarter or from the surrounding neighborhood. Secrecy, on the other hand, left women free to follow the advice of black midwives, mothers, and friends rather than that of white doctors and slaveholders. Out of concern that they might be subjected to painful and dangerous procedures, abortions, or degrading treatment, some slaves hid miscarriages, pregnancies, even the onset of labor from owners, despite life-threatening complications. When a Tennessee woman with a swelling abdomen experienced pain and other symptoms of miscarriage, she denied that she was "in a family way." Her owner called in three physicians, who consulted with one another and determined that the fetus (in its seventh month) was dead. They attempted to preserve the slave woman's health by inserting a catheter and puncturing "the bladder through the parietes of the abdomen." The patient died that night. The doctors did not admit any responsibility for the unfortunate outcome. Instead, they speculated that she "had taken something to prevent conception" which accounted for the problem or that an ulcer of the uterus had prevented it from expanding as the baby grew.[56] The woman's family and other slaves may have assessed the situation differently and cast blame according to their own understanding of proper healing and childbearing.

Such outcomes help explain why one woman in Texas continued to pick cotton after she went into labor. She did not complain, and admitted her condition to an old woman only after it was clear that she would probably miscarry. In this case, the woman belonged to a physician. She undoubtedly feared that he would interfere, even though he lived some distance away. Matilda, enslaved in Kentucky, never revealed her pregnancy before whites, although she apparently sought the help of a black woman during delivery. Planter James Old of Virginia sent for a doctor when he suspected that one of his slaves was pregnant, but she denied it. He hoped that Doctor Charles Brown would confirm the pregnancy "as soon as Possable." In Richmond, the enslaved Amy "persistently denied" her pregnancy to physician William Patteson. J. S. Chisolm, M.D., of Charleston, also encountered a case in which a pregnant woman denied her condition. When her owner became aware that her menses had ceased in March, she explained that she had taken cold. Suffering from back pain and constipation by November, the women later changed her self-diagnosis to "dropsical." Chisolm was called when the woman went into labor, assisting in the birth of an infant weighing nearly fourteen pounds.[57] Women had the sole advantage of being more attuned to their bodies than either doctors or owners, and thus could conceal information from others. Physicians' limited knowledge of pregnancy also aided slaves in this endeavor. The denial of their condition by pregnant slave women frustrated owners and physicians alike, both of whom believed they had a stake in maintaining control over slave pregnancy.

A slave woman's pregnancy presented a dilemma for the slaveholder. The pregnancy held promise of an increasing labor force in the long term. In the short term, however, concessions would be necessary—possibly in the form of shortened work hours or a lightened work load for the mother—to ensure a healthy birth. Complications of pregnancy could leave a mother disabled or dead, turning a temporary loss of labor into a permanent condition. Consequently, slaveholders and overseers alike remained on guard during an enslaved woman's pregnancy, eager to ensure that she did as much work as possible without threatening her health. By driving expectant mothers to do as much as physically possible, owners and overseers hoped to minimize the effect of pregnancy on plantation operations. At the same time desiring the birth of a new slave, they offered women medical attention for any complications that arose. By attending to the health needs of expectant mothers, they hoped to secure the next generation of slaves without ameliorating the conditions that threatened the health and safety of pregnant women and their infants.

For their part, physicians defined pregnancy as a biological condition to be managed by men of science. Within this framework, they could advocate for their individual patients without challenging broader conditions of servitude or the social order. During the antebellum era they intervened increasingly in cases of problem pregnancies, yet their tacit acquiescence in the southern social order left them little room for improving the ability of enslaved women to carry infants to term. Instead of writing treatises on the effects of hard labor on pregnancy, physicians accepted the material conditions of slavery and the social relations of power that imposed them. Rather than deploring the physical punishment of pregnant women and in some cases their reduced rations, medical men joined slaveholders in criticizing a supposed tendency among enslaved women to abort their children and thus deprive them of their rightful property.

Enslaved women approached the management of pregnancy differently. They advocated a broader approach to protecting women and their unborn babies. It was the condition of slavery that threatened women's and infant's health. More and better food, protection from physical abuse, and relief from harsh work regimens would improve a woman's chances of bringing a baby to term. By insisting that the problem was slavery, black women fashioned an indictment of southern social relations and of the approach to medicine favored by the slaveholders' medical men.

5

Childbirth

MARY WAS GREATLY AGITATED IN 1822 UPON THE ONSET OF LABOR; the midwife attending her could not control her violent flailing. Her agitation ceased about 11:00 P.M., but so did her contractions. She continued to moan and to complain of a steady pain throughout the night, however, and vomited occasionally. Twenty-six hours after the labor pains had begun and fifteen hours following the cessation of contractions, a physician arrived to take charge. Concluding that Mary had been injured by her flailing, John Overton, M.D., of Nashville, decided not to wait any longer for "nature to furnish any assistance." The accoucheur turned the infant who came into the world feet first. Soon the patient started to hemorrhage. Once again the doctor intervened, this time to stop the flow. Three days later the doctor returned to treat Mary for what he described as a tumor— most likely resulting from the accumulation of fluids. The enslaved patient was eighteen years old. She survived, but she never became pregnant again, although according to Overton she menstruated following the incident. The doctor published the story nineteen years after the events in the *Western Journal of Medicine and Surgery*.[1]

As Overton's account suggests, southern physicians and their clients were interested in more than the short-term recovery of enslaved women from childbirth. The long-range outlook for subsequent pregnancies also was of concern, as well as the woman's ability to raise her child and to labor in other capacities. Overton intended his account to serve as an anecdotal warning. Leaving women to

fend for themselves in childbirth carried certain risks. A physician
should be summoned at the first sign of trouble. Mary's owner had
waited too long, with disastrous results.

Slaveholder reliance on doctors to tend slave women at birth
grew slowly in the antebellum South. At the beginning of the nineteenth century, southerners generally considered childbirth a natural
process, which did not require interference. Yet opinion was gradually moving in another direction. Doctors in both the North and
South were using ergot and forceps to facilitate childbirth; each
could hasten delivery. Ergot, a fungus that develops on rye plants,
could restart or speed contractions that had stopped or slowed, for
example. These modern advances in medicine increased owner and
physician confidence—if not that of the slave—that doctors could
rescue women from debilitating birth experiences. In addition, doctors prescribed medications, inserted a hand into the womb to facilitate the infant's passage into the vagina, and took measures such as
bloodletting, which was thought to relax the reproductive organs
and speed labor, ease pain, and reduce inflammation.[2] Physicians
held out hope that the high mortality rate among mothers and infants resulting from complications of childbirth might be reduced by
professional attention. A slaveholder could justify the expense of hiring a doctor by calculating the profits that might ensue from a growing slave population.

For southern physicians, assisting childbirth in the slave quarter
was invaluable experience. Recent graduates from medical school
might never have witnessed a birth before and had limited knowledge of the procedures to be followed. Free women tended to shun
inexperienced doctors, so most physicians learned how to manage
childbirth in the slave quarter. When physicians penned case narratives related to practice, they often listed black women among their
first or earliest parturient patients. Some of these women may have
avoided harm or even death by the doctor's ministrations, but others

were not significantly helped and sometimes were harmed further. Bloodletting depleted body fluids. Forceps used incautiously left women suffering from lacerations. Unwashed hands spread germs that could result in puerperal fever. As one historian of medicine has observed of obstetric services in the North during the late eighteenth and early nineteenth centuries, the presence of doctors at childbirth probably did not enhance overall the well-being of obstetric patients.[3] In the South, where conditions in slave quarters were far less conducive to effective interventions, an enslaved woman's well-being would be far more problematic.

Enslaved women, their friends, and their families maintained a healthy suspicion of the male doctor and questioned whether his presence was for better or worse. Differences in social status and gendered identities conspired to alienate black women from the white physician and thus to ensure that he remained less aware of the needs of the women and their infants than did traditional attendants. In routine cases, parturient women continued to rely for help on those familiar midwives, friends, and family members who guided them through unfolding events. But when childbirth took an unnatural turn, a growing contingent of women submitted at the slaveholder's insistence to treatment by the slaveholder's physician. Childbirth was changing. No longer shaped exclusively by female folkways, it increasingly adhered to the increasingly uniform standards of a male profession.

Change did not come evenly, easily, or quickly in the quarter, because multiple persons competed for control of the birthing process. Slaves and slaveholders, midwives and medical men each had a vested interest in the outcome and so tried to orchestrate events.[4] In the contest over the management of childbirth, slaveholders and doctors together wielded considerable power to shape events; nevertheless, mothers and midwives found ways to maintain some of their preferred practices.

———

Throughout the antebellum years, granny midwives (enslaved lay midwives) attended most births in the slave quarter. Fanny gave birth to four children without difficulty, requiring no aid other than "such as could be given by the plantation nurse." Kentucky slave Delphia endured four days of labor without medical attendance even though her first pregnancy had ended in stillbirth. Kentucky physician and planter Henry H. Farmer apparently engaged no attendant for his slave Mary Farmer other than the plantation's midwife and nurse. Neither did Henry attend the birth himself, although Mary's cabin lay only three-quarters of a mile from the doctor's house. Few considered a physician's presence at a routine birth important, particularly for slaves.[5] It was assumed that women could take care of themselves as long as no complications arose.

Granny midwives were numerous and rarely devoted full time to the occupation. Clara Walker had other duties—cooking and weaving—in addition to her midwifery practice. One Alabama woman worked as a cook when she was not attending births. Another Alabama midwife did field work, cooked, washed, and ironed. An Arkansan woman not only doctored the babies and cared for other slaves who were ill—her main tasks—but completed additional plantation chores as needed. Ruthie Boyd, who worked as a midwife and nurse, also washed clothes. Midwife Judie Pulliam of Mississippi had charge of the dairy.[6]

Although some midwives only assisted at childbirth, others were healers with skills that extended to various illnesses. Fred Forbes, whose family relocated to Nebraska following the Civil War, explained that his mother "was kind of a doctor," tending women at childbirth but also other people in times of sickness. She concocted "special medicine for sore throats and colds that was used far and near." On T. B. King's plantation, known as Retreat, Pussy acted as midwife to the slaves, but she also nursed the sick slaves housed in the plantation's hospital. In Louisiana, Katy Elmore served a black and white clientele, an occupation that apparently kept her quite busy. When she was not traveling around the countryside tending women and children, she doctored the sick. Most of her time, however, was devoted to the practice of midwifery, according to a family informant.[7]

Grannies varied in their training. By far the majority learned the occupation in the manner of the enslaved Chanie Mack, whose grandmother taught her both midwifery skills and how to make medicines from various herbs found in the woods. Not every enslaved black woman who assisted at childbirth was a granny midwife. Some were family or friends, but many women eventually claimed the title "midwife" because they had gained experience by giving birth themselves or by helping others. At times an individual doctor taught a midwife to perform to his satisfaction, but generally women did the training by passing on their knowledge.[8]

For slaves, midwifery required special skills gained through revelation as well as practice. The best midwives could be identified early on by supernatural signs: children born under special circumstances—with a caul or veil (the amniotic sac) over their face, as a seventh child, or as part of a set of twins, for example—were said to understand better than others the meaning of particular events. Those with second sight perceived things of which others were unaware. Midwife Marie Campbell once explained that during a difficult labor her deceased mentor appeared to show her the right thing to do.[9] Thus, in the opinion of slaves, a doctor, mistress, or any other white person could not randomly select a woman to be trained for the role. Owners played a key part in deciding which woman might be released from other work to serve as a granny midwife, but the decision was not solely theirs to make. To be accepted in the slave quarter, a woman had to gain the confidence of other slaves by demonstrating an aptitude or calling. A woman who did not have the support of her people would not have attempted to assist in childbirth.

Not everyone born under special circumstances or with a talent for second sight grew up to be a midwife. An unusual birth or talent merely marked someone as a special person, one likely to play a role of consequence within the local community. For women, the special role often was that of midwife. Only women were expected to attend to pregnant and parturient women. Men directed special talents in other directions.[10]

Clara Walker's experience of being chosen for the role of midwife in Arkansas was no doubt typical of many others, although her training fell under the purview of a doctor. She was born with a veil on her face, which gave her the ability to see spirits and foretell the future, according to her own account. When she was thirteen, her mistress apprenticed her to a doctor to learn the art of midwifery. A major motivation was the existence of a large number of pregnant women on the plantation; however, her owner surely hoped to direct Walker's special gift along a course of which she approved as well. Children born with a caul sometimes grew up to be conjurers with power to harm as well as heal. They were viewed by some people as having power to challenge the authority of owners and disrupt relationships in the quarter. As a midwife, Walker would play a more benign, even useful, role on the plantation in the eyes of her owner. Walker worked with the doctor for five years, during which she evidently became quite skilled. Clients paid the mistress for Walker's services, earning the mistress quite a sum of money for attending both black and white women in labor.[11]

The major requirement of a midwife from the perspective of the slaveholder was that her birth procedures accorded with their notions of what was proper, which included reporting unfolding events. Walker was popular with whites in part because she understood the limits under which she was supposed to practice and always arranged for a doctor to take over when she believed she had reached them. Charles Pettigrew from 1840 to 1848 placed faith in the elderly Airy, who served not only as an occasional midwife but also as the plantation's main nurse. When the enslaved Patience gave birth unexpectedly in the middle of the night, Airy was nowhere nearby. As soon as Pettigrew heard news of the birth, he sent Airy to the plantation "in order to give Lizzy [who presumably attended the birth] directions respecting Patience's child." Pettigrew made an effort to direct the training of Airy and other midwives on his plantation, according to one of his biographers, presumably so that they could manage events to his liking.[12]

Midwives with close ties to whites and who were trusted by them had considerable freedom to travel off the plantation to do their work. Sarah Pittman's Louisiana grandmother "would put her side saddle on the old horse and get up and go" wherever she was needed, according to her granddaughter. Sarah and her cousin stayed behind to "take care of things" until the older woman returned. Jennie Ferrell's grandmother also traveled about the Mississippi countryside on horseback tending rich and poor, free and slave, white and black.[13] Those midwives who did not work closely with whites enjoyed a different type of freedom: they were less inhibited in their practice of birthing customs. Midwives who worked closely with whites had to worry about pleasing them, which usually meant adopting practices that conformed to their expectations. Those who assisted parturient women without an owner's knowledge or close scrutiny could help them make decisions about such matters as birthing position without worrying about how the owner (or the owner's doctor) would react.

It is not clear that slaves preferred a more traditional midwife over one approved by an owner. Each had advantages. While there was comfort to be found in welcoming new life in the time-honored way of ancestors, rituals might have to be conducted in secret—beyond the watchful eyes of the master and mistress—thus adding an element of stress to an otherwise happy occasion. A midwife whose practice conformed to the expectations of owners might extract more concessions from the master or mistress in the form of reduced work assignments for mother, more material resources for mother and child, and acknowledgment of the importance of the union between the parents. Part of a midwife's role was to negotiate on behalf of mothers and infants for the resources that both needed for survival. Reduced work assignments and secure family ties were considered as important as food, clothing, and shelter and were among the items negotiated on a new mother's behalf.

Whether she met the owner's approval or not, the presence of a wise woman did a lot to alleviate any apprehension that a mother and her loved ones felt at childbirth. The midwife could explain the sequence of events, tell the mother what to do at each stage of labor, and inform both parents and extended kin the best way to care for the mother and child following the birth. She provided practical advice along with explanations of customs. In one Georgia community, enslaved women visited an old Indian woman before they were confined to obtain the special charms she made to ease birth. Other midwives provided other substances to ensure a positive birth experience. Cotton root aided in childbirth by inducing or speeding labor when this seemed to be required. Birthroot also induced a birth that appeared too long delayed and speeded the process of labor. Calamus root was said to ease the pain of childbirth. Horsemint leaves were brewed to ensure the return of menstruation following confinement. Granny Sarah made her own medicines from herbs, including "red shank, cherry bark, dog-wood bark, prickly-ash roots, bamboo roots, and blackhaw roots."[14]

Many slaves believed that unusual circumstances of birth—such as the birth of a child with a caul or the birth of a seventh child— called for special rituals. Black midwife Ella Wilson in Arkansas knew that a caul required special handling. Under certain circumstances, for example, it had to be saved until it disintegrated. Maum Hagar Brown in South Carolina knew how to brew a special tea made of the caul, which prevented the child from having to face frightening supernatural forces. No white person, including professionally trained physicians (no matter how skilled), could substitute for midwives like Maum Brown, because they lacked a knowledge of the cultural beliefs that guided slave behavior and the rituals they required to channel the supernatural force for good rather than for evil.[15]

Malindy Maxwell had the misfortune to be born with a caul over the face under the supervision of a white midwife, an unusual occurrence for a slave in the antebellum South. The midwife did not know how to protect young Malindy, who throughout her life perceived disturbing forms that no one else could see. "It is like when you are dreaming at night," only it is day, she once explained. Annie Page's mistress kept the caul that covered Annie's face at birth, evidently because she understood it was supposed to keep Annie from seeing ghosts. But she had no idea of how to perform the ritual that would keep spirits at bay. The mistress turned the caul over to Annie before she was old enough to appreciate it (an indication of her insensitivity to its importance), and Annie lost it while playing in the orchard. A child so young should not have been entrusted with the precious article. As a result, Annie's visions included chilling apparitions.[16]

Lore concerning the appropriate handling of the placenta—like lore regarding the special meaning of a caul or a seventh child—invested the midwife with mystery and enhanced her authority among slaves. When the enslaved Nancy gave birth in a fence corner on the way to visit friends, she caught the baby herself, breaking the cord with her fingers. She wrapped her baby in some of her clothes and returned to the plantation in a pouring rain. Upon arrival, she sought the services of an older woman—a granny—who expressed concern that the placenta had been left behind to rot on the ground. The midwife shared her anxiety with Nancy's husband. If it remained there "his wife would gradually sink away and die." The new father immediately began the trek back to the scene of the birth, but he found nothing. Disconsolate, he reported the situation to the older woman, who reassured him that the afterbirth had probably been "eaten by bugs which would save the life of his wife." Both mother and baby did well.[17]

It was not simply the physiology of the birth that was subject to interpretation. Clara Cotton McCoy grew up in North Carolina listening to her grandmother Rowena Cotton explain the misfortunes of a white family as originating in an inappropriate response to the mistress's birth. Mistress Riah Cotton had been born the last day of March between midnight and daylight when the moon was on the wane. At the moment of birth, a cold wind blew down the chimney and scattered ashes from the hearth. Tragedies befell the mistress— the sudden death of her mother and a daughter's elopement with a Yankee—all attributable to this singular event. If only proper action had been taken, the family might have been spared.[18]

Midwives advised family members as well as parturient women about appropriate behavior at the time of birth. The rituals brought comfort and familiarity. The midwife known as Isabelle learned that a husband and older child planned to sleep in the basement during his wife's labor. Isabelle heard a voice telling him not to sleep there. The later discovery of a skeleton under the basement floor was accepted as proof of the midwife's power both to divine danger and to devise ways of avoiding it.[19] The birthing process was dangerous enough without people's coming into contact with death as represented by the skeletal remains.

Grannies continued throughout the antebellum years to assist in this fashion during childbirth. But when things took a turn for the worse, doctors were increasingly called in to redirect events. In a typical scenario, a midwife attended a Louisiana slave woman in an early stage of labor, but when her labor ceased progressing despite active pains, a doctor was called. His internal examination revealed that the infant's swollen head, too large to pass through, was "jammed in the brim of the pelvis." Considering the case urgent, the physician extracted the baby, believed dead, with scissors and the crotchet—a hook designed for this purpose. He claimed to have saved the life of the mother. It is unclear what prevented the enslaved woman belonging to Samuel Alsop from delivering her baby, but the Virginia planter considered her situation dire. "If you cannot possibly go yourself send" another doctor, Alsop beseeched the local physician. "The nature of the case will not admit of any further delay."[20]

Complications that called for a doctor's presence included hemorrhaging, prolonged labor, and the cessation of labor pains. A midwife was expected by her owner to identify the problem and summon a physician, sometimes directly but more often through the slave owner or overseer. Most midwives, however, first tried to resolve some of the problems on their own. They might attempt through massage to manipulate the infant into a favorable position for birth if the delay was due to a baby's position. They also ruptured the amniotic sac and administered herbal teas in an effort to speed labor. Doctors complained that many midwives went too far, attempting procedures for which they had no training, and complicating matters for the physician. Midwives, however, were confident of their abilities, which they learned not only from other women but also by watching or working with physicians.

Despite their grousing that midwives attempted too much, doctors did not like to be called too early in the labor. Physicians prized fees for attending to the health needs of slaves, and many southern physicians, such as W. A. Brown of Georgia, cared for more black than white patients. But obstetric cases were less desirable than others. Even if uneventful, childbirth consumed a lot of an attendant's time, much of it spent waiting. As Wooster Beach frankly noted in his medical manual on midwifery, physicians could make more money for attending sick clients than for attending a woman in labor, particularly if the labor was protracted. In addition, the many births that occurred at night robbed the doctor of his sleep and interfered with his ability to keep up with his regular practice the next day.[21]

Charles A. Hentz, who was called in 1857 to attend an enslaved woman in labor, read a magazine by the fire, slept a few hours in a "negro bed," ate breakfast with the overseer and his wife, then sat outside smoking and reading. He slept a few more hours, ministered to the patient, and ate dinner with the overseer's wife before stopping by his office in town. He returned after supper to discover that the woman had delivered the child without difficulty. In addition to time spent on the plantation, the young doctor had traveled twelve miles round trip on horseback to see her.[22] This case went smoothly; complications lengthened the doctor's commitment of time.

Doctors' fees reflected the time-consuming nature of attendance at childbirth and discouraged planters from engaging them on behalf of slaves for any but serious cases. In 1854 fifteen doctors of Powhatan County, Virginia, signed a fee schedule listing a set price for attending a birth lasting up to twelve hours. Fifty cents would be added to the bill for each additional hour. Doctors in Nottoway County, Virginia, agreed the year before to assess an additional charge for their time "at the same rate as for anything else" when obstetrical cases detained them more than twenty-four hours. A scale of fees approved by physicians in Louisville in 1859 listed twenty dollars as the charge for "ordinary obstetrical cases," but the fee increased to thirty dollars "for tedious labor requiring continuous attention more than twelve hours."[23]

Owners did not always expect to pay, and doctors did not always anticipate receiving, the same fees for attending to slave women as for attending to women in the planter's family, a fact that further discouraged them from accepting cases in the quarter. Physicians in four Texas counties hoped to receive twenty-five dollars for managing the uncomplicated birth of a slaveholder's child, but they could expect no more than twenty for attending the uncomplicated birth of a slave. The difference was even more pronounced in South Carolina, where the members of one medical society expected payment for obstetrical cases to range from fifteen to fifty dollars for slaves and from thirty to fifty dollars for others, depending on the complexity of the case. The difference in payment for lying-in services extended to institutional care. The Bellevue Hospital in Richmond bragged of its "peculiarly commodious" lying-in wards. The cost for blacks was four dollars per week, for whites five dollars. The difference reflected in part the lower status of slaves but also the lesser investment of time and energy expected of doctors and institutions caring for them. The assumption of many white southerners that black women gave birth easily and naturally helped to justify less attention from the doctor as well as the lower fees.[24]

It is not clear that physicians routinely collected the full fees recommended by medical groups. In 1834 James W. Bell charged Pettigrew ten dollars "to deliver Jinney." Fees received by John Norwood, who practiced medicine in Crawford, Alabama, were also lower than those suggested by the medical societies. In 1859 H. Waddell paid Norwood ten dollars for attending one of his slaves at childbed. H. G. Jones gave him fourteen dollars for managing the birth of a slave on his plantation, a fee that apparently included the cost of a prescription. Perhaps because of complications or because the visit occurred at night, Norwood charged twenty-five dollars for his services at the childbed of a slave belonging to a Miss Harris, but he had to accept considerably less: she paid ten. In 1855 G. Troup Maxwell collected thirty dollars from Florida planter George Jones for "attendance on Lucy in difficult labor." The difference in rates may have reflected competition among physicians. Where it was intense, doctors sometimes found it necessary to charge less than the going rate.[25] However, the difference in fees collected for attending slave births more likely reflected the relative complexity of each case and of the treatment, the duration of the attendance, and whether the birth occurred at night.

The initial fee for attending childbirth was not a physician's only source of income from obstetric cases, however. Follow-up visits and medicines could command a separate payment, whether for mother or infant. Although doctors in Richmond included visits for eight days following birth in their initial fee, others calculated each visit as a separate cost. One unnamed slave woman delivered a baby on 5 October 1859, for which Norwood was paid $10.00, but Norwood charged another dollar for his advice when he returned the next day. The doctor also collected 25 cents for each medication he prescribed. The delivery of a child to the enslaved Sarah on 15 December earned Norwood $10.00. He charged an additional $2.50 each for follow-up visits to Sarah and the baby on subsequent days. In 1833 William Henderson charged Charles Pettigrew $6.00 for delivering Molly's child, and an additional $10.00 for delivering the placenta.[26]

Physicians paid by the year to attend the health needs of slaves on a particular plantation, as many were, would have been especially eager to leave childbirth in the hands of women. Contractual arrangements were frowned upon by doctors acting collectively in professional organizations, but individual doctors entered into them nevertheless. The contracts required doctors to attend to the health needs on a particular plantation for a flat fee. The objection was that the physician would be at the beck and call of the planter "night and day" to attend "every little ailment."[27] It was best, under such circumstances, to define routine cases of childbirth outside the purview of medicine. Physicians wanted it understood that they would attend a slave at childbed only when complications threatened the health of the mother.

Monetary considerations encouraged slaveholders, as well as physicians, to leave the management of routine cases of childbirth in the hands of slaves. On large plantations, physician fees could reach significant levels over the course of a year. Masters and mistresses on smaller farms might incur fewer obstetric fees on behalf of slaves, but their limited finances might make the payment of a doctor's bill more difficult. Even the modest fees of midwives could pose problems for financially distressed farmers.

Doctors charged significantly more than midwives, a fact that encouraged slaveholders to leave women in charge of routine births. According to former slave Carrie E. Davis, "every plantation had a woman doctor," whose main concern was childbirth. Doctors were too expensive. Cora Carroll Gillam, another former slave, thought women received "good care" during childbirth in Mississippi. "They had some old ladies that stayed on the place to care for them," she explained. One was designated a midwife. Owners "didn't call a doctor unless it was something very serious," such as fever. Henrietta Murray, a former slave in Mississippi, said much the same thing. A midwife attended women at childbirth, "unless twas something special she couldn't handle," in which case a doctor was summoned.[28]

Most men who attended parturient slave women were general practitioners who attended no more than five or ten childbirths in a year. This small number neither yielded much income nor provided them sufficient clinical experience to develop expertise in midwifery practice. Only a few physicians hoped to develop a reputation for outstanding service in the field and actively promoted their midwifery skills. But if Ebenezer Pettigrew's slaves are typical, slaveholders called on general practitioners with greater frequency for complications of childbirth as the years unfolded. Greater wealth would accrue to those planters who would "patronize our scientific young men in obstetrics," opined one doctor in the *New Orleans Medical News and Hospital Gazette.* Slaves would enjoy better health, and mortality rates would fall. H. W. Wooten, who practiced medicine around Lowndesboro, Alabama, observed that obstetrical cases were beginning to form an important part of the physician's practice. Nearly "all the white women, and many Negroes," he judged, had doctors in attendance at birth in 1848.[29]

All general practitioners were expected to know something of midwifery, if not from medical lectures at least from experience and reading. This expectation explains why James Carmichael of Virginia in 1825 ordered a copy of *A Compendious System of Midwifery:*

*Chiefly Designed to Facilitate the Inquiries of Those Who May Be Pursu-
ing This Branch of Study,* by William P. Dewees, from a Philadelphia
bookseller. The book, authored by a highly respected physician who
had made a careful study of women's anatomy, disease, and childbirth, included numerous chapters outlining the latest medical
thinking on the subject of childbirth and its attendant complications. No doubt Carmichael considered it well worth the $4.50 pur-
chase price. Although letters to the doctor written from 1819 to
1830 suggest that only a small percentage of his cases related to
childbirth, planters nevertheless sought his attendance for women in
the slave quarter as well as for women in their own families when
they experienced complicated births or suffered from gynecological
problems.[30]

The challenge for doctors was to find a way to respond to slaveholder requests for assistance while limiting the time they were involved in particular cases. In what can only be seen as an effort to
resolve the problem, J. Douglass, M.D., of Chester, South Carolina,
trained one of his own slaves as a midwife, then sent her to attend
women in labor and assess their need for his services. She was to
alert him when the situation grew dire. In one case, for example, she
sat with a slave about five or six hours until hemorrhaging began, at
which time she summoned Douglass.[31] The situation held advantages beyond simply saving the doctor's time. It helped assure that
any care a patient received before the doctor's arrival met with his
approval. Slaveholders also were reassured that any health measures
undertaken on the woman's behalf accorded with standards acceptable to slaveholding society generally.

The South Carolina woman whose hemorrhaging brought
Douglass to her childbed suffered from placenta previa, a condition
in which the placenta partially or completely covers the opening of
the cervix, causing bleeding and interfering with birth. Placenta previa was life threatening for both mother and child. Douglass felt
"compelled to resort to force and turning." He also administered a

"full dose of ergot" to restart the labor pains, which had ceased. He kept administering small doses throughout the day until at last the child was delivered dead.[32]

Because bleeding was not always a sign of placenta previa, the doctor's treatment in such cases might begin conservatively. Cornelia, a slave woman seven months pregnant, did not appear to be in any real trouble when R. D. Arnold of Savannah first saw her, according to his later testimony. Her symptoms consisted of "bearing down pains" and bleeding. For these the doctor prescribed bed rest, along with "gallic acid" (used as an internal astringent) and "cold acidulated [soured or acidic] drinks." When she began to bleed more profusely the doctor realized that this was a life-threatening case of placenta previa, which prompted him to act more boldly. He reached into the uterus and pulled out the placenta. "Nature" delivered the child sometime later, he said.[33]

Physician James W. Fair attended a case of placenta previa in Louisiana in early 1861. The enslaved Mary had been in labor for twenty-four hours by the time he arrived. After pushing the placenta back and delivering the child, Fair tied a bandage around the mother's abdomen, which he hoped would help expel the placenta. The doctor cut the cord, attended to the dressing of the child, and waited until he was able to pull the placenta away using slight traction. Fair prescribed laudanum (a tincture of opium) and stayed two more hours before leaving. Mary's child survived, and so did Mary, who apparently credited the doctor with saving her life. A similar case attended by M. J. Greene in Alabama ended in the death of the child. The mother was hemorrhaging when Greene arrived. After consulting with a colleague, the doctor decided to hasten the birth with the use of ergot and external pressure to the womb. Another twelve hours went by before delivery was completed.[34]

Placenta previa was not so common that doctors became accustomed to managing it, a fact that prompted Douglass to describe his case in the pages of the *Charleston Medical Journal and Review*. In forty-five years of medical practice, Douglass encountered only four women with the condition. Yet he and other doctors were expected to handle any cases that developed among their clientele. Douglass recounted his experience, he said, to "relieve the anxious embarrassment of obstetricians" when they confronted placenta previa in their own practice.[35] His frank admission offers insight into not only the limits of medical training but also the complications of the southern doctor's practice and the burden placed on him to know something about all types of medical matters.

Intervention during labor by medical men became more likely and drastic when hemorrhaging occurred but also when the mother's labor ceased or lasted so long that the chance of a successful vaginal delivery appeared slim. Prolonged labor resulted from a variety of conditions, ranging from the unfavorable position of the baby to a rigid cervix. Doctors first tried conservative measures—some in the manner of a midwife. This is not to say that physicians remained inactive, however. Having been called to the bedside by a concerned owner or overseer, they were expected to do something. For the most part, this involved managing the parturient woman's purportedly excitable nature and controlling her diet and excreta. In this sense, the southern doctor's approach was more akin to what one historian of medicine has termed "expectant" treatment, rather than "active" care. Whereas the active mode, in the words of a northern practitioner, was aimed at "checking or rendering the disease safer, or of arresting it at once," the expectant approach required the doctor to watch and allow the disease to run its natural course, while removing any "obstacles which may hinder the method of nature."[36]

Only when the situation appeared ominous did doctors employ ergot, forceps, or other bold measures that were considered to be standard treatment. When W. L. Sutton of Kentucky saw Judy in 1847, her pains were "trifling" and widely spaced, as they had been all day. He administered "teas, &c.," and only when these did not work did he give ergot, which soon produced the child. A Mississippi woman labored for four days assisted only by a midwife before William E. Brickell was called to her childbed. By then she was fearful and expecting to die. Even so, the doctor limited his actions to ascertaining that the child was not dead and repositioning the infant for a vaginal delivery. When this proved impossible, he and another doctor called in as a consultant agreed to remove the child with instruments. The mother survived the ordeal; the infant did not.[37]

Doctor Henry R. Frost of South Carolina was called by a midwife in 1838 to attend a woman, aged twenty-five and in good health, whose labor seemed to be progressing normally except for its duration. At first the doctor took no action. The woman had already been given castor oil and bled "a small quantity" by someone else. The midwife was agitated, but he considered her concern unwarranted and left the patient for the night under her care. Lack of significant progress by the following morning prompted the doctor to reopen a vein and bleed more. Frost next consulted another doctor, who concurred with this approach. Bloodletting continued. The following day Frost resorted to forceps and ergot, but this did not produce the child either. He tried next to draw off urine, in the belief that an extended bladder was interfering with labor's progress. Finally, the decision was made to forfeit the infant's life for the sake of the mother's. Its "head was perforated"; that is, a craniotomy was performed—a procedure in which the fetal head is broken to reduce its size and allow its extraction through the birth canal.[38] Treatment had escalated over time as the doctor saw that less drastic measures were proving ineffective.

When confronted with a parturient woman who did not dilate sufficiently to allow her infant to pass through the cervix, J. Y. Bassett of Huntsville, Alabama, in desperation and probably fearful of having to perform a craniotomy, opted for a different course of action. He used a long, narrow knife (a bistoury) to nick the cervix in two directions. "The parts yielded under my finger," he later reported, and "there was no further tearing." The premature infant had already died in the womb. The woman, who seemed at first to improve, also died from the ordeal.[39]

When Samuel Hogg arrived at the prolonged labor of a Tennessee woman, he learned that the midwife had already tried to speed the labor by rupturing the amniotic sac. Hogg extracted a pint of blood. He also "gave her an opiate, and directed that she should be allowed to rest." She slept for about three hours. When she awoke, her labor pains again proved insufficient to deliver the baby. Hogg extracted more blood before returning home. Summoned again the next morning, he "drew blood a third time." The baby was soon born, proving to Hogg—if not to modern readers—the worth of his chosen therapy.[40]

Doctors read about these and other treatments in medical texts and journals or heard about them through lectures or consultations with other physicians, then practiced on their patients. Carthon Archer, of Henrico County, Virginia, first heard about spirits of turpentine as a means of exciting uterine contractions in an article published by the London Lancet. Believing the published report that it worked better than ergot in some cases, he tried it on two women— one black and one white—both of whom benefited, he said. Although Archer did not state which case occurred first, the fact that most of his discussion focused on the slave Catharine suggests that she was first or at least more important in the development of the therapy. Catharine was in labor with her sixth child. The baby was clearly dead, but the mother appeared to be doing well. For a time, Archer left matters to nature. However, after a while the pains grew weak and irregular, and an exam revealed little progress. A turpentine enema proved just the thing, he said: she was soon and safely delivered of a stillborn baby. The other case involved a "lady" in labor with her second child, both of whom survived.[41]

Doctors tried every method they could to facilitate a vaginal birth because no satisfactory alternative was available. When vaginal deliveries proved impossible, slaveholders and physicians could contemplate a caesarean delivery—a highly risky operation that in and of itself threatened the life of the mother—or a craniotomy—a procedure that took the life of the child to save the mother. British medical authority W. Tyler Smith, whose lecture on the subject found its way into the southern medical press in 1857, warned that neither caesarean sections nor craniotomies should be resorted to except under extreme circumstances. Instead doctors should try more conservative measures: inducing premature labor, turning the child, and delivering by forceps.[42]

Almost always, craniotomies were preferred to caesareans. Caesarean sections were little practiced in the antebellum era because they usually resulted in the death of mother, child, or both. Atlanta physician W. F. Westmoreland in 1856 performed a craniotomy on a black woman in labor when he realized that the infant's position was not favorable for a vaginal birth. He first tried to turn and deliver the child, who presented by the neck and shoulder. He succeeded to a degree, but the birth went no further than the leg (to the knee). After consultation with another doctor and "several ineffectual efforts to deliver," Westmoreland decided "to amputate the thigh already delivered." To complete the procedure, he broke the thorax, then the head, which was perforated through the base. The woman died just three hours following the procedure.[43]

One Alabama doctor apparently felt that he had no other choice but to attempt a caesarean when confronted with a woman with abnormal genital development. The nineteen-year-old enslaved mother had been burned severely as an infant over her abdomen, thighs, and perineum. The resulting deformity precluded a vaginal delivery of the child alive or dead, in the opinion of attending physician Augustus Lilly. "Astonished at the novelty of the case," Lilly tried to cut through the scar tissue but did not succeed. A colleague, F. E. H. Steger, arrived on the scene at this point and completed the surgery. Steger closed the woman's abdomen and checked the woman the next day and again two days later. Mother and child were doing well, he reported in the pages of the *Nashville Journal of Medicine and Surgery.*[44] Nothing is known of how the patient or her child fared beyond this. Perhaps the reporter did not want to know the all-too-predictable outcome of such surgery or assumed the prognosis without saying.

Caesarean sections were considered risky in the early nineteenth century because mothers often died from infection or bleeding. The operation posed a risk to infants as well. If performed too early, the infant would be premature. Insufficient development in the baby could pose a danger in and of itself. But even infants at full term were at risk. There was danger that they would suffer a severe laceration and bleed to death or be permanently injured. Even if not severe, a cut could introduce an infection. Most infants born through caesareans have difficulty breathing. Although most recover in a couple of days, they breathe faster than other newborns. Faster breathing uses glucose at a faster pace than normal, which can make for a problem. In addition, the infant is subject to injury upon removal from the abdominal opening, especially if the opening is not made large enough. One of the more common injuries is to the hand, hardly a minor concern for a slave expected to perform physical labor.[45]

Despite the risks, doctors retained an interest in caesareans, as evidenced by such sensational stories as "Successful Case of Extraction of a Living Child by the Caesarian Section, after the Death of the Mother" and "The Caesarian Section Successfully Performed by a Negress While Drunk," both of which appeared in the *Nashville Journal of Medicine and Surgery* in the early 1850s. The second article concerned a black midwife who reportedly cut open the abdomen and womb of a woman whose birth was preceding naturally "and took therefrom a living child." The mother was said to have recovered with no ill effects other than "a slight incontinence of urine."[46]

Louisiana physicians led the nation's doctors in performing caesarean sections before the Civil War, all of which were performed on slaves. Because free women declined procedures performed by inexperienced practitioners (particularly unproven ones), doctors learned by treating enslaved women, who had less say in medical matters. In Donaldsonville, a young French doctor, François Marie Prevost, who had left Haiti following its revolution, performed the operation sometime between 1820 and 1825 upon a slave woman whose malformed pelvis (probably the result of rickets) made vaginal delivery impossible. Although the doctor had only rudimentary instruments at hand, both mother and infant survived. When she became pregnant again, he performed a second caesarean, once more with a happy result. These outcomes notwithstanding, the procedure was dangerous for both the mother and the child. In 1825 another slave woman died as the result of a caesarean performed by Prevost, although the infant lived.[47]

Prevost was not the only physician performing caesareans in the state. In 1830 Charles A. Luzenberg performed a caesarean on a woman whose infant was dead in the womb. Two New Orleans newspapers reported the operation, which did not save the life of the slave—its stated purpose. Subsequent operations met with mixed results. A study of nineteenth-century caesareans by a physician of the era indicated that fifteen operations in Louisiana saved the lives of nineteen slaves: eight children and eleven mothers.[48]

Most planters concerned with preserving the life of the mother first and foremost apparently considered caesareans too risky. The operation was only rarely undertaken even in antebellum Louisiana. The small number performed elsewhere in the South during the period seem to have been regarded primarily as experiments. When in 1855 the enslaved Maria appeared unable to deliver her child because of an occluded vagina, her Virginia doctors waited until the next day before performing a caesarean operation in the hope that nature might rectify the situation and render the procedure unnecessary. They admitted that the operation "afforded barely a possible hope" for the mother to survive and performed it only when they

became convinced of the "certain death" of both mother and child in
its absence. The mother survived the six-minute operation for only
six days. Attending physician William G. Smith attributed her death
to "the inevitable consequence of the original cause of all her sufferings, the occlusion of the vagina." Physicians in Louisville listed caesarean section among the services they provided when they adopted
a fee scale in 1859, an indication that at least some doctors there
were presenting the operation as a viable if only last-resort medical
service. The charge of $200, which put it among the most expensive
of medical procedures, suggests there was not a lot of competition
among doctors to perform the procedure.[49] The high fee would have
discouraged planters, as well as others, from agreeing to the surgery.

The difference in status and race of the women who underwent
caesareans and those who did not suggests that enslaved black
women were more apt than free white women to be exposed to risky
treatment. In addition, they were more likely to be attended by inexperienced doctors. It is difficult to say exactly how the physician-
assisted birth experiences of black and white women may have
differed in other ways given that no two documented cases were ever
exactly the same. However, two cases reported to the members of the
Atlanta Medical Society in 1856 are enough alike to suggest a general hypothesis. Both concluded with stillbirths that followed prolonged labor due to the difficult presentation of the infant. J. G.
Westmoreland and W. F. Westmoreland (brothers) attended both, in
consultation with other doctors. The physicians expressed "a good
deal of solicitude" for the white woman, referred to in the record as
Mrs. W——. They acted to relieve whatever discomfort she was experiencing and to ward off convulsions through bleeding and the administration of chloroform, the latter a relatively new treatment.
They "carefully watched the progress of the labor" and ruled out any
attempt to turn the child or introduce forceps. In the case of the
black woman, identified only by her first name—Jane—no chloro-

form was used to ease her pain. Nor was she bled. And her child was delivered "with the aid of the blunt hook."[50]

The doctors' behavior suggests that they were more concerned about the comfort of the white woman; hence their greater efforts to manage her pain. Black women were thought to have a higher pain threshold. At the same time, the different treatments may have reflected a perception that blacks did not tolerate bloodletting as a therapy as well as whites. Generally bloodletting preceded the administration of chloroform. It is also possible that culturally ingrained responses on the part of the doctors influenced their treatment of the women. Although blacks were considered more susceptible to harsh drugs than whites, medical schools generally did not teach that medical treatment should differ for blacks and whites. However, prevailing thought among nineteenth-century white Americans held that Europeans and people of European descent were more civilized than Africans and people of African descent and that civilization took its toll on childbirth experiences. For example, one author of a medical text maintained that "*the duration of labor* [was] much shorter in savage than in civilized life, in hot, than in cold countries," thereby implying that the suffering of free white women surpassed that of enslaved black women. Southern doctors shared and reinforced this belief through their writing and their bedside behavior, as did physicians from other places. Eminent obstetrician William P. Dewees of Philadelphia blamed "civilization" for the suffering of women of European descent; famed Scottish physician James Y. Simpson held "savagery" responsible for the supposed absence of pain among the "uncivilized."[51] Such unsubstantiated beliefs would have encouraged doctors to develop greater sympathy for a white than black woman at childbirth, which in turn helped to justify in their minds the different treatment afforded each.

By the 1850s, anesthetic agents (chloroform and ether) were beginning to come into use to eliminate the pain of childbirth, but they appear to have been employed more commonly for free white than enslaved black women. Their use for this purpose was not without controversy, however. Doctors disputed whether pain was helpful—a necessary part of the healing process. Reports from the United States, England, and France suggested that women might die from the inhalation of chloroform and ether or that the infant might be harmed. Some people believed that labor pains played a role in regulating contractions in parturient women and promoting a mother's tender feelings for the child. Eliminating the pains retarded the birth and exposed the child to possible neglect. Others rejected anesthesia on religious grounds: God ordained pain, and to alleviate it was to tamper with his grand plan for humankind. Yet treatment of females with chloroform had reportedly been successful not only for childbirth but also for headaches, uterine cramps, uterine disturbances, convulsions, and vomiting during pregnancy, although there were detractors of its use even in these cases. *The Stethoscope* in 1855 reprinted an article from the *Edinburgh Journal of Medical Science* advocating the use of chloroform to inhibit convulsions during pregnancy and labor with an added editorial warning: although chloroform could be administered during pregnancy for appropriate purposes, patients were better served by "copious venesection" (bloodletting).[52]

Doctors did not tend to use chloroform in slave births to relieve the mother's pain, but they employed it on occasion for other reasons. Widely regarded as a miracle drug that might relieve any of a number of symptoms, its appeal for heroic practitioners lay in its drastic physiological effect. Kentucky physician J. V. Withers, for example, tried "chloroform by inhalation" when confronted with a convulsing slave in labor. He hoped to shorten the convulsions. The patient (and her twins) died, despite treatment with calomel, turpentine, castor oil, ergot, bleeding, cold water, and a mustard plaster. J. Y. Bassett applied chloroform in an attempt to relax a rigid cervix so that an Alabama slave could deliver her child. Doctor Cenas used it for the same purpose in Georgia.[53]

Physician John Butts of Mississippi made no attempt to disguise the experimental nature of the treatment he afforded nineteen-year-old Amelia using the anesthesia. She was nine months pregnant, slightly dilated, but the mouth of her uterus was hard and unyielding. After examining her vaginally, he placed his ear upon her abdomen. Hearing no heartbeat, he decided to deliver the fetus manually as soon as the enslaved woman was sufficiently dilated to allow the infant's passage. Adhering to standard procedure, he bled her for some time in each arm before pains began to occur regularly. He waited for five hours before administering chloroform (by handkerchief) to the woman, who lay in an epileptic state. When he removed the handkerchief, spasms occurred, so he decided to keep Amelia sedated until she delivered. Meanwhile the doctor broke the amniotic sac with his fingers, grabbed one of the baby's feet, and pulled. It took about half an hour to deliver the dead child. Butts stayed long enough to deliver the placenta, than left to attend other duties. He had used half a pound of chloroform and left more in the hands of a black nurse with instructions to administer the drug as needed. Reflecting on the experience, Butts maintained that the anesthesia had saved the woman's life and advised colleagues to follow the same procedure in similar cases.[54]

It is easy to see why slaves preferred midwives to physicians as birth attendants. Doctors aligned themselves closely with the interests of the slaveholders, who called them only in the most adverse of cases. Unfavorable outcomes came to be associated with their medical practice in part because doctors had little experience with the procedures they attempted on slave women. One doctor did not even try to disguise the great peril his treatment involved. When he decided to employ forceps to deliver a Kentucky woman suffering convulsions during labor, he announced in advance that the procedure would probably "prove fatal." Her parents heard the doctor's prediction and watched as he delivered not one but two babies, both dead. The mother died too.[55] Perhaps they were desperate enough to try any measure that held out hope for their daughter's recovery. More likely they had no say in the matter and watched the drama unfold to their ultimate grief and horror.

Slaveholders, physicians, and slaves all wanted women and their infants to survive, but slaves also hoped to experience birth according to their own understanding of proper practice. They saw birth as more than a physiological episode. Events that occurred during pregnancy and childbirth had meaning that required interpretation and in some cases action. Doctors called late to a complicated birth understood the case as a pathological development. When the midwife was a slave, she guided the birth according to the beliefs and assumptions that gave meaning to life in the quarter. She understood each event as part of the personal story of the mother, the infant, and extended kin across time. The doctor whom planter Charles Pettigrew called to attend three enslaved women experiencing difficult labor bled them all—an action hardly favored by the women or their people, in part because the procedure, while expected to evoke a physiological response, did not address the woman's social and spiritual state.[56]

Everyone in the slave quarter understood that childbirth posed general dangers, and granny midwives prepared in advance for the experience of birth whatever its course. To slaves, white men appeared to wait for a crisis and attempt to manage it after it was already too late. Physicians seemed insensitive to the dangers posed by all births, focusing instead on particular and infrequent problems. They dismissed fears on the part of the mother and instead focused on a narrow range of concerns taught in medical schools and texts.

As soon as "she knew herself to be in the family way," Harriet "believed something was wrong." When the doctor arrived, she confided her fears, but the attending physician, J. E. Manlove, dismissed

them as typical of the anxiety women sometimes felt at such mo-
ments. He offered no means of ameliorating the danger sensed by
Harriet. Before delivery, one Kentucky slave confided in the "old
lady" who attended her that she had a foreboding of evil to happen
during her confinement. The midwife reported the mother's misgivings to the doctor who arrived later to take over the case because of
the onset of convulsions. The doctor, recording the incident in the
pages of the *Western Journal of Medicine and Surgery*, described the
woman's apprehension as unusual, suggesting thereby that enslaved
women did not commonly express such fears to physicians. The doctor's strategy was to divert her attention much as one would with a
child—an approach opposite that employed by the majority of midwives. Grannies listened carefully to the fears of women and offered
explanations for them, along with strategies to ward off the danger,
thus providing a sense of security and confidence. The Kentucky
physician boasted later of his success. The patient became "lively and
talkative," he said, as though this were evidence that her fears had
been overcome. Perhaps it was this tendency to divert attention
rather than to deal with concerns directly that led all southern
women—not just black women—to prefer midwives to doctors at
childbed.[57]

Women who wished to leave childbirth in female hands had
means of ensuring that much of its management remained so. Physicians did not usually remain with a patient for the time-consuming
duration of labor. J. E. Manlove in Tennessee "retired to the dwelling
house" shortly after his arrival at the childbed of Harriet, whose
labor unfolded in the kitchen. He instructed "one of the attendants"
to summon him after the woman "had four or five strong pains."
Samuel Hogg stayed with one woman several hours, but departed
when birth seemed not to be imminent, leaving directions that her
"attendants" (most likely a midwife, relatives, perhaps friends) let her
sleep. Charles H. Hentz took time out from one birth to visit his
office, and the woman he was attending had her child during his

absence. The midwife in contrast stayed with the mother, doing whatever she could to make the birth a positive experience, including cooking, cleaning, and watching the mother's other children if that was necessary. The enslaved Jennie Butler, who assisted a physician in cases of childbirth, said that doctors did not do any real work. They visited in the parlor and left the patient in the hands of the assistant until trouble arose.[58] The unwillingness of doctors to remain with women throughout labor gave midwives and other women considerable latitude in their work of birthing babies.

Because the presence of friends and family helped ensure that events would go as mothers wished, whenever possible women nearing confinement arranged to be close to loved ones. The slave woman Matilda Green somehow managed to obtain permission to stay with her sister Eliza Thompson King when she gave birth to a daughter in July 1860, even though they lived on different plantations. The fact that Green's husband was working at the Virginia estate where King lived must have factored into the decision that allowed the sisters to be together. Georgia rice planter James Hamilton Couper expected parturient women to give birth in the hospital he had constructed on his farm, but few women did so. Instead, they "contrived to be taken by surprise at home," according to Couper.[59] They could avoid reporting to the hospital as the slaveholder ordered by feigning the sudden onset of labor.

The element of surprise was a major aid to slaves in their efforts to maintain control over childbirth. No one could predict exactly when contractions would begin, including the mother. Ellen Cragin was born in Mississippi just before or during the Civil War. Her mother, "a great shouter," was attending a religious meeting when she felt her first labor pains. She returned quickly to the cabin, and Ellen was born that night. Frank Fikes's mother did not recognize labor as such when the pains began. She had eaten the first watermelon of the season and attributed her pains to that. After consuming a piece of calamus root to ease the pain, "behold I was born," her son reported. Nancy, an enslaved woman living near Redbone, Georgia, gave birth in a fence corner four miles from home. She had planned to visit friends on a neighboring plantation when labor pains overtook her and left her no choice but to give birth alone. Jane Brown gave birth in the Arkansas canebrake after she and her husband ran away. Violet Aldredge was born while her mother was being transported for sale in a speculator's drove. Pleasants gave birth in a Virginia prison, much to the consternation of her jailor, who lamented the "trouble & additional Expense." She had been captured after running away from her owner, and she bore her child while awaiting his arrival to reclaim her.[60]

At times, women were working when labor began. Cornelius Cross was born in a sorghum field. Millie Evans' mother pulled fodder until about an hour before her birth. Mattie Curtis gave birth to some of her children in the field. North Carolina slave Rosetta also recalled women who gave birth in the field, like the cows. Kenyon Morps earned a reputation for meanness in Georgia because he kept women working "right up to the last minute" before their confinement. As a result, the women on his place gave birth in the field and in fence corners, rather than in the cabin as preferred.[61]

Doctors employed by slaveholders were hard pressed to insert themselves where they were unwanted, because they could not predict when labor would begin. Owners might decide in advance to summon a physician for a parturient woman, but doctors commonly did not know when to come unless some slave initiated the call. Even when women found themselves confronting an owner's directive to send for a particular attendant, they might wait so long that the doctor arrived after the baby's birth. One South Carolina physician waited for hours at a slave woman's childbed only to discover "to his astonishment" that the woman had given birth earlier in the field, a fact she chose to conceal. Slaveholder James M. Torbert evidently did not know of a birth that occurred on his Alabama plantation until two days afterward, and the slave Matilda kept her

pregnancy secret from her overseer "until a few minets before the
burth of the child." John Harris in 1814 summoned a doctor for one
of his slaves after a midwife informed him of a possible complication
following birth, but the Virginia planter could not state with certainty exactly when the woman had delivered her child.[62] A desire to
control the birthing experience no doubt explains the reticence of
these slaves to inform owners about the births.

For slaves who wanted to manage childbirth to their liking, the
site of birth became a subject of concern. Enslaved women commonly gave birth in the cabin, a setting that allowed them a say in
how events unfolded. North Carolinian Mattie Davis, who gave
birth to some of her children in the field, noted that she had a granny
for the others, all of whom were born in the cabin. She liked giving
birth in the cabin because she could better take measures to ease the
pain. William Pope Brown's mother gave birth to her son in a one-
room hut built of hand-hewn logs and daubed with grass and dirt to
protect the inhabitants from the wind and rain. Barney Alford was
born in Mississippi near the Louisiana state line in a small log house
built in back of the kitchen where his mother worked as cook. Lizzie
Dorgens gave birth in a frame house that joined the kitchen. Because she was the cook, she lived with her family in the two rooms
attached to the outbuilding. Hattie Newbury in North Carolina gave
birth in a room above the storage area for feed and seeds. This was
where the enslaved family lived. Emma Countee Wilson and all her
brothers and sisters were born in a log cabin situated in the backyard
of her owner's house. Informant Harriett McFarlin Payne explained
that everything happened in the one-room cabins inhabited by
slaves: "birth, sickness, death."[63]

A small number of slave women gave birth in the owner's home,
a setting that allowed the mistress, master, or other members of the
slaveholding family to oversee the birth. Alice Rawlings was born in
her owner's Texas home, Milton Starr in the Arkansas home of his
master. Betsy Vann gave birth in her master and mistress's bed. She

was weaving nearby when labor began, and the birth occurred quickly; the mistress may have concluded that she had no choice but to direct her to the closest bed. Planters with sizable slaveholdings sometimes maintained "sick houses" or hospital buildings where slaves were expected to give birth according to the owner's idea of appropriate procedures. James Hamilton Couper's hospital, mentioned earlier, had four wards, one of which was specifically for "lying in" women. Hospitals were not the rule, however.[64]

When black women gave birth in the quarter without white supervision, they decided such procedures as the position assumed at birth, but when doctors or slaveholders were present, they expected the women to yield to their advice. In Arkansas the unattended Elsie Jones gave birth outside while hugging a tree, presumably in a standing position. A Tennessee slave with the aid of an old slave woman gave birth in a sitting position. Physician Charles A. Hentz found a woman laboring on the floor of her cabin. But Betsy Vann gave birth according to her mistress's idea of the proper position—lying in bed. Whether she would have chosen this position if her mistress had not been present is unknown.[65]

Simply giving birth in the cabin as opposed to the owner's home or hospital did not guarantee slave women the privacy to do as they wished. Owners and overseers often attended childbirth in the slave cabin or visited periodically to see how labor was progressing or at least asked particular persons to report its progress. At times, a mistress served as midwife to women on the plantation. This practice was rare, however, and some mistresses took note of slave births only from afar, visiting with more or less frequency depending on their own experience with motherhood, the availability of other women on the plantation to help, other obligations, and personal inclination. In Arkansas one mistress merely brought corn bread and the pot liquor left from cooking peas to the cabin where the new mother lived. Such visits could be motivated by genuine concern for the new mother, or they might reflect the mistress's sense of obligation as embodied in the paternalistic ethos that characterized the South. If perfunctory, the visits were brief and infrequent. Tryphena Blanche Holder Fox visited her slave Susan only twice in two weeks following the birth of Susan's son. In a letter to her mother, Fox made clear her aversion to the custom whereby mistresses visited new mothers: "I . . . hope I shall hardly see her during the time."[66]

On larger plantations the mistress might designate a woman to act as midwife and report any problems that arose at birth. Pussy regularly reported slave births at Retreat plantation in Georgia to her mistress Anna Matilda King, as well as the health of newborns and their mothers. In November 1852, Pussy sent word to King that Sarah's baby, ten days old, would not nurse. Pussy thought that the infant suffered from lockjaw. King's response reveals the social, emotional, and psychological distance that separated mistresses who took a hands-off attitude in caring for slaves: "One thing seems certain we are never to grow *rich* by the increase of our negros." She counted her loss "almost as severe a blow . . . as it is to poor Sarah." King was not without compassion for slaves she knew well and liked, however; when the children of two favorite house servants died, King expressed a deeper sense of regret.[67]

The need for goods by the mother and child ensured that mistresses were informed of births and kept abreast of the mother's and baby's well-being, because mistresses usually controlled the distribution of clothes, blankets, and other domestic supplies. After Sarah gave birth to a baby while her mistress was out, Rhina and another slave, Maria, looked without success for the necessities, which no doubt included a layette for the child. Upon the mistress's return, she found Rhina at the door anxious not only to tell her about the birth but also to obtain the items that Sarah required to care for her child.[68]

The mistress's frequent presence at the childbed of a slave suggests that the home remedies developed by and for white women were applied to black women. For example, thyme supposedly

speeded childbirth, fatherfew (also feverfew) was said to strengthen
wombs, and motherwort was good for women's disorders in general.[69] Of course, it is difficult with hindsight to sort out what folk
remedies had their origins in Europe, Africa, the West Indies, and
North America. It seems likely that Euroamerican, Afroamerican,
and Amerindian women shared folk cures as they came into contact
with one another, each one accepting or rejecting specific agents depending on their apparent efficacy, the woman's preexisting prejudices, and the ease with which substances could be obtained.

Midwife Victoria McMullen, known to most people as Hetty,
was of mixed race. The oversight of her physician owner and her
blood ties to her owning family probably encouraged members of
the slaveholding community to view her as a suitable birth attendant
for both black and white women. Her mixed African and Amerindian ancestry would have persuaded members of the enslaved
community to trust her midwifery skills. Given the tendency of
slaves to ascribe special status to children born of multiple births, the
fact that McMullen was a twin may have further enhanced her reputation for healing within the slave community.[70] Through her ancestry and clientele, McMullen demonstrated that the folkways of
different ethnic groups might be blended or shared by women of different social standing.

The physicians who arrived to treat complications of childbirth
joined a drama already in progress, one largely under the control of
women. When E. F. Knott arrived at the Manly plantation to assist
Jane with a difficult labor, he derived the case history from Aunt
Winney, an "old servant midwife" who informed the doctor that regular labor pains had begun about two o'clock that morning and had
grown stronger over time. Also, Jane had experienced "facial Neural-
gia" for several hours before the onset of labor, and she had not
moved her bowels even though she had been given a laxative. Doctor
Samuel Hogg arrived after the midwife had ruptured the amniotic
sac with her finger without good result. He had been summoned

because labor pains had ceased. Hogg blamed the woman's problems on the midwife—not because she had ruptured the membrane (he probably considered this standard procedure), but because she had engaged in "excessive handling," by which he apparently meant she had tried to manipulate the infant into position for delivery.[71]

Mistresses, who usually took an interest in the obstetric and gynecological needs of slave women, summoned doctors on their own and monitored physician-prescribed therapies. At times the mistress even suggested procedures to be followed. Doctor Thomas H. Todd found it necessary to consult with the mistress of the enslaved Prissa, who gave birth to a stillborn child in September 1839. Prissa had not expelled the afterbirth. She was in pain, and her mistress was much alarmed. Todd advised the use of castor oil to stimulate the bowels, which he thought would produce the afterbirth. After two or three bowel movements, Prissa was resting easily, but she still had not expelled the placenta. In his account of the case, Todd wrote: "*we* resolved to leave the case for the night to nature. At 10 o'clock next morning *we* gave her a dose of pills containing equal parts of calomel, rhuebarb and aloes," again in the expectation that further bowel movements would bring forth the placenta.[72]

The situation in which mistresses summoned and even directed doctors in their work represented a reversal of gendered roles that many physicians found troubling. More typically in the patriarchal South, men expected to determine the behavior of women. The mistress of a Tennessee woman called in a physician for a slave who had been in labor for forty-eight hours. She made clear that she wanted ergot administered to speed the labor and expel the child. The doctor apparently felt he could not counter her order. Against his better judgment, he administered the drug, but only after what he later called "a little *diplomatic* quackery." He diluted the drug and threw some out while the mistress's back was turned.[73]

An editorial in *The Stethoscope* excused such deception—or prudence, as the editor termed it. The patient or the patient's family (presumably this included slave owners) not infrequently requested more medication or faster or different treatment. In such cases it was perfectly permissible for the doctor to order some harmless concoction.[74] By giving themselves permission to commit subterfuge, physicians found a way to accommodate "tampering" without the risk of alienating a client. They also preserved a sense of pride. In a patriarchal society, men needed a means whereby they avoided the appearance—at least to themselves—of serving at the beck and call of women, even when the social order seemed to demand it.

Intervention at the birth of a slave was not limited to mistresses and midwives, of course. Masters and overseers also tried their hand at managing the birth, in part to save the expense of the physician's fee. Indeed, a complete lack of formal medical training did not prevent men from intervening in childbirth. Slaveholders with no medical training could follow advice on managing childbirth published in medical books for home use or have their overseers do so. John G. Gunn intended that his popular *Domestic Medicine*, which described procedures for childbirth, be used in slave states. *Popular Medicine; or, Family Adviser,* by Reynell Coates, also covered childbirth under the heading "diseases of women and children." It, too, was promoted as useful in situations where physicians were not readily available, including plantations.[75]

Planter A. C. Philips of Alabama took a week in 1846 to read in its entirety a medical text called *A Compendium of the Theory and Practice of Midwifery, Containing Practical Instructions for the Management of Women during Pregnancy, in Labour, and in Child-bed,* by Samuel Bard. The author, a New York physician, intended his "concise, cheap book" to be accessible to the lay public, as well as to medical students and physicians. The principle behind Bard's book was that the best practices were time-honored ones rather than innovations of the day. In particular, Bard worried about the increasing "use of instruments, and the introduction of the hand into the womb" because when practiced by unskilled men they posed rather than

resolved problems associated with birth. Nevertheless, by the publication of the book's third edition in 1815, Bard found it necessary to
add a fourth chapter on prolonged and difficult labor, which included a section on using instruments in delivery, thereby suggesting
that some laypeople were undaunted in tampering under the most
difficult of circumstances. Philips recorded the births of his slaves in
the page margins of Bard's book, an indication that he consulted the
manual whenever one of his slaves had a child.[76]

Overseers not only treated the health complaints of slaves generally but also occasionally intervened in childbirth. Typically, they
hoped to keep slaves in the fields as long as possible and only reluc-
tantly acknowledged sickness; even the onset of labor might not be
enough to convince an overseer of the need to excuse a woman from
work. However, the fear that a woman or infant might die from
complications of childbirth motivated most to summon a physician
in the face of difficulties. Thomas Seddon's overseer informed him
when one of the women on the plantation experienced a difficult
labor, prompting the Virginia planter to summon a doctor immediately. To have done otherwise would have left the overseer vulnerable
to criticism for any negative development. The manager of President
James K. Polk's Mississippi plantation found it necessary to reassure
his employer that the death of an infant had not been due to his
failure to call for help. Rather, the mother had failed to notify him
of her condition until it was too late to issue the summons, he
explained.[77]

As with other health problems, physicians expressed unhappi-
ness at being called too late in cases of childbirth. Although doctors
summoned to attend complicated deliveries complained about the
tendency of owners and overseers to try home remedies before calling for professional aid, their major concern was with the practices of
the midwives, who saw the parturient woman before the doctor arrived. Some seemed to attempt more than their skills allowed. Doctor M. Marsh of Louisiana charged that midwives harmed infants by

using force to deliver them: "Instead of *assisting* nature, they attempt to usurp her." The *New Orleans Medical News and Hospital Gazette* carried numerous reports of midwives who supposedly tore the uterus from patients, causing death. In Georgia, attending physician Rowan Green blamed the death of a slave infant on "rough and improper management" by the midwife. Doctor Thomas H. Todd of Tennessee blamed retention of the placenta by several of his patients on the midwife in charge of the cases.[78]

Physician T. P. Bailey, of North Santee, South Carolina, blamed the midwife for the deaths of twins he helped deliver in 1858. Delia gave birth to the first of her twins in the "ordinary way," but the second presented by the arm. In an effort to expedite the birth, the midwife pulled on the appendage, making matters worse. On his arrival, Bailey found the shoulder and arm wedged "in the interior strait of the pelvis." With great difficulty, he inserted his hand and turned the child, who delivered feet first. The child did not thrive, a fact that the doctor ascribed to the midwife's poor handling: "The arm was so much injured that I think this in a great measure contributed to its death." In the same year, Bailey oversaw the stillbirth of twins to Tenah. He attributed the death of the first-born to natural means, but the second death he believed due to the midwife's effort to extract the child, who presented by the arm. In yet a third case of twin births the following year, the doctor took credit for a successful outcome. Like the other sets of twins, the second child presented by the arm, but this time the doctor was on hand soon enough to save the situation.[79]

All of these cases involved slaves and focused on the *practices* of granny midwives rather than their *employment*. When it came to white women, some doctors argued that only doctors should oversee childbirth. "On plantations, of course it cannot be expected that the physician is to be called in to every case of natural labor" among slaves, physician William E. Brickell of Mississippi acknowledged, but "amongst white persons . . . the 'granny' should really be nothing more than the nurse, her every step being under the guidance of the physician." In the case of enslaved women, grannies might still oversee routine births, provided a physician was called at the first sign of difficulty. Of course physicians did not wish to eliminate the granny's assistance entirely, as Brickell's words attest, for they were loath to carry out many of the mundane tasks associated with childbirth themselves, especially aftercare. "If we could only get these old grannies to acknowledge that they only know how to receive and dress a baby," Brickell continued, it would be to the slaveholder's profit and doctor's relief.[80]

Differences in social status, as well as notions of what constituted appropriate procedures in childbirth, impeded the ability of white doctors to work effectively with black midwives. The midwife might relate the facts of the case upon the physician's arrival: what had gone wrong, which procedures had been followed, and why the doctor had been called. More often, owners relayed this information. White men found it difficult to take direction from a woman, a black, or a slave. Midwives encompassed all three attributes; consequently doctors neither valued nor followed their opinions. Samuel Hogg went out of his way to expose what he regarded as the midwife's ignorance in contrast to his own superior knowledge when he penned an article for the *Western Journal of Medicine and Surgery*. The midwife had advised a craniotomy in what appeared to be a hopeless case. Hogg instead bled the woman. The baby was born alive sometime later. Maintaining that the situation was not "novel or particularly striking," Hogg proclaimed his medicine superior to the ministrations of the female attendant.[81]

The choice of birth attendant was not between modern medical men and meddlesome midwives, as Hogg would have it. Although they pointed with pride to medical practices that they thought improved the mother and baby's chance for survival, in truth physicians did not always produce positive outcomes. Mortality and morbidity rates for mothers and infants in the slave quarter remained high despite doctors' involvement in troublesome childbirth cases. Some part of the invective physicians directed toward midwives no doubt originated in their own susceptibility to charges of incompetence. Thus, physician criticism of midwives can be seen as defensive. "In the name of common sense, and in a true spirit of justice," Brickell implored, "if the physician is to be the responsible person in these cases . . . let him have the conduct of the whole matter," as if to say that this strategy would resolve the problem of death and illness among women and infants in the slave quarter.[82]

At the same time that doctors criticized midwives, they excused their own shortcomings. Indeed, physicians of the nineteenth-century South were more candid than modern physicians in admitting medical error. Doctor E. B. Haskins failed at first to diagnose a case of puerperal peritonitis (a particularly deadly form of childbed fever), which took the life of a woman in Tennessee. He wrote about the events in the pages of the *Western Journal of Medicine and Surgery* to alert fellow physicians of the need to take seriously the abdominal pains in women who had recently given birth. Physician T. P. Bailey discussed in the *Charleston Medical Journal and Review* six cases of childbirth involving nine infants (including three sets of twins). Six of the children had died. Bailey attributed one death to natural causes, two to the midwife's rough handling. He readily attributed one death to injury he caused by the use of forceps. His inability skillfully to insert the second blade of the forceps had resulted in the woman's death.[83] Doctors seemed to think that they were owed understanding for their own failures. With additional experience, they would learn to manage childbirth better. The granny, it seemed to them, stood in the way of professional advancement. If she would step aside in all but uneventful cases, doctors would have a free hand in developing procedures that would benefit all women. Physicians did not wish so much to replace the midwife in the slave quarter as to limit her services so as to enlarge their own.

The effort by medical men to usurp some of the midwife's duties at childbed mirrored the trend by slave owners to insert themselves more and more into the personal lives of slaves. Less overtly, slaveholders had already extended their control over childbirth in the quarter by taking over some traditional functions of the midwife. In the colonial era midwives had operated in the public sphere by noting births and deaths and providing opinion as to the nature of illness and injury. They might examine a woman and offer testimony as to whether she had engaged in intercourse after a charge of sexual abuse, for example. And in the case of unmarried women, she might at the time of birth be relied upon to elicit from the parturient woman the name of her child's father. Black midwives performed no such public function. Because the woman's owner presumably would welcome the addition of the child to his plantation and assume financial responsibility for his or her upbringing, no need existed to establish paternity upon the birth of a slave, at least from the owner's perspective. And acknowledging children of mixed race or sexual abuse raised more questions about sexual relations across the color line than slaveholders wanted answered. Some black children grew up without knowing their father's identity because it was better for all concerned to have no one speak about their paternity. Martha Mays, born a slave in Georgia, never knew anything about her father. Evelyn Jones never knew anything about her father except what her mother revealed, and this did not include his name or status.[84] Reliance on granny midwives suited the purpose of the master, who did not always want details of sexual relations recorded.

Denied literacy by virtue of her status, the slave midwife could play no public role in the announcement of births or deaths outside the quarter. Instead, each slaveholder assumed responsibility for maintaining vital statistics according to his or her own notions of usefulness. Planter and physician James Ritchie Sparkman dutifully recorded in his farm record book the time enslaved women reported quickening and the time they gave birth. In December 1857, for example, Ritchie reported that three women on his Birdfield Plantation felt life. Hannah, who reported her pregnancy on 1 December, bore a daughter on 25 April; Violet, who experienced quickening on 20 December, gave birth to a son on 22 June; Nanny also gave birth to a boy in June—on the second—after reporting her pregnancy on 25 December. Miscarriages and stillbirths also were recorded. In 1858, for example, June experienced quickening on 10 January and miscarried on 7 February.[85] Sparkman's choice of information reflected his interests as a farmer: Which workers would be laboring at reduced capacity? When would they need to be excused from field work? As a physician, he no doubt assumed that he could spot any women who were shamming by noting who should have given birth in which month. Many planters, Sparkman included, kept records of slaves born each year. Valuable property, they were tallied up in farm journals much the same as livestock. Some children were listed alongside the names of fathers, but others were not. Granny midwives in contrast produced no written records, although they no doubt etched the circumstances of each birth in memory.

———

The different assistance offered enslaved mothers by regular physicians and granny midwives reflected their different understandings of what could go wrong during childbirth. For slaves—indeed for most people throughout history—childbirth represented a time of vulnerability for the mother, the child, and the larger community. One purpose of birth rituals is to protect everyone from danger. Thus, people in all times and places tend to resist changing birthing practices for fear that harm will come to those involved; only someone steeped in the cultural customs of a society can advise those living there, people believe. This attitude explains why enslaved women consulted birth attendants familiar with life in the quarter even after the physician arrived on the scene.

Doctors defined their services narrowly and in terms that resonated more with the inhabitants of the "big house" than with those of the quarter. They held out hope that high rates of maternal and infant mortality might be reduced through an improvement of techniques to start or speed labor or retard hemorrhaging. Slaveholders responded by calling them when trouble developed during labor, but black women—patients and midwives—remained skeptical of their services. Both preferred that the birthing process remain in more experienced, female hands. Medical practice was changing, however, and doctors were becoming interested in women's health in general. Medical men were gradually intruding into women's domain, not only during but also after birth.

6

Postnatal Complications

In 1814 John Harris, slaveholder of Albemarle County, Virginia, summoned physician Charles Brown to the bedside of "a woman delivered of one child a day or two past." Because she complained very much, Harris asked the doctor to "come with speed"—after stopping by the post office to "bring my news paper."[1] No record reveals what the patient's problem entailed or what services Brown rendered, but the case illustrates an important aspect of medical practice in the South during the early years of the new nation: slaveholders who hesitated to hire a physician to attend an enslaved woman during labor might welcome the doctor when complications arose after birth. Clearly, Harris thought the woman in question required medical attention and he was willing to pay for it, although he did not consider the case urgent enough to do without his mail. In the decades that followed these events, other planters acted to ensure the continuation—even expansion—of slavery through attention to human reproduction in the slave quarter. Determined to perpetuate a population of bonded laborers, they followed Harris' example and sought the services of a physician when complications following childbirth threatened the health of enslaved women.

Childbirth was a dangerous time for women and infants. All too often a birth ended in tragedy—the death or disability of the mother or child. Because proper recovery was crucial for a woman's ability to bear more children and return to productive labor, masters, mistresses, and overseers watched new mothers carefully for signs of trouble in the hours and days immediately following childbirth. Anxiety impelled them to consult medical men when trouble arose. Physicians were to alleviate the immediate danger, but doctors went beyond this role to explain why the problem had developed in the first place. Improper management by lay midwives and mothers appeared to them a frequent cause. Neither seemed to understand proper procedures for giving birth or caring for newborns. Nature or providence played a role in delaying the delivery of the afterbirth, spreading puerperal fever, and jeopardizing an infant's health, but ignorant black grannies and mothers abetted both. The key to managing difficult slave births was to summon professionally trained men—scientific men with knowledge of anatomy—at the first sign of trouble.

Tragic developments were keenly felt in the slave quarter, of course, but physicians reserved much of their sympathy for the slaveholders who summoned them and paid the bill. A Georgia physician and planter warned that improper medical care during or following childbirth would "prove nothing but a source of misery and suffering" to the woman but would also render her "a useless burden" to her owner because she would be incapable of performing either reproductive or productive labor. Failure to call a physician at the first sign of distress could result in debilitating "diseases peculiar to women."[2]

Like owners and physicians, slaves feared improper management of birth's aftermath. They defined improper procedures differently, however, and blamed ignorant white men for many ills. To be sure, natural or spiritual forces might thwart the recovery of new mothers, but doctors further complicated matters—sometimes by attempting extreme procedures and often by rejecting the traditions and rituals that ensured a good birth. Enslaved women formed their own interpretation of events, which differed from that of physicians and their slaveholding clients.

Aftercare in the slave quarter was largely under the purview of black women even when a doctor attended a birth. Midwives stayed with new mothers a week or more to help them care for the infant and to see that they recovered from the ordeal of parturition. James Henry Hammond directed that the midwife on his plantation attend a new mother and infant for seven days following delivery. Daphney's owner, a rice planter, expected the midwife to help a new mother for a fortnight following the birth of a child and instructed his overseer to release her from other work accordingly.[3] Even if the child was stillborn, the midwife would remain with the grieving mother to render aid and comfort.

During this period, midwives worked with new parents and owners to ensure that women followed customs and had time from work necessary for recovery. They used the roots and herbal cures favored within their community, along with measures of a more spiritual nature. They also offered advice on daily activities. For example, a certain time might have to elapse before a new mother would be permitted to work around water. Former slave Minnie Hollomon said that seven weeks had to go by before women who had given birth could safely "put their hands in a washtub."[4] Laundering was difficult labor, and this precaution might have been intended originally to lighten the woman's workload after childbirth; however, by the antebellum era the admonition had become embedded in the lore that surrounded aftercare in the slave South.

Many women complained of having inadequate time for recovery from childbirth before returning to arduous field work. Although most women were assigned a week or more of lighter work following childbirth, Mary A. Hicks of North Carolina said that some never had this time for recovery; she had known them to leave the field, have a child, and "be back at wuck de next day." Ophelia Whitley of North Carolina recalled similar situations in which women who left the field to give birth were expected to be back at work the next morning. This requirement was unusual, she admitted; but the fact that it existed at all galled slaves, who considered time for recovery from childbirth important for mother and child alike.[5]

Clara Jones, who gave birth to five children in quick succession, fainted in the field the day after her fifth child was born. Her master, Felton McGee, kicked her in anger and decided on the spot to sell her. Growing up, Eustace Hodges heard Jones (her mother) describe how each of two successive owners treated her following childbirth. The second, Rufus Jones, proved better than McGee in that he called a doctor and allowed her several days of bed rest following a birth. Most slaveholders fell somewhere between the two in allocating resources for recovery from childbirth. Typically slaveholders excused new mothers from the most arduous work for about a month following the birth of a child. So common was the practice that one physician's wife described it as "the law." This was not time spent idle. Rather the women engaged in lighter-than-customary tasks while they breastfed and cared for their children. Some women carded cotton or spun thread while they recovered, for example. On the cotton plantation belonging to Bennet H. Barrow in Louisiana, "sucklers" (women who were breastfeeding infants) performed a variety of tasks, from drying cotton to spinning to planting peas. After weeks of recovery, they might be put to hoeing and picking cotton, but the expectation was that they would do less work than before. Barrow understood that the amount of cotton picked on any given day reflected the situation of the women, some of whom could not be expected to pick their best. There were enough men like McGee around, however, to be cause for concern among slaves.[6]

Rosaline Rogers recalled mothers spending only two or three days in bed following delivery before returning to their usual tasks in the field. In North Carolina, Hanna Clay lost only three days from work following childbirth. She carried her baby on her back wrapped in a red blanket, and when the baby needed to nurse, she would slip the blanket around so that the infant could breastfeed while she continued to pick and hoe. On her plantation in Georgia mistress Frances Sutton required a new mother to return to hoeing within two weeks of giving birth. On Kenyon Morps's Georgia plantation, women had only one week to recover from childbirth before being sent back to work, a practice that earned the master a reputation among slaves as a "mean man."[7]

Occasionally the period of aftercare was punctuated by a crisis in the health of the mother or child. In such a case, the doctor might be summoned for the first time to the slave quarter. Doctors who were not deemed essential at a routine birth were sometimes called specifically to assist with a problem in the delivery of the placenta and membranes—the afterbirth. Midwives were not expected to attempt manual extraction, a procedure reserved for the doctor. Physicians also were brought to the plantation to treat cases of childbed fever and other gynecological problems, to determine why infants had died, and to examine children born with severe disabilities. Generally they did not stay long; they made an appearance, took some action, and left orders for other caregivers to follow. As with childbirth, doctors (and slaveholders) were unwilling to invest large amounts of time tending patients after birth. Because they generally received pay according to the time they spent, owners preferred to have them devise a plan of treatment that left most of the aftercare to black midwives, nurses, friends, or family. At the same time, lower fees than those assessed for other medical services discouraged doctors from remaining long with patients even if they had been inclined to do so.[8] Slaveholders and physicians each tended to be satisfied with the arrangement. Any grousing tended to be directed at female patients and attendants for not following orders.

Physicians routinely complained that neither patients nor caregivers could be counted on to comply with their orders.[9] The fact that physicians frequently arrived well after the onset of a crisis, even days late, suggests that slaves were reluctant to have them involved.

The poor outcomes they achieved made slaves skeptical that doctors could do much to turn a serious situation around. Many preferred their own methods of managing a crisis, some of which mirrored those of doctors. Anyone could induce evacuation of the bowels in an attempt to dislodge a placenta. And midwives did not limit their efforts to actions that might be taken by a doctor.

As with childbirth, doctors blamed midwives for doing more than their skills allowed when dealing with complications. On two occasions, one in 1839 and the other in 1840, Thomas H. Todd found fault with two midwives who had broken off the cord in attempts to remove the afterbirth.[10] Doctors complained that such actions put them in a difficult position. They were charged with improving a situation, but only after "tampering" rendered their procedures ineffective.

Henry R. Frost, who performed a craniotomy on the fetus of a South Carolina woman on 14 September 1838, returned to see the patient on each of the next three days and grew concerned at her slow rate of recovery. She complained of fever and sweating, and "there was considerable discharge from the vagina." Frost prescribed an astringent injection on the nineteenth. Only then did the doctor examine her internally, whereupon he was shocked to discover what appeared to be "a mass of hair, in short pieces, of an inch to two inches in length." Frost was at a loss to explain what it was, although he wondered if it was "an abortive effort of nature in the projection of twins."[11] More likely the mass was a concoction the midwife inserted to stem the hemorrhaging of the hapless woman. The incident suggests that slaves engaged in indigenous practices following delivery despite the involvement of the slaveholders' physicians.

Deliberate adherence among slaves to traditional practices frustrated doctors, but so did the inadvertent failure of other people to follow the doctor's orders, including at times the owner. William M. Boling, of Montgomery, Alabama, in 1843 treated a woman who had given birth to a stillborn child. She was hemorrhaging and had retained the placenta. "After making some ineffectual efforts to induce uterine contractions, I was compelled to leave her, to attend other pressing engagements," the doctor reported. He pulled "the detached edge of the placenta through the os uteri, and left it acting the part of a tampon" to stem the bleeding. He also left orders with the woman's master to administer ergot and directed that "some powders, composed of sugar of lead and opium . . . be given in case the flooding should again become profuse," but only if the hemorrhaging was unaccompanied by pain. The master misunderstood. He gave her ergot, and when she began bleeding again with "pretty severe pains," he commenced giving the powders. The doctor discovered the error when he returned the next day. To his great relief, the mistake resulted in no long-term harm to the woman (at least in his estimation).[12]

Doctor E. F. Knott, called to attend the enslaved woman Jane, saw to the expulsion of the placenta; applied a compress saturated with a mixture made of balsam extract, olive oil, and the white of an egg to her internal organs; and wrapped her belly with a bandage. At that point he retired to enjoy "the most perfect rest and quietude." He visited Jane the next day, ordering castor oil and leaving "general directions as to cleanliness, strict regimen, and a wash of tepid water and sweet milk to be thrown up the vagina, as a detergent, three times daily, and a decoction of red oak bark to be used immediately after it as an antiseptic, together with" instructions on how to keep the breasts soft and bowels open. His goal was to regulate Jane's bodily functions to ensure a well-ordered recovery under the care of her family and friends. He did not examine her again but received word over the course of a week or two that things were going well for Jane and her baby. The mother had abundant milk, and her child was healthy. He had served in a crisis, but once normalcy was achieved he was no longer needed. One woman following childbirth developed a headache of enough magnitude to preclude her sleeping or even resting. When "the usual remedies" failed to bring relief, the doctor returned to produce a blister on her shaven scalp and prescribe something to move the bowels. She convalesced slowly after the physician left.[13]

One of the most common reasons doctors were called after delivery of an infant was retention of the afterbirth. In normal births, the placenta and membranes are dislodged and expelled shortly after the baby's appearance. If the placenta was retained long, the slave owner or the owner's designated agent might call for a doctor's aid at this stage of birth. Of course some doctors who arrived in time only for the delivery of the afterbirth had been summoned earlier but inadvertently arrived late. Other doctors were called only after a lengthy lapse of time. Whatever the circumstances of their late arrival, many of the stories told about birth by doctors centered on this final stage of delivery.

Cases of adherent placenta (in which the placenta fails to detach or only partially detaches from the uterine wall) were relatively rare; one Kentucky doctor claimed to have seen only one in twenty-eight years of practice. Retention of the placenta because of the premature contraction of the uterus was more common, however. The same Kentucky physician described for readers of the *Boston Medical and Surgical Journal* nine of the cases he had encountered over his decades-long career. The condition was common enough that he rarely left the delivery of the afterbirth entirely to nature, but rather helped it along. He had permitted only a dozen or so patients to deliver the placenta on their own since beginning his career as a University of Maryland medical student.[14]

Doctors had few means of assisting when the afterbirth was not promptly expelled, and they disagreed about the efficacy of the methods. Most waited as long as possible for nature to take its course, sometimes for hours or even days, except when hemorrhaging occurred. In that case, they acted in haste. To facilitate delivery, doctors typically rubbed the abdomen and gently pulled on the cord. Next they administered ergot to stimulate contractions. If the problem persisted, a hand could be inserted in an effort to dislodge the placenta. The course of action could be shortened by skipping the ergot if the situation was dire. When S. Henry Dickson found an infant already dead and the mother's life endangered, the doctor immediately inserted his hand in an attempt to remove the placenta. But generally physicians acted conventionally; they attempted to stimulate contractions and waited as the woman's fate unfolded. Medicine had done all it could; the woman's future was in the hands of God or nature, depending on the doctor's religious sentiments and understanding of physiological processes.[15]

If doctors did more, they customarily fell back on the standard measures of bloodletting and the use of purgatives as a way of speeding the delivery to conclusion. Doctor L. Faulkner, of Halifax County, Virginia, was summoned to a slave quarter twelve hours following the birth of an enslaved child because the afterbirth still had not been expelled. He concluded that a portion of the placenta was adhering to the uterine wall, informed the master of his suspicion, and asked to consult with another doctor. Permission granted, the two medical men waited with the new mother for some hours, each taking turns holding the placenta in the hope that an opportunity would present itself whereby it could be drawn out. They administered ergot to start contractions that they hoped would expel the afterbirth but without the desired effect. Various treatments were tried on the exhausted patient, including bloodletting, poultices, "tepid fomentations to vulva," leeching, and an enema. (Fomentations were poultices intended to convey heat and moisture.) Days went by. The doctors visited periodically, leaving directions with the nurse about how to continue treatment in their absence. Four days after her baby's birth, the mother reported the afterbirth discharged. Unconvinced that her claim was true, the doctors continued treatment for two more days. Although there was some talk early on of letting nature take its course in this case, the periodic return of the doctors to the mother's childbed to perform ever-more-aggressive measures

demonstrated their belief—and no doubt that of the slaveholder—
that the situation required action. Faulkner ceased visiting on the
seventeenth day, presumably because the owner believed that no
more could be done for her. The mother's condition remained critical, and she eventually died.[16]

The enema Faulkner prescribed represented a long-standing
method used to expel a tardy afterbirth by midwives as well as by
doctors. In the early 1840s Thomas H. Todd of Tennessee employed
cathartics intended to force the evacuation of the bowels and consequently (he hoped) the placenta and membranes. He tried the
method with three women (his brother with a fourth) before writing
up the experiences for publication. It produced positive results in all
four cases—or so he claimed. In the first case, planter Richard Ellet
asked Todd to attend a twenty-eight-year-old slave who had given
birth to her first child without expelling the placenta. She was exhausted but not hemorrhaging. The doctor began conservatively. For
a few hours, he employed "friction and pulled gently upon the cord
only." When that did not work, he "administered the ergot, with
the view of exciting uterine contraction," but this did not produce
the desired effect either. He next tried to insert his hand to remove the afterbirth, "but here again I was doomed to meet another
disappointment; as the soft parts had by this time contracted so
much, that any attempt to introduce the hand, however slow and
firm it might be, entirely failed." He next resolved to administer the
purgative. The subsequent movement of the bowels appeared to produce the desired result.[17]

Bolder and desperate doctors sometimes went beyond such standard protocol to employ more innovative methods intended to dislodge a retained placenta. Doctor W. L. Felder in South Carolina
stumbled on what he considered a new treatment for "adhesion
of the placenta" when the "usual way" of handling a case failed to
produce the desired result. Called to remove the placenta from a
hemorrhaging slave woman who had given birth three or four days

previously, the doctor achieved success (or thought he had) by applying a sponge soaked in watered creosote. By the time he wrote his account of the case for the January 1853 issue of the *Nashville Journal of Medicine and Surgery,* he had performed the procedure twice, first on a white woman, next on the black woman mentioned here. If a similar case occurred, he informed readers, he would experiment by injecting the creosote directly into the blood vessels of the cord.[18]

Felder initially tested the procedure on the white patient in November 1839. He had attended her for one and a half days before she gave birth. Her child had been delivered by forceps, and she experienced severe hemorrhaging soon afterward. Felder applied friction over the abdomen and pulled on the placenta. He next inserted his hand into the uterus in an effort to tear the cord away. When that did not work, he gave the patient opium and a lead compound (used as an astringent), followed by ergot to excite contractions. Still the afterbirth was not expelled, so Felder tried his hand again. All of this failed to produce the desired result. Then he introduced the creosote-soaked sponge. The hemorrhaging soon stopped, and the doctor was able to pull away the placenta using force.[19] It is not clear that the sponge stopped the bleeding and allowed the placenta's removal, but the doctor believed it had.

Felder's case involving the slave occurred eight and a half years later. This time he was not present at the birth but was brought to the plantation three or four days after the child's delivery. The period of elapsed time between this birth and the arrival of the doctor was especially long. Doctors complained that any delay retarded their ability to improve the situation and that a delay of this duration could prove fatal. In this case, hemorrhaging was severe, and the patient was exhausted. After pulling on the cord, the doctor inserted his hand and felt the afterbirth firmly attached to the uterine wall, much as had occurred with the white woman treated previously. Skipping the step of employing ergot, he immediately determined to use the creosote, this time without the opium or lead compound.

The patient experienced "no inconvenience," according to the doctor, by which he apparently meant she felt no pain, although the basis for this conclusion is unclear. Manual removal of the placenta would have resulted in considerable pain for the patient. Felder ordered oil, rest, and a bland diet before leaving her bedside firmly convinced that the creosote had worked in this case and would in all similar situations.[20]

Although regular physicians throughout the nation purported to disdain an approach to healing in which treatments were developed ad hoc during the day-to-day experience of the practitioner, doctors like Felder unabashedly recounted in the pages of medical journals and by word of mouth their own medical testing of newly devised treatment. Southern doctors, like men of the slaveholding class, attached great importance to reputation. Southerners admired men who were bold of action: decisive, independent, and in command of the situation. Doctors tried to act accordingly. Reluctant to admit failure, uncertainty, or reliance upon others, they attempted in desperate obstetric cases all that they could within the framework of standard medicine and their own understanding of the individual patient's condition.

Doctors needed to take action when called for complications following childbirth, but action did not always produce the desired result. Complications such as retained placenta were frequent enough that physicians could not avoid them over the course of a career, but they occurred with such irregularity that doctors had little opportunity to gain expertise in handling them. When standard procedure failed, the decision about whether to attempt a bold or innovative procedure was up to the doctor in consultation with his slaveholding client. Enslaved patients had little if any say in the development of the plan. A doctor could implement treatment only if the patient cooperated, however. He based his decision to go ahead with therapy on his assessment of the situation, including the patient's ability to withstand the plan of care and willingness to go along, both important considerations.[21]

Doctors were driven in part to innovate in cases of retained placenta because the efficacy of standard treatment was in doubt. W. L. Sutton complained specifically of the course of treatment recommended by physician William P. Dewees (author of an influential medical text called *A Compendious System of Midwifery*). Dewees thought that ergot should be used in an effort to expel the placenta before the insertion of the hand. The problem, Sutton explained, was that the contractions produced by the ergot made the latter procedure difficult and dangerous for the doctor. He had once injured his hand this way while attending a black woman named Judy, and it had taken two months for his hand to heal. Only if the ergot failed to produce strong contractions should the doctor consider introducing his hand, the Kentucky doctor advised.[22]

At times the doctor left the scene of birth believing everything was well, only to be recalled because of puerperal or childbed fever, a condition that claimed the lives of many new mothers in the days before the germ theory was established. At other times the doctor was called only after a new mother had developed symptoms of the infection. No sure cure existed. An element of desperation sounded in the correspondence of Virginia planter A. A. Morson, who sought medical assistance for one of his enslaved women showing signs of the fever. She "has just been attacked with alarming symptoms after delivery of a child," he wrote. He gave no other details for why the doctor's presence was promptly required. Presumably the doctor would know what to expect without them.[23]

Puerperal fever is a severe bacterial infection that occurs chiefly in a woman after childbirth, usually because she has been subjected to unsterile birthing procedures or less frequently because placental fragments have been left in the uterus. It originates in the uterus and generally involves a significant invasion of the bloodstream by the microorganisms responsible for the infection. Symptoms include fever, rapid pulse, uterine tenderness, and a malodorous vaginal discharge. Today doctors strive to avoid infection by such measures as maintaining a sterile environment, keeping internal exams to a minimum, and ensuring that the uterus is completely clean following birth. Neither nineteenth-century physicians nor midwives understood the role of germs in contagion, and the importance of a sterile environment was only beginning to occur to some. Physician efforts to extract a retained placenta greatly increased the possibility of infection and no doubt added to the number of women suffering from puerperal fever.[24]

Having become convinced by reports from European and U.S. doctors that puerperal fever was spread by contagion, Oliver Wendell Holmes published evidence in 1843 that birth attendants carried the infection from patient to patient. The article in the *New England Quarterly Journal of Medicine and Surgery* was reprinted and widely discussed, but many readers were skeptical of the doctor's finding. By the early 1850s, his thesis that physicians were implicated in the spread of the disease was under attack. Debate about causes of and cures for childbed fever occurred throughout the United States and in Europe. Charles D. Meigs, a prominent physician in Philadelphia, for one, led the condemnation, which served to stir further discussion of Holmes's ideas.[25]

Most southern physicians—like many other doctors—adamantly denied any responsibility for puerperal fever. The thought that doctors might be the origin of disease did not fit into their concept of standard medical narratives, which featured practitioners boldly curing grateful patients. Even when his treatment produced no cure, a doctor was reluctant to admit the fact. To acknowledge that disease had got the better of him was to admit the limits of his authority. With regard to the cause of puerperal fever, doctors affiliated with the Louisiana State Medical Society rejected outright the idea that physician practice could spread "contagion as absurd in the extreme."

Instead they attributed the disease to "rough usage by an ignorant midwife" and to the prolongation of the lochial discharge that normally follows childbirth. Virginia physician C. R. Harris also repudiated the notion that doctors might communicate the disease to patients in accouchement. When nine women died of puerperal fever in Augusta County, the country doctor pointed out that none of the afflicted mothers had been attended by the same person, at least to the doctor's knowledge. Harris treated eight of the nine women while attending parturient women who never contracted the fever, offering this circumstance as further proof that the doctor did not play a role in spreading the disease. Only slowly did some doctors begin implementing the recommended sanitary precautions when they attended women at childbirth.[26]

Meanwhile southern medical men debated other preventive measures. Noted physician John P. Mettauer thought the administration of a purgative shortly after birth prevented the fever's development and touted purgation in both South Carolina and Virginia medical journals. Mettauer, who served as professor of the principles and practice of medicine and surgery in the Medical Department of Randolph-Macon College of Virginia, urged other doctors to experiment with his plan. Its appearance in the Virginia journal provoked a response from Goodridge A. Wilson of Richmond, who believed that purging might cause the disease rather than ward it off. To support his position, Wilson told of two women, one black and one white. Both of the new mothers had been purged but died anyway. Wilson, like Mettauer, relied on traditional heroic means of cure, bleeding "as far as the patient's strength would warrant," blistering, and applying fomentations. Wilson chastised Mettauer for generalizing too much about the practice of medicine. No one treatment worked for all patients.[27]

Far from settling the issue, Wilson's communiqué to the Virginia medical journal only elicited more on the subject from Mettauer, who now felt compelled to refute Wilson's claim that the organs of gestation and labor required rest following the delivery of a child. The fact that neither doctor recognized contagion as the origin of the fever suggests that the attitudes of Harris and the practitioners affiliated with the Louisiana medical society on the topic were far from unusual.[28]

Cases of puerperal fever were common enough that most physicians expected to encounter them. Each was left to develop his own cure based on written texts, word of mouth, and experience. Readers of one Virginia publication learned that brewer's yeast might work, but the advocate of this remedy—who originally submitted the cure to the *Boston Medical and Surgical Journal*—admitted that his only source of knowledge was his own practice; "it is a purely *empirical* remedy," he acknowledged. In 1858 Medicus (perhaps a pseudonym) Ransom, of Murfreesboro, Tennessee, encountered "a much greater number of cases of this kind" than he usually met. He reported five women (three black and two white) suffering from the condition to members of the Rutherford County Medical Society in an effort "to compare notes" among the members. As his narrative reveals, he rejected the notion that birth attendants might be culpable in spreading the fever, doubted the efficacy of standard methods of treatment, but harbored a reluctance to eschew the latter in favor of another approach.[29]

One of Ransom's patients—an eighteen-year-old slave—had developed general symptoms of illness on the fifth day following the birth of her first child. The doctor was not called for another two days, however. Upon arrival he bled the patient "to faintness," administered calomel (which worked as a laxative), Dover's powders (an opiate), oil, "fomentations to the abdomen, and stimulating frictions to the extremities." Seeing no improvement the following day, the doctor repeated the bleeding, calomel, and Dover's powders. Similar measures were taken the next day, only now the woman received "opium enough to keep quiet." The day after, the doctor resorted to a blister and an enema, together with the same medicine and fomentations. At last the woman began to improve, though very slowly.[30]

Barely two weeks later the doctor again found himself confronting a case of childbed fever in the slave community. A similar routine again produced positive results in his estimation. The thirty-five-year-old mother recovered following a round of bleeding, calomel, and poultices, only in this case the doctor supplied opium from the time of his arrival.[31]

About a week later Ransom encountered his first case in the white community. The doctor began the now-familiar treatment, but with one variation: he added tincture of veratrum (American hellebore), a substance that would have purged the bowels, induced nausea and vomiting, slowed the heart, and lowered blood pressure. When the woman's condition worsened instead of improving, the doctor suspended the veratrum temporarily, then restarted it "in such doses as the stomach will bear or the pulse demands." The doctor kept up the regimen for three more days; on the fourth the "patient sank very rapidly . . . and died at night."[32]

A few weeks later Ransom encountered yet another case in the white community, when a woman developed "all the usual symptoms of puerperal fever" on the fifth day following the birth of her third child. Ransom embarked on the same plan of treatment, expecting to increase the dose of veratrum gradually until "either the pulse is reduced to sixty or seventy, or she is sickened by it." This time the woman recovered.[33]

Months went by before Ransom was called to treat another case of the fever. The patient this time was black, and the doctor began by "bleeding to faintness," which was followed by the usual calomel and oil, supplemented now with sulphate of morphia, a narcotic intended to reduce pain that, much like opium, can induce a half-sleep state. He also "ordered the veratrum as in the last case," as well as an enema. This treatment worked as before, and the doctor reported her as "convalescent" when last he saw her.[34]

Ransom was at a loss to account for the large number of cases in the area, which he said occurred "nearly upon a line" that extended eight or nine miles through Murfreesboro. The women did not appear to share the same attendant, and childbirth had proceeded easily and naturally for all, although in the first case the attendant had removed the placenta by hand. Although he used veratrum in only three of the cases and one of the patients who received it died, Ransom's faith in its therapeutic value had grown, along with his faith in bloodletting. "I have not used this remedy [veratrum] as a substitute for bloodletting," he emphasized. Such a course of action would have been too risky. It was better to apply new and old remedies simultaneously. Thus, empiricism supplemented rather than supplanted standard measures as doctors sought a cure. In fact, one reason Ransom and other doctors recounted a series of cases in print was to stimulate discussion among colleagues of little-understood medical phenomena.[35]

So-called heroic medicine had many defenders in the antebellum South, although it was losing favor elsewhere. C. R. Harris recognized that physicians were divided on purgatives in cases of puerperal fever and that the doubters reflected skepticism in general about the invasive methods associated with the approach to healing. He nevertheless leaned toward them. A doctor should keep the patient's bowels clear if for no other reason than to eliminate gas that could prove quite troublesome to the patient, he believed. Harris expressed particular faith in bleeding. Death was staved off only "by prompt, bold and energetic treatment early after the attack," usually between twelve and thirty hours after onset of the fever. Bleeding begun late was "of no benefit, but had rather a tendency to some extent to hasten the fatal termination." To support his position, Harris cited the case of a white woman who he said survived because of the large quantity of blood extracted from her. Taking a lesser amount would not have worked.[36]

When symptoms of childbed fever appeared, Mettauer also fell back on measures involving decisive and vigorous action. Called to a case in the early 1850s, the doctor bled the patient to the point of fainting. He next administered medications intended to have her vomit and excrete copious amounts. Fomentations and blister plasters were applied. He fed his patient ice and iced water and also packed the woman's vagina with ice to reduce her fever, which he said proved to be a fine remedy. The doctor kept up his attendance for some time, seeing her twenty, forty, and fifty-eight hours following his original visit. "Perhaps in no other disease but puerperal fever would such apparently ultra, bold or rash treatment have been justifiable," he wrote. The regimen reportedly warded off death—in this case the enslaved woman remained alive. A secondhand account sometime later described her as feeble, however.[37]

The favorable outcomes described by Mettauer, Ransom, Harris, and other doctors notwithstanding, many women who contracted puerperal fever did not recover. Harris, who practiced medicine in Augusta County, Virginia, reported an epidemic from the fall of 1850 through the summer of 1851 involving three-fourths of the women who delivered children in this period. Of the thirty-six who were afflicted, seven died and twenty-nine recovered.[38]

As with other forms of illness, doctors complained that a delay in diagnosis contributed to the death toll. E. B. Haskins, of Clarksville, Tennessee, was called to see an enslaved woman with a swollen and painful abdomen. Nothing unusual had occurred during the delivery of her second child, except that she complained of stomach cramps right afterward. Instead of summoning Haskins immediately, however, someone—probably the midwife or her owner—gave her laudanum in an attempt to alleviate her symptoms. Upon arrival the doctor tried bleeding, opium, and poultices all in one day, but her health declined and she died five days after giving birth.[39]

Slaveholders delayed calling a doctor for a variety of reasons:

custom, cost, a location distant from a doctor. Perhaps because childbirth was considered a natural occurrence not requiring medical intervention except on rare occasions, people were especially prone to
trying home remedies before resorting to a physician. Harris considered the custom whereby doctors were called to the childbed only
under unfavorable circumstances especially egregious with regard to
childbed fever. In the absence of early symptoms, the doctor was unlikely to arrive in time to save the woman's life once she contracted
the illness. It was best, he insisted, to have doctors in attendance at
all stages of birth.[40] This degree of attention was unlikely, however,
especially for enslaved women, whose birthing traditions were well
entrenched and entailed little expense to the owner.

Because the disease took many lives—black and white—in the
countryside, rural doctors were keenly interested in developing a
cure. White women in particular appeared to suffer, according to
statistics from Kentucky collected by physicians for 1853. In that
year, forty-three deaths occurred from this cause, thirty-one among
white and twelve among black women. The compiler of the statistics
considered neither the proportion of black and white woman in the
population at large nor the rate at which each group of women contracted the disease. Instead, he merely noted that numerically puerperal fever was more of a problem in the white community than the
black. To modern statisticians the figures are flawed, but for southern
practitioners they reinforced the urgency of solving the problem.[41]

In 1856 J. Boring, professor of obstetrics and diseases of women
and children at the Atlanta Medical College, acknowledged that
"few subjects have excited greater interest in the profession" than
puerperal fever. Although it is impossible to prove Boring's claim,
the record shows that southern medical school students and their
professors considered childbed fever a topic worthy of study. Ten
graduates of the Medical College of South Carolina wrote dissertations on puerperal fever in the 1840s, thirteen in the 1850s. Two of
twenty-six 1851 graduates of the medical college located in Rich-

mond also wrote dissertations on the subject. Of the forty graduates of the Atlanta Medical College in 1856, at least eight wrote dissertations on diseases of women, including one on puerperal fever. In 1856 the *Atlanta Medical and Surgical Journal,* founded by faculty at the Atlanta Medical College, sent physician and editor W. F. Westmoreland to Europe, where he observed and reported the latest in medical techniques for treating a wide range of medical conditions, including puerperal fever.[42]

Childbirth posed a danger not only for mothers but also for infants. Infant mortality ran high among enslaved people, and slaveholders hired doctors periodically to examine infants who were stillborn or who had died shortly after birth. Thus, some doctors who had no role in an infant's delivery arrived in its aftermath to determine the cause of death. They, along with owners, tended to place the blame on poor parenting rather than on the limitations of medicine or the conditions of slavery. Some went so far as to charge mothers with deliberately destroying children. Just as slaveholders worried that midwives would conspire with pregnant women to induce abortion, so they worried that midwives and their female patients would carry out infanticide. The limited evidence supporting the charge suggests that slaveholder fears on this score were unfounded; yet their suspicions led them to enlist physicians to ferret out cases. Once more doctors employed professional expertise to preserve slaveholders' interests in human property.

Infanticide was a chargeable crime, even for a slave. In Georgia magistrates investigated the enslaved woman Lucy, whom they suspected of smothering her newborn and conspiring to conceal the act with the aid of the midwife who attended the birth. Both Lucy and her attendant at first denied the fact of birth. A physician brought in to examine her determined otherwise, and a search of the plantation premises by farmhands soon recovered the decomposing body of a baby. In the face of this compelling evidence, Lucy and her attendant had no real choice but to change their story; they now insisted that the girl had been stillborn. Following the mother's admission of the birth and deceit, the magistrates convicted Lucy of concealment rather than of infanticide. They imprisoned her for eight days and ordered "corporeal punishment to the amount of ninety stripes." These were to be administered over a period of two or three days rather than all at once, presumably so as to avoid inflicting permanent physical damage upon the woman.[43]

Another sensational case of infanticide appeared in the pages of the *Western Journal of Medicine and Surgery*. In 1853 Kentucky physician W. L. Sutton was directed by the Scott County coroner to investigate the death of a newborn black baby found at the house of P. Gillgin, Georgetown. The child had been discovered in the privy. The mother, Susan, denied that she had thrown the infant there or that she had even been pregnant. Matilda, a black woman, testified that she had retrieved the child from the privy and knew that Susan was the mother because she had helped deliver the afterbirth. Susan eventually admitted maternity but maintained that the child had been born "whilst she was sitting on the hole in the privy." For her action, "Susan was committed for further trial; baled [that is, bail was set], and then sent down the river [sold]." An attorney argued that Susan was not guilty of infanticide, but Sutton cited the child's inflated lungs as physical evidence that the baby had been born alive. He also argued that the infant had been injured in a manner that could not be accounted for solely by the fall into the privy. Other, nonphysical evidence included Susan's original denials of pregnancy and of giving birth.[44] Perhaps in this case the mother was guilty of infanticide; however, many whites were all too ready to believe that black women had a tendency to kill their infants through negligence if not deliberate murder. A small number of cases like this one fueled their suspicion.

Members of the owning class interpreted stories of women maintaining secrets about the birth of babies as evidence that enslaved women could not be trusted to care for children or even tell the truth about pregnancy and childbirth. When interviewed in the 1930s by government workers, former slave Tom Mason of Mississippi repeated a story of attempted infanticide that allegedly occurred right after the Civil War. The black mother was said to have thrown the infant into a well to drown, but the baby landed on a crevice of some kind, and its cries attracted a rescuer. Mason in repeating the tale made clear he was not the original source. He had heard the story from white people: "plenty good whitefolks" could corroborate the events, he said.[45] His intention may have been to emphasize the truth of the story by citing believable witnesses. Racist attitudes held by many Americans at the time of the interview attributed greater veracity to white than to black people. In fact many whites continued well past emancipation to believe that black women could not be trusted to tell the truth or to raise their children well.

Fact blended with fiction not just among masters and doctors but also among white women. Their gossip reinforced the idea that black women might in fact go so far as to injure infants deliberately. During the Civil War, Elizabeth Scott Neblett of Texas, for one, repeated rumors of infanticide that had been circulating in her Texas neighborhood. Supposedly two black sisters had given birth to infants fathered by the same man and then hired someone to bury both babies alive. Neblett heard that not only the man and the two mothers would be hung but also "the old woman" who had attended the births. Even as she repeated the story, however, Neblett acknowledged misgivings about its veracity. "A part of this is no doubt false," she wrote.[46]

Rumors of infanticide and even the murder of older black children proliferated generally within the white community. In 1831 a Missouri jury convicted a nineteen-year-old mother of murdering her baby girl by poison and smothering. The verdict was overturned by an appellate court, which found the original indictment to be defective, and the case was never retried. More widely known is the case of Margaret Garner, whose actions were fictionalized in Toni Morrison's novel *Beloved*. Garner in 1856 fled her Kentucky home for freedom with her husband, Robert, their four children, and Robert's mother, Mary. When it became clear that they were about to be captured, Garner turned on her children with a knife and succeeded in decapitating her two-year-old daughter. Northern abolitionists seized on the incident as a means of protesting slavery after Garner made statements that she would rather see her children dead than returned to bondage. Garner herself was sent back into slavery and died of typhoid fever two years later. Considerable publicity attended these events. The experience is nevertheless notable in its singularity. Enslaved mothers did not typically murder their children, Margaret Garner notwithstanding.[47]

Stories of infanticide circulated in the slave quarter as well as in the white community, but the enslaved tellers of such tales reshaped the narratives to suit their different understanding of who was to blame, who had been victimized. The aggrieved party was not the slaveholder at risk for the loss of valuable property or even society bent on justice in the wake of a horrendous crime. Instead the stories circulating among slaves centered on the grieving mother who lost her children through the crime of slavery. Slaveholders and overseers appeared as villains. Former slave Caroline Longacre, born in South Carolina, told of a woman who vowed never to let her owner sell more of her children. He sold three when they were between one and two years old. When her fourth child was about two months old, she poisoned the infant. "I just decided I'm not going to let old Master sell this baby," she reportedly declared.[48]

The possibility of the accidental—not deliberate—death of children through smothering haunted enslaved mothers, who on rare occasions told stories about such events. One story concerned Tabby Abbey, born in Richmond and removed by her owner to the deep

South, who was said to have fallen asleep while nursing her baby and accidentally smothered the child when she rolled over. Far from intending this outcome, she nearly went crazy with grief as a result, according to the black informant who recounted the tale.[49] The circulation of this story may have represented the enslaved community's effort to defend mothers against the charge that they deliberately murdered their children. Slaves treasured sons and daughters and looked for ways to keep families together. The notion that mothers did not have strong bonds to their children was used by whites to excuse the severing of black family ties through sale.

Slaves told other tales of infanticide and murder that taught very different lessons from those of slaveholders and doctors. Parthenia Rollins recalled hearing of a sale in Kentucky in which a slave trader rejected a young woman because she had a baby to tend. Her owner beat the infant to death to facilitate the mother's sale. In the end, the slaveholder gained nothing monetarily, because the woman developed epilepsy and her former owner had to refund her purchase price. According to Rollins, the origins of the disease lay in the grief the woman experienced over the loss of her child.[50]

Former slave Josephine Smith told of a woman who died three weeks after giving birth to a child. She was slated for sale in New Orleans and was marching there as part of a coffle of slaves assembled by a slave trader when she fell in the middle of the road. It was August, when the heat was intense. The drivers of the coffle had allowed the slaves to rest a while in the shade. The woman begged for water, which a passerby provided. But when the coffle resumed its trek south, the woman fell and died. She was buried beside the road. No one knew what happened to the baby, who had been left behind on the previous owner's plantation. Emma Countee Wilson, born in Texas, told of witnessing such a separation in her childhood. A woman whose baby would not stop crying was accompanying a parcel of slaves intended for sale. The overseer of the coffle ordered the woman to rid herself of the child, which was laid by the side of the

road. Traders thought nothing of selling a baby or small child away
from its mother, according to former slave Stephen Williams. They
looked upon it as "taking a little calf away from a cow."[51] The separation of mothers and infants was a special cause for concern among
slaves, because infants did not thrive without a mother's milk in the
days before sterilization of bottles became common.

Doctors told different stories about infant mortality. The parting
of mothers and infants through sale did not command their attention, even though separation put infants at risk. Everyone understood that separation from mother practically ensured the infant's
death unless a wet-nurse stood in for her. Yet doctors took no notice.
Abnormalities at birth, on the other hand, garnered the doctor's attention. Severe disabilities negated the worth of a slave in the eyes of
a slaveholder; owners viewed severely disabled enslaved children as
disappointments if born on their own plantations, as curiosities if
born on the plantation of someone else. Doctors shared in the view
that the children represented a curiosity, but their interests reflected
at least in part a quest for an understanding of nature and its aberrations. Termed "monsters" or "monstrosities" by physicians and members of the larger society, these infants—dead or alive—were put
on public display within the white community. Slaves must have
watched in horror as children were taken from parents, sometimes
to educate, at other times to amuse, medical practitioners and laypeople. They regarded the child not as the result of faulty congenital
development but as a sign requiring cultural interpretation. As discussed earlier, special circumstances of birth frequently signaled a
spiritual gift that had to be managed correctly. Failure to do so could
have negative consequences.[52]

Whereas doctors poked, prodded, discussed, and displayed abnormally developed infants, mothers tried to comfort them for as
long as they lived and grieved when they died. One doctor who attended the birth of a "double-headed monster" in Louisiana took the
infant boy from the enslaved mother soon after he died. He wrote an

account of the events surrounding the baby's birth for a French-language publication before passing the "specimen" to another doctor who drew the infant's picture and wrote a description in English for the *New Orleans Medical News and Hospital Gazette*. For the physicians, the significance of the birth lay in the opportunities it presented for the study of pathology and professional enhancement. The mother viewed the birth quite differently. She comforted her son, who cried at birth (he lived for twenty-six hours), by feeding him at her breast. The inability to observe customary funerary rites related to the baby's passing must have compounded the distress of the mother (as well as of her relatives and friends), who, having lost the infant once through death, now lost the child again through body snatching. There would be no grave to decorate according to custom, no ceremony to mark the journey of the deceased "home."[53]

In this particular birth, their different responses reflected the very different emotional investment of the mother and doctor. The woman experienced the birth—its opportunity to nurture and its tragic ending—as a part of her own life story. The event was not an isolated episode, but one that linked her to other people, an important rite of passage. As a man of science and learning, the doctor discounted the emotional and cultural meaning of the moment for the mother. A difference in status no doubt helps explain the different responses of doctor and mother. As a member of the ruling class, the doctor would have been accustomed to discounting the feelings of slaves. The mother, in turn, did not care about the doctor's reputation or about advancing the knowledge of a medical profession that answered to slave owners rather than to enslaved people.

The birth of a "monster"—an extraordinary phenomenon—catapulted a physician to fame. Such was the case with J. E. Manlove, who attended the birth of Harriet's fifth child. The enslaved Harriet had a premonition that something was wrong from the moment she realized she was pregnant. Manlove at first dismissed her concern as typical of the generalized anxiety experienced by many parturient women. Uncertain as to which part of the infant presented, the doctor inserted his index finger as far as he could, but he could not determine whether he felt fingers or toes. He continued to examine the presenting parts periodically, but the farther the birth advanced, "the greater the doubt and the more impenetrable the darkness that surrounded the case," Manlove later said. At first his inability to determine the infant's position proved a source of embarrassment for the doctor. Only gradually did it dawn on him that the fetus was "one of those freaks of nature which are occasionally met with." By then, the labor had lasted twelve or fifteen hours. Another six hours elapsed before a strong uterine contraction coupled with the doctor's tug produced a "monster, which, so far as I know or believe, is without a parallel in the records of obstetricy," Manlove wrote in 1859.[54]

News about the birth of a severely disabled enslaved child spread through private conversation and correspondence as well as through medical journals, meetings of medical societies, and public display. Since there were no precautionary measures that could protect against birth defects, its circulation served only to heighten fears among expectant mothers, including white women. Slave mistress and physician's wife Tryphena Blanche Holder Fox in 1861 wrote to her northern mother about the birth of such an enslaved child in her husband's medical practice. The woman "after a terrible ordeal gave birth to a child without any brains or top to its head. It only breathed a few times." Fox confessed that the event had aroused fears about her own impending motherhood.[55]

In their explanations of physical abnormalities physicians tended to fall back on nature or the idea that a mother's experiences during pregnancy marked the child. In this sense, a disability represented a more severe type of mother's mark than those discussed previously. A doctor known in the record only as Perry attended a Tennessee slave woman in labor who gave birth in her cabin to a child described as having the characteristics of a human and of an elephant. The infant died, and fellow physician J. W. B. Garrett assisted with an autopsy. Perry preserved "the skull, heart, end of the nose, with some other parts," which he planned to give "to some medical institution." The mother's labor had not been difficult. She had previously given birth to several children, who were not malformed. Garrett gave this account of what had gone wrong: "During the first stages of her pregnancy . . . she had been much frightened by seeing for the first time, and very unexpectedly, an elephant belonging to a traveling menagerie, which was passing through the country. I leave it to you, sirs, who are better able to decide than myself, to account for this singular malformation. There is only one way in which I can do so; and this is in the inexplicable sympathy said to exist between a mother [and] foetus."[56]

Such explanations for severe malformations were by no means limited to those of black babies. Shortly after the Civil War, J. K. Hamilton, of Stone Mountain, Georgia, described the "peculiarities" of a stillborn white child encountered in his medical practice who, among other abnormalities, had the umbilical cord attached to its head and a stump for an arm. Knowing that the father had served in the late war and lost an arm through amputation, Hamilton speculated that the deformity might have originated in "maternal imagination" if not caused by the infant's changing position at a crucial point in development or by a "defect in the germ."[57]

E. C. Moyer had no explanation other than "spontaneous generation" for what he witnessed. Slaveholder Steven Harvey called Moyer to examine an infant slave girl in 1842. The baby had been born with an enlarged abdomen. She survived, but now at age two she had caught an inflammatory fever that was making the rounds of the slave quarter. According to the master and mistress, an opening had occurred in the child's abdomen, which had grown larger with the fever. Offensive matter drained from it, including locks of hair. The child appeared emaciated and suffered from diarrhea.[58]

Doctors' interest in disabled children reflected a genuine desire to understand complications of childbirth. All physicians—not merely those practicing in the South—took a special interest in "monsters," especially conjoined twins. The *Boston Medical and Surgical Journal* noted in 1855 that doctors in Georgia possessed a corpse of slave children joined together at birth. A country doctor from Cass County, Texas, wrote to the editor of the *Nashville Journal of Medicine and Surgery* about delivering a case of conjoined twins, the children of Liz, a slave of mixed race. He hoped to hear from other doctors of similar experiences. *The Stethoscope* carried news of stillborn Canadian conjoined girls, which the editor had picked up from *Nelson's American Lancet*. Exhibition of the most famous of the twins—the so-called Siamese twins born of Chinese parents in 1811—occurred in cities ranging from Quebec to London to Boston, and reports of them circulated in Canadian, European, and U.S. medical journals.[59] Doctors used the pages of southern medical journals to report the cases and to elicit discussion about their cause. Their interest forced enslaved parents to worry about the public display of living children as well as dead ones.

Slaveholders sometimes took it upon themselves to showcase live slave children whose development in utero had resulted in unusual features. The editor of a New Orleans medical journal in 1858 boasted that the city presented numerous opportunities for viewing such "monstrosities." These included Milly and Christina, born into slavery and described by the editor as about six years old, black, bright, active, and joined through the fusion of their sacral bones.[60] The popularity of their exhibition is evidence that the public at large shared with doctors a callous disregard for the sensibilities of black parents and children; or perhaps it is more accurate to state that doctors shared the cultural assumptions of the dominant white class, which failed to empathize with black parents or children when infants suffered severe disabilities.

The North Carolina twins were on exhibit for years. In 1852

their owner displayed them in Richmond. At that time they were accompanied by their mother, described by a doctor who saw her as "a
very stout negress, aged 31 or 32, very fat and of large frame and
pelvis." P. Claiborne Gooch, physician and editor of *The Stethoscope
and Virginia Medical Gazette*, explained to readers of the journal that
the twins were the result of her third pregnancy. Gooch had obtained permission from the white woman who owned the slaves to
interrogate the mother and examine the babies. The mother described her labor as "usual, brief, and easy."[61]

Gooch's examination of the children found them healthy and
lively. One child was larger than the other, he observed. Between
them, they had only one anus, but Gooch suspected that it bifur-
cated only half an inch from the opening. The mother reported that
both girls strained whenever one had a bowel movement. Each girl
had a clitoris, but Gooch believed there was only one vagina, despite
the assertion of another Virginia doctor, Professor C. P. Johnson,
who claimed to have discovered two. Gooch urged all doctors near
Richmond to conduct an examination of the twins and expressed
hope that the babies would live and learn to sit and walk. "A most
curious example of nature's freaks," the girls would "afford illus-
trations of physiological laws which are as yet unknown, or at least
unsettled."[62]

Although the owner of the North Carolina twins allowed Gooch
to gawk, probe, and quiz the girls as he wished, the doctor confined
his concerns about their welfare to their handling by the mother.
The children were clearly thriving, yet Gooch said she handled the
twins "awkwardly, and seems to have little idea of managing them."
To breastfeed them, the mother had to lie first on one side and then
the other.[63] He never questioned the wisdom of the slaveholder's
public display of the girls for profit.

Doctors termed such examinations important to the advancement of medical science. The editor of the *New Orleans Medical
News and Hospital Gazette*, a physician, was frustrated when in 1858

the owner of Milly and Christina denied him "the privilege of probing or catheterizing" the children to determine if there were two bladders. The editor had conducted an intimate examination that had revealed one anus but separate genitalia and urethra, but apparently the slaveholder drew a clear line beyond which the doctor could not probe.[64] Perhaps the children refused to cooperate or cried at so much handling. By this time they apparently had been separated from their mother, for they were accompanied only by their owner and a black nurse.

In the case of stillborn or short-lived infants, doctors were eager to obtain "specimens"—both those that appeared to have developed normally and those that had not—to add to their personal collections or to round out the anatomical holdings of the region's burgeoning medical schools. Charles A. Hentz, for example, obtained for his personal collection "a foetus of 3 or 4 mos—, enveloped in the unbroken membrane, or *caul*," which he brought home after attending a slave woman who had miscarried. While a student, Hentz received as a present the body of a black baby wrapped in newspaper. Happy to accept, he dissected the infant and placed the heart and other internal organs in the college museum. He much preferred having the infant to the bones of a large black man who had been dissected by his class. Hentz won the man's bones by lottery, as was customary among the medical students. He gave them away, however, because they were too large and difficult to clean. Student Hentz possessed the bodies of other stillborn infants, one of which had been given to him by a professor who hoped he could preserve its heart and head. Although Hentz thought the infant too badly decomposed, he tried to preserve the parts, but without success. By the following January Hentz had acquired the body of yet another infant, which he began to dissect. He hoped "his little subject" would not "be injured by the warmth & moisture of the weather" and regretted that lectures left him little time for this type of work. Despite a busy schedule, he found time that term to prepare two specimens for the school's museum: a gall bladder, presumably of an adult, "& the bladder of an infant showing the umbilical arteries."[65]

So great was physicians' desire for malformed infants that even white parents stood in fear of body snatching. Virginia physician M. Emanual helped deliver a white child in August 1851 whose biological aberration made it difficult for the infant to excrete waste. Consequently, the infant died four days after birth. Immediately following the doctor's initial departure, the parents buried the infant in an undisclosed location to prevent the physician from taking possession of the body. Emanual, in fact, had intended to return for the body. After learning that he would not have access to the "specimen," the doctor used the pages of *The Stethoscope and Virginia Medical Gazette* to lament the difficulty country practitioners encountered in getting "a post mortem examination" and in obtaining "parts for preparations."[66]

Hentz's desire for the bodies of infants and fetuses was not restricted to black ones. While practicing in Cincinnati, he was called to the childbed of an unmarried white cook who had given birth to a boy. She regarded her situation as disgraceful and had somehow managed to conceal her pregnancy. Hentz found the infant dead upon his arrival. Believing he had been summoned on a routine sick call, he was surprised to learn that his expected role was to take the body away. Although Hentz understood that the case was a matter for legal inquiry, he nevertheless accepted the body and "made some very nice dissections and preparations with it." Everyone involved in the matter "thought it was erring on the side of mercy," he wrote later in an effort to justify his action.[67]

A white woman had a say in what happened to her baby, at least relative to black women. When "a case of monstrosity" occurred in New York in 1859, the attending physician "offered large inducements to the parents to allow" the doctor "to preserve this most

remarkable specimen." The offer was of no avail, however, as the
Catholic parents insisted that the infant be buried in consecrated
ground.[68] Enslaved mothers, fathers, extended kin, and friends had
less of a claim to their dead children in the eyes of southern physicians and society generally. Doctors looked to the slaveholder for
permission to dissect or preserve infants in various stages of development for their own edification and the admiration of colleagues.
When Lucy, Susan, and other black mothers concealed childbirth or
hastily buried infants in a manner similar to the white women described here, they met with little sympathy or understanding from
doctors or slaveholders, who were quick to accuse them of infanticide, rather than of protecting infants from body snatching or insisting on a particular type of burial as occurred with white parents.

Because doctors took pride in acquiring physical specimens, normal or abnormal, to satisfy individual curiosity and professional enlightenment, a market developed for aborted fetuses and the bodies
of dead infants. The bodies of severely disabled infants were especially prized. Possibly some medical students or practitioners supplemented an income through the procurement, preparation, and
subsequent sale of bodies or body parts. The Philadelphia firm Bullock and Crenshaw published a catalogue that, among other things,
listed the retail value of various anatomical preparations, including
fetal heads and fetal skeletons, worth two and seven dollars respectively. Heads of children "during 1st and 2d dentition" sold for eight
dollars each. An entire fetus "disarticulated, within a Frame" sold
for ten.[69]

Southern doctors who wished to collect their own "curiosities"
rather than to purchase them could order from Bullock and Crenshaw the instruments, jars, and chemicals needed for dissecting and
preserving body parts. A complete dissecting kit, including a case,
cost $3.50. By contrast, surgical instruments for practicing mid-
wifery were relatively expensive. A pair of forceps, a vectis (similar to
a single blade of the forceps and used to speed the passage of the

fetal head during labor), a crotchet, a pair of perforating scissors, and a blunt hook together with a leather case were priced in the same catalogue at $10.00.[70]

Medical schools placed an emphasis on dissection so that doctors could gain familiarity with anatomy. Regulars considered knowledge of the body important in establishing their credentials. They claimed superiority over other practitioners, including midwives, by virtue of their anatomical knowledge. When complications of childbirth arose, doctors presented themselves as educated men of science who knew about fetal development and the female body, as opposed to lay practitioners who relied on superstition and lore.[71]

Dissection proved popular with students throughout the nation, but public opposition made bodies difficult to obtain. The aversion of slaves to dissection was widely remarked upon by physicians, as was the general aversion to dissection found in society at large. As a result bodies were often obtained illicitly. At the Louisville college attended by Hentz, the sexton of the graveyard supplied most of the bodies. After helping to bury cadavers, he clandestinely retrieved them from the cemetery. Sometimes fresh bodies were so scarce that the doctors had to help. Students, too, might assist, as Hentz did on a number of occasions. Other medical schools also obtained cadavers through grave robbing. Black bodies made up a disproportionate number of those stolen.[72]

Medical colleges required bodies not only for dissection but also for their museums. Professors of medicine considered a school's museum important for instructing a new generation of physicians, as well as for the continuing education of doctors already in practice. Medical societies also collected specimens for the continuing enlightenment of members. Black bodies and body parts were publicly displayed more often than white ones. For example, doctors affiliated with the Richmond medical society studied organs removed from blacks five times during the period January 1853–June 1854. During this time they also discussed diseases of whites, but no body parts from these patients were brought to meetings for examination.[73]

Slaves also found autopsies appalling, as did members of society at large. When an "epidemic" of puerperal fever struck one Virginia community and seven women died, doctors applied for permission to perform postmortem examinations. They gained access to only one corpse. The opposition of slaves to autopsies was widely known and well documented, so much so that owners often denied permission for their performance for fear of arousing resentment and possible trouble among their slaves. Objections from slaves stemmed in part from the importance they attached to caring for the body after death and the fear that physicians would abscond with bodies or body parts. Slaves also considered the goals of autopsies and the questions asked by doctors in performing them irrelevant to their interests. Autopsies were performed to further medical knowledge, satisfy curiosity, and settle legal disputes between owners. In 1844 a slave woman about to give birth was sold as "sound." Three days later she lay dead. What had caused the death? An autopsy was performed to determine whether a preexisting condition was the cause and whether the buyer or seller "ought . . . to be the loser," a question not likely to be of interest to the woman's family and friends.[74]

Slaves did not oppose all autopsies but rather held their own ideas of how and why to conduct them. After the enslaved Grace was buried, questions arose about the cause of death. The doctor said she had died from uterine hemorrhage, but some of her friends believed that she was about three months pregnant and had been poisoned. The body was disinterred and an autopsy performed. Doctors concluded that Grace had not been poisoned. Indeed, she was not even pregnant but rather had died of uterine cancer.[75]

Slaves carried out their own style of postmortem examination in which they explored questions about social relations and the conditions of enslavement. Rachel Conrad's infants were killed by conjure when a woman (the children's Aunt Sarah) grew jealous of the favoritism shown the children by the mistress. After the baby brothers died, an autopsy by slaves reportedly revealed the presence of frogs in each of the children, said to have been implanted by the aunt and the cause of the children's demise. Former slave Hattie Austin, born in Georgia but living in Texas at the time of her statement following the Civil War, described an autopsy performed on her owner's plantation that proved, she said, that slaves were poorly fed.[76]

Slave questions about the cause of death resembled those asked about the cause of disease: the status of the body was to be understood as part of an unfolding story concerning social relations past, present, and future. In contrast, physicians narrowed their focus in autopsies seemingly to concentrate on physiology, but the questions they asked, even the cases they considered, also reflected the concerns of the planter class or their own sense of what would further medical knowledge. An autopsy performed on a slave boy who died at age sixteen in Henry County, Virginia, reportedly revealed not only the cause of his death but also that "he had been well fed and clothed," according to one of the doctors involved in the proceeding—a finding likely to elicit skepticism in the slave quarter.[77]

Descriptions of doctors who pickled or paraded malformed children lent credence to charges of infanticide directed against slaveholders and doctors by slaves. Most doctors who collected specimens of severely disabled children were careful to note that the child had been stillborn or had lived only a short time. Hentz described the infant he had received as a gift while a medical student as having been "born dead." But slaves knew that doctors took an interest in dead infants and worried that they would use medical knowledge to kill an infant or hasten its death. Former slave Ellen Betts recalled that when a slave woman in Louisiana gave birth to a baby with two faces, the doctor first purchased the infant from the slaveholder, then killed it and pickled "it in a jar of brandy." Catherine Brown, who had lived in slavery, believed that slave stealers would murder blacks to sell the bodies for dissection. Former slave Drucilla Martin maintained in later years that enslaved women who gave birth in the field or on the road were forced to leave certain infants to starve or be eaten by hogs. William Yager of Virginia was left for dead after his mother died during childbirth. No one thought the sickly infant would survive. Abandoned under a tree—with the knowledge of the attending physician, according to Yager's testimony—he surprised everyone by thriving.[78] Some of the children who ended up in whole or in part on the dissecting tables and museum shelves of medical schools were the remains of miscarried, stillborn, or sickly infants whose enslaved parents were left to mourn them without a ritual burial.

Slaves blamed the failure of infants to thrive or survive on inadequate time for baby care. Lou Williams, speaking after her enslavement in Texas had ended, told of sick babies who had to accompany mothers to work. The women would carry them to the fields in baskets, lay them under the cotton stalks, and tend to them as best they could. "Lawd, Lawd, honey!" Williams lamented; those were "awful times."[79]

Allowances of inadequate time for breastfeeding evoked impassioned words from former slaves. Denied the opportunity to feed infants as often as they liked during slavery, some mothers tried to sneak away from work to give a child an additional feeding. If caught, they were punished. A Texas woman was whipped for coming from the field without permission to nurse her infant. A Tennessee mother was more fortunate. When she was discovered in the quarter with her infant, her mistress only threatened punishment should she try to do the same again. On Barrow's Louisiana plantation, the enslaved Candis apparently wanted to breastfeed her infant more often than the master allowed. By his own admission, he stopped her four times in one day from attempting to leave the field for this purpose. Peggy Perry described a heart-wrenching situation in which she was unable to suckle her newborn infant. The overseer would approach her in the field to tell her when it was time to return to her cabin to breastfeed. She was allowed only fifteen minutes— not enough time to walk there, nurse the baby, and walk back. In despair, the new mother would leave the field, sit alone, and pray that the infant would soon die and end her misery as well as his.[80] Fugitive slave William Wells Brown expressed in a poem the anguish of mothers who feared that work regimens would deprive their infants of needed nourishment:

> The morn was chill—I spoke no word,
> —But feared my babe might die,
> And heard all day, or thought I heard,
> —My little baby cry.
>
> At noon, oh, how I ran and took
> —My baby to my breast!
> I lingered—and the long lash broke
> —My sleeping infant's rest.[81]

The fear expressed in the poem that infants suffered for the mother's work regimen was common among mothers if not doctors.

———

In the eyes of physicians, complications after birth in the slave quarter largely entailed physiological processes requiring professional skills. The services they provided slaveholders ranged from treatment for such occurrences as retained placenta and puerperal fever to certification that enslaved mothers—not slaveholders—were responsible for the high rates of infant mortality that characterized the slave population. They attempted to further medical knowledge of human reproduction and to enhance professional reputations through empirical practice (even as they remained reluctant to give up the standard invasive measures characteristic of medicine) and through the study of human development, especially its idiosyncrasies.

Enslaved people defined complications of childbirth more broadly than either physicians or slaveholders. Apprehensive about the ability of women and infants to survive childbirth, slaves wanted help, physically and spiritually, to protect and care for mothers through pregnancy, childbirth, and the postpartum period. Slaves wanted time to recover and to care for their children. When infants did not thrive, they sought to observe funerary rituals and to express grief in accordance with the conventions of the slave quarter. They were skeptical of the ability and willingness of the slaveholder's medicine man to help them. He not only shared the slave owner's biases but also posed a risk of his own.

7

Gynecological Surgery

MARY, A BLACK WOMAN BORN IN LOUISA COUNTY, VIRGINIA, WAS about age thirty when she was purchased by a slave trader who hoped to make a profit upon her resale. Before he could collect a coffle of slaves and start for the lower South, however, Mary began hemorrhaging. The trader arranged for her to be treated by a local retired physician, and she seemed fine for a time. Soon after her sale to a Mississippi planter, she began trickling urine through her vagina, evidence of a vesico-vaginal fistula (a tear in the wall between the bladder and vagina). An examination revealed that the Virginia doctor had inserted a gourd into her vagina to stem the flow of blood and facilitate her sale. Mary underwent at least six surgeries in an attempt to repair the fissure caused by the gourd. Finally New Orleans physician D. Warren Brickell pronounced her cured in 1859. He minced no words in criticizing the medical care she had received previously. It amounted to "flagrant abuse of her by one who claims to be a medical man."[1]

By the late 1850s doctors were treating surgically certain gynecological disorders of enslaved women. The operations were novel and often of uncertain worth. Enslaved women who participated in early experimental treatments were helped or harmed more or less depending on the procedure's state of development, the skill and scruples of the surgeon, his definition of what constituted "normal" and "abnormal" vaginal organs, as well as his definition of "cure." The

patient had little to say in the matter. Instead, slaveholders and surgeons decided which women were the best candidates for surgical
procedures. By 1849 Alabama physician J. Marion Sims had developed an operation for the repair of vesico-vaginal fistula, and the
search was under way for a means of correcting other problems
termed "disordered organs of generation." Although all women ultimately would benefit from surgical advances, the goal for slaves was
more immediate: to correct any aberrations that impeded a woman
in performing reproductive and productive labor. The most ambitious and innovative of surgeons hoped to pioneer cures for "diseases
of women" that would earn fame and fortune as well as eliminate
suffering among all classes by exploring new treatments with captive
patients. However, breakthroughs in maternal care and mortality
beyond surgery to correct obstetric fistula would not come until the
introduction of antisepsis in the 1880s, sulphonamides for the treatment of puerperal fever in the 1930s, and the development in the
1940s of other drugs to contract the uterus following childbirth to
prevent bleeding and reduce infection.

Negative stereotyping of enslaved black women by slaveholders
and southern doctors shaped surgical practice in the antebellum
South and encouraged doctors to use untested or unfamiliar procedures on black women rather than white, enslaved women rather
than free. This approach in the end fostered a certain recklessness
that did not make for responsible medicine. The common assumption was that black enslaved women existed for the benefit of a white
ruling class. Doctors were concerned for their patients, but their
concern was constrained by their support for slavery and their belief
that a black woman's destiny was to serve her owner. E. R. Mordecai,
M.D., of Mobile, summarized this principle succinctly when he described the outcome of an operation he performed upon sixteen-
year-old Sally to repair a tear resulting from childbirth: she "became
a useful servant, led a comfortable existence," and once again became
pregnant.[2] Thus, surgeons worked with slaveholders to maintain the

economic definition and worth of black women in the South, a strategy that made southern medicine distinctive.

Medical men were most likely to carry out surgical experimentation on women who were perceived by owners as incapable of contributing to the production and reproduction processes of the plantation. As long as women could work or bear children, owners were reluctant to subject them to operations that held out little hope for cure. But some women appeared unlikely to do either, and these women were at times subject to surgery of uncertain worth. Nathan Bozeman (a pioneering gynecological surgeon who operated in Alabama) tested a surgical technique that eventually brought him a measure of fame on eighteen-year-old Kitty, who had developed a vesico-vaginal fistula following an embryotomy during a difficult labor. Given her condition, she was unlikely to return to field work or to become a mother. She was bedridden for two months following the procedure, which mutilated the fetus in utero to allow its removal. After this period of recovery she spent most of her time sitting on a stool with a hole in the seat—designed so that the urine could drain from her vagina. She was racked by pain.[3] Her owner no doubt calculated that he had little to lose financially by granting Bozeman permission to operate. Doctors who carried out experimental procedures were often willing to absorb the cost of the patient's care.

Slaveholders were interested in correcting "disordered" vaginas in enslaved women. Their reproductive capabilities represented an important asset. The ability of antebellum surgeons to cure gynecological problems was at best inconsistent, but, operating in a different social context from that of the North or Europe, southern surgeons cooperated to ensure that gynecological conditions did not negate a woman's worth to her owner.

In the antebellum era, overwhelming numbers of southern physicians continued to use traditional measures such as bloodletting, blistering, and dosing with powerful medications. Only a small number explored surgery as a corrective for women's reproductive disorders. In the days before anesthesia, surgical experimentation was not easy. Those doctors who did experiment simultaneously maintained faith in more traditional measures. Instead of replacing older therapies, they supplemented them with more invasive and more drastic surgical options.

Black women responded in different ways to the surgeons who sought to right wrongly configured reproductive organs. Some suffered pain from untreated conditions; others endured surgical procedures. The difference reflected their medical condition, the willingness of the slave owner to submit the slave to surgery, the skills and knowledge of the physician, and the patient's inclination to disclose serious medical problems to her owner and cooperate with the owner's physician.

————

Only the boldest of doctors performed surgery, which was regarded as a separate medical specialty in the antebellum era even though some general practitioners engaged in it. Of necessity, surgeons were "strong, fast, forceful," and "relatively inured to the screams and struggles of the patient," who until the 1850s endured operations without anesthetic. Doctor John Bellinger, operating in 1835, had no sooner made an incision to remove an ovarian tumor than he had to halt the operation momentarily; the patient, who "screamed and struggled violently," had to be subdued before he could continue. J. Marion Sims, after achieving fame for his surgical technique, observed that "it required great nerve to be a good surgeon" in the days before anesthesia subdued the patient. The doctor would "gouge and chisel and work away," all the while urging the patient to hang on.[4]

Not until the late antebellum period was anesthesia used with any frequency to facilitate surgical procedures, and even then it was not employed with any consistency. This situation obtained even though opposition to the use of anesthesia for surgery never reached the height of opposition to its use for childbirth. As with childbirth, opinions varied about the role of pain and the effects of chemicals on recovery and the body generally. Chemical anesthetics had been around for many years. Ether had been known since at least the sixteenth century, if not before, and nitrous oxide since 1772. Both had been shown to relieve pain in surgery, and by 1831 chloroform had been discovered to do the same. Nevertheless, physicians hesitated to use anesthesia. One fear was that anesthesia might work not to relieve pain but only to paralyze the patient so as to prevent her from expressing agony. Knowledge that some patients died as a result of anesthesia added to anxiety about its use. Doctors were unsure how much anesthesia to administer, and they were unaccustomed to dosing patients with the large amounts necessary for sedation. Perhaps the administration of ether (introduced for surgery in 1846) or chloroform (introduced for surgery in 1848) would increase hemorrhaging or retard recovery.[5]

When they administered anesthesia, surgeons did not do so solely to ease patient comfort but also for their own ease in operating. It eliminated the problem of the struggling patient; indeed, it made some surgeries possible that otherwise could not have been attempted. W. L. C. Du Hamel acknowledged to the Pathological Society of Washington, D.C., in 1855 that chloroform and ether had been solely responsible for the development of certain difficult and dangerous operations which could not be managed with an active patient. Black women, however, seemed to doctors and other white people more inured to pain than white women. In 1817 the *London Medical and Chirurgical Review* maintained that "negresses will bear cutting with nearly, if not quite, as much impunity as dogs and rabbits."[6] Such thinking encouraged surgeons to subject black women to painful treatment with a lesser degree of concern about pain than they had for white patients.

Enslaved women had their own reasons for avoiding anesthesia. Ether and chloroform were feared by the population at large in part because they were said to give the doctor too much power over an

uconscious patient. Patients often preferred remaining awake because doing so allowed them to monitor medical treatment and
protest erroneous or unreasonable measures as they occurred. Anesthetized patients could be subjected to careless or reckless treatment
at the doctor's will. Even worse, they might be raped or become the
victims of other crimes, including euthanasia. In a telling metaphor,
the Philadelphia-published *Presbyterian* likened "etherization" to
"enslavement."[7] Women whose ability to control their bodies was already circumscribed by enslavement may have welcomed any opportunity to protect themselves from medical abuse, even if it meant
enduring severe pain.

Enslaved women had little choice but to submit to the surgical
procedures recommended by doctors and approved by owners. Con-
ditioned from birth to avoid direct confrontation with whites, they
were ill equipped emotionally or physically to resist overtly, and outright physical resistance was generally ineffective. Two of the women
Bozeman treated for vesico-vaginal fistula fought him fiercely but
unsuccessfully in an effort to prevent the operation.[8] Once an owner
and doctor agreed on a course of action, a slave was hard pressed to
avoid it, particularly if she was in pain or debilitated.

Silence concerning health conditions generally proved a more effective method of avoiding unwanted medical attention. Countless
women pursued this strategy, among them the enslaved Kitty. When
she developed abdominal pain from an unspecified cause, physician
S. B. Robison not only prescribed medication for her but also returned the next day to ensure that she was recovering. He left, apparently satisfied that she was. In fact Kitty was in great pain and
exhibiting a high fever, but she kept the seriousness of her condition
to herself, or at least confided exclusively to healers, family, and
friends within the slave community. Only by chance when he was
called back to the plantation to see a boy living near Kitty did the
doctor subsequently realize that she remained critically ill. Apparently having experienced once the doctor's approach to a cure, Kitty
was determined at all costs to avoid a repetition.[9]

Enslaved women, who sometimes suffered in silence to avoid the owner's medical regimens, devised their own cures for "female complaints," according to former slave William Edwards, a self-described root doctor from Georgia. Edwards declined to say exactly what these complaints and treatments were. He may not have known, since healing of ailments related to reproduction generally fell under the purview of women. But his brief reference suggests that black women treated reproductive problems among themselves even into the twentieth century, when Edwards made his statement. In the 1930s former Texas slave Teshan Young still knew how to treat a variety of illnesses with herbs and other plants she gathered in the woods. These included "Red Shank" boiled into a juice for "female trouble."[10]

Doctors could hardly be expected to treat conditions kept secret from them, and black women largely refrained from discussing gynecological difficulties with doctors or any other white man. Instead they turned to familiar figures: midwives and other women of the slave quarter. Keeping obstetric fistulas private was next to impossible, however. And women who suffered the condition might have welcomed attention from anyone who held out hope for a cure. The condition manifests as urinary and fecal incontinence. The woman suffers not only the obnoxious odor and general discomfort but also social ostracism and the knowledge that she will probably not become pregnant again. The offensive smell repels social contact, limiting opportunities for marriage and childbearing. In addition, the trauma to the pelvic floor inhibits fertility and correlates with a high percentage of stillbirths.[11] Because women were valued highly by slaves and slaveholders precisely because they became mothers, they suffered socially and psychologically as well as physically.

Women healers focused on alleviating the discomfort caused by obstetric fistula. Doctors staked their professional reputations on cure, not palliative care. They hoped for positive outcomes, even in the most desperate cases, and celebrated medical breakthroughs. The greatest cause for celebration stemmed from the development of a surgical repair for vaginal tearing. Both vesico-vaginal fistula (a tear that occurs in the wall separating the vagina and bladder) and recto-vaginal fistula (in which a tear occurs between the vagina and the rectum) were debilitating conditions. When the enslaved Caroline suffered from a recto-vaginal fistula in the early 1840s, no corrective procedure was available. Delphia, who developed a vesico-vaginal fistula later in the decade, was more fortunate. A slave of Robert Howard, an Alabama physician, Delphia gave birth to her second (and what would be her last) child in August 1849 after four days of labor. Childbirth was natural, in the sense that no physician attended the birth, although it was unnatural in that it lasted so long. Normally birth occurs ten to twelve hours after the onset of labor. Her baby was big but healthy. During her prolonged parturition, Delphia developed a tear between her vagina and bladder. Doctor Nathan Bozeman decided to correct her problem using the surgical technique developed earlier that year by J. Marion Sims. At first Delphia could retain fluid for only two or three hours, but within a matter of days her situation improved. The surgery, though still experimental, was successful if painful.[12]

Obstetric fistula often results from obstructed labor. Either the fetal head is too large, or the pelvis is too small or misshapen, or the baby's position is such that it cannot pass through the pelvis. In all cases, contractions push the baby forward into the pelvis through which it cannot pass, causing damage to the soft tissue. The problem is seen more often in very young women than older ones because a woman's pelvis continues to grow until she achieves full physical maturity, although certain older women are at risk as well. It also occurs more frequently among certain ethnic groups, including some in Africa. It is possible that enslaved women of African descent exhibited the condition more frequently than other women in the South. The size of the pelvis varies among women of different ethnicities, and certain African women have been found to have relatively shallow pelvises. If the condition is left to resolve on its own, maternal death sometimes results. Almost always the infant dies and decomposes, finally passing through the pelvis if the woman survives the ordeal. It is impossible to state how often obstetric fistulas from this cause occurred in antebellum slave quarters, but it is clear that the condition exists today in epidemic proportions in sub-Saharan Africa, where modern obstetric services are unavailable to assist in cases of obstructed labor.[13] Most likely it was prevalent in the slave quarter.

A misshapen pelvis can have its origins in poor nutrition as well as other conditions. In severe circumstances, poor nutrition can result in rickets, causing skeletal deformities, including a malformed pelvis. Because their bodies are still growing, teenage girls who become pregnant compete for nutrients with their fetuses. The average age of first birth among slaves was nineteen or twenty, which meant that many enslaved women had children in their teens. As youngsters, slaves frequently spent time locked in dark cabins while mothers worked in the field or completed other chores about the plantation. They were thought to be safer there than roaming about on their own, but in the process they were deprived of sunshine. Not all had access to milk and other foods rich in calcium, phosphorous, and vitamin D that would have prevented rickets. In adulthood, pelvic deformities caused by rickets posed a hindrance to the passage of an infant through the birth canal. Other possible causes of pelvic malformation included diseases other than rickets, congenital anomalies, and fractures or other physical trauma.[14]

An additional source of vaginal tearing was damage to tissue from the use of pessaries (prescribed by doctors to keep a prolapsed uterus in place). A doctor's inexperience or ineptitude with instruments used in delivery—forceps, catheters, and the tools of craniotomy— was yet another. Nationwide, the number of vaginal injuries declined as physicians became more skilled in the use of forceps. Meanwhile women suffered from doctors' awkward attempts to rectify a problem. Caroline, mother of two, suffered from a vesico-vaginal fistula caused specifically "by the use of the perforator" during a craniotomy performed in the delivery of her second child. She submitted to an operation and survived both the original injury and the failed surgery intended to cure it.[15]

Doctors of the day did not always understand or even entertain the relation of women's reproductive health to poor nutrition and poor medical care. They recognized pelvic deformity, however, and understood it and prolonged labor as leading to vaginal tearing. J. Marion Sims described cases of vesico-vaginal fistula that resulted when the cervix did not dilate sufficiently during parturition to allow the passage of the infant's head. Other practitioners attributed cases of vaginal tearing to rigid perineums and distended bladders, which also interfered with the infant's passage.[16] The midwife came in for her share of criticism. Any adverse consequence of childbirth could be and often was attributed to her bungling the birth.

Doctors termed obstetric fistula a physiological defect of nature. Cure—not cause—became the subject of medical inquiry. A woman with a malformed pelvis who could not bring a baby to term was of special concern because she would still have the same pelvis at the next birth. The same was true of a woman whose pelvis was too small to allow the passage of the infant. Physicians employed different means of measurement to determine the size of a "normal" pelvis against which the "abnormal" might be gauged. European women were judged to have the highest rank of pelvis; other women were aberrant by definition. This attitude prevailed despite the widespread belief that European women did not necessarily experience the easiest births. Doctors explained the discrepancy by stating that the size of the baby's head (too large) was the problem in childbirth, not the pelvis.[17] Southern doctors who ignored the problems presented by an enslaved woman's malformed or too-small pelvis put the women and their children at risk, and not incidentally the economic welfare of the slaveholder. Yet until 1849 there was no known treatment other than identifying the problem and inducing labor before the fetus was developed fully, and this approach posed risks of its own in an age when premature babies rarely thrived.

Operating in Alabama, Sims successfully repaired a vesico-vaginal fistula in 1849, and over the next decade the subject excited considerable attention. Doctors could treat the condition without fear of reprisal because patients did not generally die of the condition or the treatment. A branch of the Medical Society of Virginia debated the nature and treatment of vaginal tearing into the night during a summer meeting in 1852, demonstrating both the keen interest evoked by the condition and the possibility of a cure. Less than a decade later an editor for the *Atlanta Medical and Surgical Journal* marveled that "several new methods of operating have been proposed within a few years."[18]

Sims's success in treating vesico-vaginal fistula came after four years of multiple experimental surgeries performed on Anarcha, Betsey, and Lucy, three enslaved women, always without anesthesia. Slaves were an important part of Sims's early medical practice, although unlike many contributors to southern medical journals he usually did not identify his patients as slaves in his writings. He did not merely treat slaves; he also owned them. According to the federal census of 1850, Sims claimed seventeen slaves when he lived in Montgomery, Alabama, twelve of whom were female. Some were patients; others were assistants. At least some of the patients may have been purchased for the express purpose of experimentation.[19]

Sims operated first on Anarcha. She was just seventeen and living on a plantation located only about a mile from Montgomery when birth pains began. After three days of labor with no child to show for it, the attending physician asked Sims to help with the case. Although he had little experience with instruments, Sims offered to deliver the child using forceps. Five days later Anarcha exhibited signs of recto-vaginal fistula, probably the result of prolonged labor due to obstruction but possibly because of Sims's intervention. At the time, many doctors attributed obstetrical tears to inexperienced physicians wielding instruments. The incident did nothing to dampen Sims's enthusiasm for forceps, however. Although he acknowledged that the physician's efforts might be at least partly responsible for tearing, early use of forceps at birth was more likely to prevent than to produce the condition, he maintained.[20]

Sims soon acquired two more patients, Betsey and Lucy, who—like Anarcha—also developed vesico-vaginal fistulas in giving birth. Although Sims knew of no cure for the condition, he took them on as patients and advised local planters to send other enslaved women suffering from vaginal tearing to his Montgomery hospital. He planned to treat them under the watchful eye of local doctors, whom he invited to witness whatever procedures he devised. When operating he used a crude speculum of his own creation. Anarcha underwent thirty surgeries in three and a half years.[21]

By Sims's own admission, Anarcha, Betsey, and Lucy suffered at his hands. When he first attempted an operation upon Lucy, a sponge he was using adhered to her bladder. Sims forcibly pulled it away. The patient's agony was "extreme"; "she was much prostrated, and I thought she was going to die." Lucy required months to recover from the ordeal.[22]

Sims eventually designed a cure. But even as he continued his experiments on Anarcha and other enslaved women, he envisioned a larger clientele. "I thought only of relieving the loveliest of all God's creation of one of the most loathsome maladies that can possible befall poor human nature," he once wrote—language that white men used restrictively to describe women of their own race. The procedure needed to be perfected first, however. He remained for a time in Alabama operating on enslaved women. In 1852, several years after his first successful surgical repair, he moved to New York City, where he achieved fame and fortune for his continuing efforts to correct surgically obstetrical fistula among white women.[23] His achievements eventually catapulted him to the presidency of the American Medical Association and later the American Gynecological Association. Today he is known to many as the "father" of modern gynecology.

Sims's use of black bodies to perfect procedures eventually performed on white women suggests that he did not consider race important physiologically. Women's bodies were the same. It was the sensibilities that in his view separated white from black women. While experimenting on black women, Sims regarded anesthesia as unnecessary. Yet when he began performing the surgery on white women, he found it indispensable. His different treatment of black and white patients may have reflected a belief among physicians (and whites generally) that black women tolerated pain more readily than did white women. Or perhaps free women, having more choice in the decision to undergo surgery, demanded it as a condition of their submitting to the knife.[24]

Black women may have suffered through the operation without outwardly displaying the same degree of discomfort as white women because years of living in the South had taught them to display the demeanor whites demanded of them. Anarcha, according to Sims, "never murmured" a word about his previous failures, even as he placed her "on the operating table for the thirtieth time." Enslaved women learned from childhood to avoid criticism and punishment by playing the part of an agreeable, subordinate servant before members of the owning class. Those women who endured the ordeal—surrounded by the onlookers Sims invited to witness the procedure—would have understood the role Sims wanted them to play. They apparently acted the part of the docile patient to the satisfaction of all present. No anesthesia was deemed necessary. Then, too, they may not have had an option. They were enslaved, and their affliction was both physically agonizing and socially isolating.[25] Sims's medical offices may have been the only place where they were truly welcomed.

Sims later downplayed the importance of enslaved women in the discovery of his cure for vesico-vaginal fistula. He wrote about his enslaved patients in vague language, as if to disguise their role in his early medical research. He also shifted the blame for having experimented upon black women by insisting that the slave cases had been thrust upon him, and he justified his experimentation on black women rather than white by maintaining that they tolerated pain more readily.[26]

Other, lesser-known physicians and surgeons tried to perfect cures for vaginal tearing similar to those of Sims. Both Nathan Bozeman in Alabama and John P. Mettauer in Virginia operated on vesico-vaginal fistulas. Bozeman began as an assistant to Sims in Montgomery, but Mettauer's surgical success predated that of Sims. Like Sims, Mettauer tested his method on at least one slave woman. He published his findings in the 1840s, but his technique never gained for him the degree of fame that Sims achieved.[27]

Bozeman publicly admitted the experimental nature of his work, which represented an attempt to improve upon Sims's technique. In an account written for publication, he described "four successive cases requiring seven operations" in which he applied the button suture—the procedure for which he achieved professional acclaim—to four African American women, all apparently enslaved. In the first case, a woman had developed a vesico-vaginal fistula following the birth of her child. She had been delivered by instrument following forty hours in labor. The unnamed woman "came under" Bozeman's charge shortly afterward. The procedure developed by Sims was tried without success, and the patient's health declined. Bozeman thought it best "to allow her to return home." After regaining her general health, she came under Bozeman's care again. He performed surgery a second time; once again it failed. He was about to give up when the idea of the button suture occurred to him. "I immediately determined to subject the case [woman] to an experimental trial," Bozeman recalled. By the time Bozeman published news of his success, he had performed the operation seven times. He did not expect the medical profession to adopt his technique "without further trial," but rather urged colleagues to employ the procedure to determine whether it had "an indisputable claim to superiority over all other[s]."[28]

Bozeman eventually became a competitor and critic of his former teacher and claimed that the majority of operations Sims performed in the South for vesico-vaginal fistula were unsuccessful. Bozeman told a tale of a young slave of uncertain age whose master sought help from the surgeon in repairing a tear originating in bladder surgery also performed by Sims. Sims's inability to repair the tear had led the master to Bozeman. The younger surgeon also accused Sims of performing ten botched operations on one of Sims's own slaves, whose obstetrical fistula the senior doctor had never been able to repair. By then, Sims had publicly denounced Bozeman for stealing his technique, and Bozeman may have been motivated by the intense rivalry that developed between the two. Sims went so far in his effort to refute Bozeman that he actually operated on white women in the North using Bozeman's "button suture" solely to prove the procedure a failure.[29]

Generally, medical practitioners of the day cited the techniques of both Sims and Bozeman as useful. Most were willing to grant Sims credit for being first in devising a successful treatment, but Bozeman had adherents. An editorial note in the 1856 *Atlanta Medical and Surgical Journal* pronounced Bozeman's "button suture" superior to Sims's "clamp suture." Bozeman's was simple and applicable in most cases, it protected the edges of the tear, it could be used in cases in which there were multiple fistulas, and the same level of exactness was not required in positioning the points.[30]

Bozeman, who remained in the South throughout his career, not only boasted unabashedly of perfecting a cure for the dreadful condition called vesico-vaginal fistula but also of improving fertility in the slave quarter. In 1855 the surgeon discussed Delphia's case as a problem of infertility. Bozeman implied she had not conceived because she had no control over her flow of urine. Dinah, another of

Bozeman's patients, had developed a tear eighteen years before he encountered her. In the interim she had become pregnant "quite a number of times," Bozeman stated. All but one pregnancy ended in miscarriage, however.[31] Bozeman's description of Dinah did not comport with the prevailing idea of women suffering from obstetric fistula. Most women were not expected to become pregnant. Bozeman's account was no doubt meant to emphasize that women such as Dinah would bear children and bring them to term if only the button suture were utilized.

Sims's and Bozeman's successes in treating vesico- and recto-vaginal fistula encouraged imitation, though not necessarily with the same outcome. Robert Battey, of Rome, Georgia, reported his experience with the operation "after the manner of Sims, as modified by Bozeman" to members of the Medical Association of Georgia in 1859. The patient, an enslaved mother of two known only as Caroline in the record, survived the operation, which Battey himself termed unsuccessful. She retained urine when lying or sitting, but "it dribbles when [she is] upon her feet," he admitted. Although the tear was "found in better condition than expected" following the procedure, Battey confessed that to "complete the cure" he would need to perform another operation.[32]

Despite a high incidence of negative outcomes in the early years of the operation's performance, many antebellum doctors came to consider vesico- and recto-vaginal fistula treatable conditions. After suffering from bladder disease for twelve years, a black woman spontaneously discharged a urinary calculus (stone) through the walls of the bladder and vagina, with a vesico-vaginal fistula resulting. Joseph W. Smith, the Virginia physician who attended her, called this event an example of "the great recuperative and conservative powers of nature," which came to her rescue when science failed "to perform her duty." Of course, the woman cured of one condition—the bladder disease—now experienced another, but Smith considered the incident fortunate, since the fistula was "within the pale of a successful operation."[33]

In addition to the cures by Sims and Bozeman, there was one by Parisian M. Nelaton, whose procedure was reported to the readers of the *Atlanta Medical and Surgical Journal*. In 1856 its editor, W. F. Westmoreland, was traveling in France and sending back his observations about medical practice for publication. Nelaton's method— "the figure of eight suture"—was not new, but Westmoreland offered it as an alternative to Sims's and Bozeman's methods in the belief that the more resources available to doctors, the better the chance that they would effect a cure in a particular patient. Westmoreland did not advocate the use of Nelaton's method in all cases, but he thought it might be suited to specific situations. The style of surgery chosen to repair a vaginal tear should be based on the particulars of the case and not on the predilections of the surgeon, Westmoreland believed.[34] Doctors should know how to perform more than one operation for the condition.

Westmoreland described Nelaton's method as follows. Three suture pins with threads attached were inserted, just as in an ordinary wound. "A ligature passed around the pins in the form of a figure 8" brought the edges of the tear together. A catheter collected the urine. After five days, the first pin was removed by tugging on the string; the two other pins remained two more days before being extracted by the same method. Two weeks later the catheter was removed. Apparently Westmoreland considered his brief description clear enough that doctors familiar with the other techniques would have no trouble following his directions. It was not unusual for medical publications to lay out surgical procedures in this manner for others to follow. Indeed, one self-help medical manual insisted that laypersons could perform such complicated procedures as correcting a child's harelip and inserting catheters merely by following written instructions.[35]

Shortly after Westmoreland's article was published in the *Atlanta Medical and Surgical Journal*, yet another method of repairing a vesico-vaginal fistula appeared in its pages. This one, picked up from the *Virginia Medical Journal*, described a method used by one Doctor Bertel. His cure involved pinching and crushing the mucous membrane of the vagina. It had been tried on a fifty-year-old woman (it is unclear whether she was black or white) who had suffered for fourteen years from a tear that developed during "a laborious delivery." Bertel held off in describing the instrument he used. He promised to reveal this later after he made his notes "more presentable and scientific." Other southerners experimented with alternative methods of fixing a vesico-vaginal fistula: both Moritz Schuppert in New Orleans and C. W. Fenner in Memphis practiced on enslaved women.[36]

Debates over the relative value of surgical cures for vesico-vaginal fistula persisted through the 1850s. In the opinion of the *Atlanta Medical and Surgical Journal*, by 1857 Bozeman's button suture was rapidly gaining favor over Sims's procedure. Two years earlier a reader of the *New Orleans Medical News and Hospital Gazette* had defended Sims's approach in a letter to the editor. Sims's method for repairing a recto-vaginal fistula was superior to another that had recently been reported in the journal's pages, the letter writer remarked. It was astonishing that the woman survived the alternative surgery. Most likely she would suffer complications should she become pregnant again. The woman's survival despite the ill-conceived surgery represented a triumph of nature over malpractice, he concluded.[37]

Doctors who treated women for obstetric fistula regularly reported success, but it is not clear that the women in these cases were always cured. Sometimes subsequent pregnancies reopened tears, and repeated operations were often necessary, even after Sims's technique had been judged effective. A subsequent pregnancy could put the patient's life in danger. Sally, a sixteen-year-old slave, was "torn to pieces" when her first child was born. She developed a fistula, which was operated upon using Bozeman's method. The cure was incomplete, however. Another small tear was soon discovered. This, too, was repaired, but anxiety grew as another accouchement drew near. There was a pelvic malformation, and the previous operation had rendered the vagina rigid.[38] Both conditions presaged a prolonged labor.

Although surgeons interested in women's ailments focused most of their attention on the repair of obstetric fistula, other gynecological problems were thought to require corrective surgery. Most of these were attributed to complications of childbirth, but others stemmed from infections or represented medical curiosities, the latter a vague term that encompassed a wide range of congenital birth defects and other physical idiosyncrasies found in all social groups. Doctors performed surgery on enslaved women to correct these specific problems, though none so frequently and successfully as that to correct vaginal tears. The goal was always to repair "disordered" vaginal organs. Alabamian A. G. Mabry tried to correct an occlusion of the vagina. The patient had given birth twelve months earlier. At that time she developed a fever, which the doctor attributed to an inflammation of the womb. Although she appeared to recover from the infection, she suffered intense pain at the return of each menstrual period. After a year of this agony, Mabry was asked to examine her. It was then that the closing of the vagina was discovered. Unable to detect an opening large enough to admit a probe, he commenced treatment by making incisions into the dense, inelastic tissue that connected the walls of the vagina. He introduced bougies (thin cylindrical instruments) to keep the passage open, but "owing to some bad management the incisions healed up," and he found it "necessary to repeat the operation again and again." After several operations a bougie was introduced successfully and kept in place by a bandage, resulting in "a perfect cure."[39] So it seemed to the doctor, although it might not have to the patient.

The enslaved Maria also suffered from a closed vagina resulting in painful menstruation (dysmenorrhea) and presumably stemming from an abortion followed by a "violent inflammation of the mucous membrane of the vagina." The two doctors who examined her in Virginia determined that she required an operation, but they were unsure of their own skills and unwilling to perform it. They advised Maria's master to send her to Baltimore, where she might have the appropriate procedure. Her Virginia master followed their advice, but the Baltimore surgeon did not find her a suitable candidate for the surgery. He sent her home with her vagina still uncorrected.[40] Some doctors evidently knew their limitations and were unwilling to risk surgery where the outcome was doubtful.

When physician Alban S. Payne first saw Clary in Fauquier County, Virginia, he assumed that she was pregnant, but she was later found to be suffering instead from an "inadequate" vagina. Clary was forty years old and had given birth to fifteen children, all still living. Her menses had ceased, and she suffered pains similar to those of a woman in labor. A vaginal exam satisfied Payne that she was not again pregnant, and her medical history—recounted by the patient herself—revealed a miscarriage about nine or ten months earlier. Her period had not returned, and she felt poorly, particularly at the time when menstruation would normally have occurred. The doctor quizzed her about coitus: it was always painful and very unsatisfactory. As for work, she could perform chores except for about four to eight days around the time her menses would normally appear. The pain she felt at this time of month was worse than the pain of childbirth, according to her account. By the time Payne arrived on the scene, she had been treated with laudanum in large doses (which afforded no relief) and purgatives (which made her feel somewhat better).[41]

Realizing the complexity of the case, Payne consulted the doctor who had treated Clary previously. He responded that a miscarriage had occurred about a half an hour after his arrival at her bedside. Because the placenta had not detached on its own, the doctor had inserted his hand in an attempt to remove it. At first there was no more flooding than usual, but about an hour and a half later she began to hemorrhage profusely—a condition the attending doctor attributed to the patient's "own imprudence in turning over abruptly several times." Eventually it ceased following the patient's taking medication and having cold cloths applied to the abdomen.[42]

Payne now discovered that he could insert his finger into Clary's vagina only about one inch. A rectal exam revealed a tumor about the size of a fetus at full term. Another doctor was brought in, and the two doctors decided on immediate surgery as the only hope for relief. The situation, however, proved less desperate than they had feared: the tumor shrank on its own, the patient's suffering diminished, and the doctors proposed putting off the operation until the woman's next menstrual cycle. Nevertheless, fearing the pain of her next period, the patient insisted on going ahead, according to the doctor's account.[43]

The doctors began the operation to release "the accumulated menses of some nine or tenth months"; this measure afforded immediate relief. So rapid was Clary's recovery that it was difficult to convince her to remain in bed for four or five days as the doctors recommended. She suffered from heavy bleeding (menorrhagia) at the next menstrual cycle, but this "readily yielded to the proper remedies." In a subsequent visit Payne measured Clary's vagina. On finding its "length four and a half inches" and its width adequate to admit "the passage of the index finger from its entrance to the os uteri," Payne pronounced it "altogether . . . a very passable vagina."[44] The surgery was a success.

When confronted with a person whose genital organs did not conform to male or female standards, antebellum doctors proposed surgery to define the individual as one sex or the other. In this they were emulating northern and European medical men of the nineteenth century who were classifying such cases as either male or female in an effort to eliminate an ambiguity that they could neither understand nor accept. In Mecklenburg County, Virginia, a slave described as of doubtful sex drew the attention of physician S. H. Harris. Upon examination the doctor declared the unfortunate to be a hermaphrodite (a person in which ovarian and testicular tissue coexist). After making a subsequent exam, colleague William D. Haskins disagreed. Although the slave considered himself to be a man, dressed in men's clothing, described himself as having a penis and erections, and expressed a desire for a sexual relationship with a woman, Haskins declared the individual a woman. From outward trappings, he appeared to be "a woman dressed in man's apparel," Haskins wrote. He was small of stature and had a delicate frame and broad hips. His walk was not the "firm, strong, elastic step of manhood." The slave also exhibited mammary glands, although they were not as well developed as one would expect to see in a mature woman, the doctor opined. Female sex organs were present, and the slave menstruated, but not regularly.[45]

The male sex organs "presented a very curious condition of things," according to Haskins, who dismissed them as inauthentic. The slave appeared to have "a dwarfish penis . . . about an inch long and half an inch in diameter," he wrote, but the appendage might be a clitoris. As for the slave's claim of having erections, "all anatomists have described [the clitoris] as consisting of erectile tissues like those of the penis, and subject to similar orgasms." The slave had been "taught from childhood to look upon himself as a male, [and] now in imitation of others, deports himself as such to the other sex." This was "a case of occlusion of the vagina, accompanied with hypertrophy of the clitoris," Haskins explained. By way of a cure, he proposed an operation, but the slave adamantly refused to cooperate once he learned "that it would entirely change his assumed sex, and make him a woman."[46] Apparently his owner did not insist on the procedure.

In 1851 *The Stethoscope and Virginia Medical Gazette* reported another case of "doubtful sex," which reflected the doctor's interest in genitalia. William M. Broocks, of North Carolina, described a slave known as Martha belonging to a man from Pittsylvania County, Virginia, who presumably gave his consent to Broocks's investigation. The woman had been married for three or four years but had never menstruated; possibly this circumstance explains why the doctor had been called to examine her the previous year. She was assumed at first to be suffering from suppressed menstruation (amenorrhea). The doctor noticed right away an "entire absence of . . . breasts." Suspecting malformation of the genital organs, he examined her "both by the sight and the touch" and confirmed that she had no uterus. She had a vagina, but also a penis with a foreskin. Martha reported "little or no desire for copulation, and did not enjoy it, and it sometimes gave her pain," the doctor reported. Although Broocks did not propose a surgical repair, his reporting of the case illustrates that the medical profession's fascination with pathological conditions extended to unusual or ambiguous sex organs of African Americans. As has been shown in the previous chapter, black slaves, like this woman, were especially vulnerable to doctors' probing, experimental treatment, and public discussion. According to one study, the Virginia medical press in the 1850s more often published accounts of medical curiosities involving sex organs or serious congenital birth defects among blacks than those among whites.[47]

In 1823 a case of doubtful sex surfaced in Virginia that as far as can be determined was never reported in any medical periodical. This involved a "lady," never married, whose condition was revealed at her death at the age of seventy-two. Attending physician William S. Fife described the case in a private correspondence with colleague James Carmichael in the hope that he would share information about the condition; however, Fife mentioned the case to no one else. When it came to ladies or other members of the white community, doctors were expected to keep secrets.[48] When it came to blacks, however, publication of the most intimate case details was permitted. This circumstance made slaves much preferred as patients for experimental procedures; intimate medical knowledge could be shared publicly without fear that the doctor would be criticized or told not to return to the patient's bedside. No white person recognized a slave's right to privacy.

There is no indication that slaves defined as "of doubtful sex" by doctors were under pressure in the slave quarter to alter their sexual identity. The rarity of the condition ensured that it was of no concern to the enslaved community. A similar attitude prevailed among slaveholders. Doctors, however, promoted the idea of surgery to serve their own professional goals much as they did the display and collection of severely disabled children and other of nature's aberrations. They expected to learn from the study of hermaphrodites, correct the condition, and thereby impose their own standard of normality. They no doubt anticipated that a measure of fame and fortune would accrue to the surgeon who devised a cure. Although slaveholders were not interested in promoting surgery to correct genital organs of doubtful sex, they did not oppose physician attempts to right perceived deviations. Both slaveholders and doctors valued regularity and order when it came to women's reproductive organs.

Virtually all societies practice some form of surgery, but slaves in the antebellum era appear to have been an exception, a fact that can be established more by the absence of evidence than through corroborative documentation. Physicians in the antebellum South almost never encountered women whose genital abnormalities resulted from the kind of cutting rituals associated with puberty rites of passage in parts of modern Africa, for example. Those few physicians who encountered evidence of them failed to recognize the practices for what they were, a fact that in itself serves as evidence that ritual cutting was quite rare. Doctor F. E. H. Steger in Alabama consulted with another physician concerning a nineteen-year-old woman whose health appeared good but who was unable to deliver her child vaginally. After examining her female anatomy, Steger was at a loss to explain what he saw, because it did not accord with any medical narrative he had previously encountered. He observed scarring with "no development, whatever, of the labia externa, or mons veneris . . . nor even the slightest trace, or indication, by which we would infer they ever existed." The opening to the vagina appeared more like a "smooth incision" of about one and one-quarter inches. He thought that the woman might have been severely burned as a child or that the anatomy might reflect a congenital deformity. The doctor would have asked the woman's mother for an explanation, but he found that she had died. As an alternative, he presented these and other details to his colleagues, asking them to speculate about the origin of the young woman's abnormal anatomy.[49] As far as can be determined, no response was forthcoming, an indication that other doctors were as unsure about the cause as Steger.

Over the course of his practice physician S. Henry Dickson encountered three cases of "obliteration of the vagina." One involved a ninety-year-old woman born in Africa. Her vagina had only a small opening—sufficient, the doctor said, for inserting a probe. The second was "an old lady" whose condition was similar to that of the first woman. The third was a young married woman; her vaginal problem could be accounted for by "inflammation of the womb and its appendages, after a protracted first labour." The "old lady" also had experienced a severe inflammation following childbirth, which the doctor thought might account for her condition. The African woman's state was inexplicable, however; she "could give no history of the affair at all." The condition had not occasioned the doctor's visit and was discovered by chance when the doctor examined her while treating "a stone in the bladder."[50]

These two cases of possible deliberate cutting notwithstanding, surgical correction of the enslaved woman's vagina was under the purview of white men. The genital surgery suggested by the cases could have been performed in Africa as a means of controlling a woman's sexuality.[51] In the African diaspora, the control of black women's sexuality devolved upon elite white men who exercised power through law and custom. Instead of restricting sexuality, however, the surgical alteration of a woman's "organs of generation" by the slaveholder's doctor was intended to ensure the owner access to the woman's vagina. Through surgery, black women's sexuality might be managed to serve the slaveholder's purpose.

By the late antebellum era, most white Americans North and South believed that blacks were inferior, and certain southern physicians set out to prove that inferiority by pointing to physiological differences in the races. One of the leading proponents of racial difference was Josiah C. Nott of Mobile, who did much to popularize a school of ethnology holding that different geographic zones produced different species of humans. Samuel A. Cartwright, who practiced medicine in the Natchez area, was another leading advocate of this view, the "logic" of which suggested that blacks possessed unique physical characteristics calling for physicians specifically trained in treating their health problems. Nott's and Cartwright's followers considered their findings to be supportive of slavery's continuation and of southern nationalism.[52]

The theories of Nott and Cartwright represented an elaboration of the medical theory of specificity, which held that individuals were best treated by a doctor who knew the idiosyncrasies of the person. Not only was it desirable that the doctor know the patient, but the doctor would preferably be familiar with medicine as practiced in the patient's locality (climate). This is considerably different from the philosophy prevailing in modern medicine, in which the physician might not know the patient but may instead rely on abstract data in deciding treatment. In the South, doctors did not always know individual slaves, but they cited among their credentials for treating them a supposed ability to understand their general character and habits. "Is it not natural that we should better understand the treatment of [blacks]—than should those who have never had anything to do with them?" H. R. Casey inquired rhetorically in the pages of the *Savannah Journal of Medicine*. When a hospital for slaves opened in Charleston in 1860, its proclaimed advantages—as touted in the pages of the *Charleston Medical Journal and Review*—included the opportunity it afforded medical students to study "the personal and race peculiarities of the African, as influenced by our climatic and industrial conditions."[53]

Despite such calls for recognizing racial difference, the majority of southern doctors practiced medicine as if women were anatomically all alike. The therapy appropriate for one patient generally worked for all, with the possible exception of bloodletting. The social status of the patient mattered when it came to such important issues as access to medical care, subjection to experimental treatment or inexperienced doctors, and sensitivity to pain. As one historian of southern medicine has observed, grand theories of difference in racial pathology and physiology were "not useful in a livelihood where usefulness was the touchstone."[54] If this attitude prevailed in medicine generally, it prevailed even more in reproductive medicine, which somehow seemed more grounded in nature than did other fields of study.

Because most women—indeed most females—experienced pregnancy and childbirth, obstetric and gynecological cases seemed close to nature and less influenced by race than other factors. Physician E. M. Pendleton of Sparta, Georgia, maintained that "the general laws of nature" ensured that females of different races and species bore and nurtured offspring. An article first appearing in the *Dublin Quarterly Journal of Medical Science* and reproduced in the *Edinburgh Quarterly* and *The Stethoscope* went so far as to liken the physiological changes that occurred in women during labor to the changes experienced by cows and guinea pigs.[55] When it came to understanding parturition, species was not a significant factor, at least in this doctor's eyes. The equating of female birth experiences across lines of race and class reflected this kind of thinking about physiology. Doctors did not need different medical protocols for women of different status.

The ideas of Cartwright and Nott may not have found wide acceptance by southern doctors, whose patients included slaveholding and enslaved women, but they may have helped call into question the applicability of southern medical findings to people living outside the region. Southern surgeons and physicians who hoped to publicize their findings more broadly in the northern states and Europe were careful to avoid any implication that procedures developed through the treatment of blacks could not be applied to whites. In writing about his success in using button sutures to treat vesico-vaginal fistula, Bozeman gave no indication that a surgeon would need to know the peculiarities of race or personality in order to provide effective treatment. J. Marion Sims, who moved his practice from South to North, took a different approach. He must have worried about the growing school that promoted the idea of difference in medicine for a black and white clientele. He not only avoided any mention of the role played by slaves as research subjects in his first medical experiments, but he also substituted white for black patients in the woodcuts that originally illustrated his articles. He took care to term his triumphal discovery of a cure for vesico-vaginal fistula an honor "for my country." National—not regional—pride had spurred his research efforts, he declared.[56]

Yet Sims's clamp suture had been developed in a society that allowed early trials to occur on captive patients without anesthesia. Sims's Atlantic world colleague, Edinburgh obstetrician James Y. Simpson, relied on Sims's innovations for treating his own patients, but he publicly expressed disdain for the manner in which the American surgeon developed them. Simpson, who pioneered the use of inhaled chloroform in obstetrics, contrasted Sims's experimentation with his own. His own trials, Simpson maintained, had been performed on pigs that had been anesthetized.[57]

Simpson may have been motivated by concern for the plight of slaves in the American South or by concern for human subjects generally. Experimentation on patients was constrained by medical ethics to such an extent that it was known to retard the use of anesthesia by surgeons, who feared charges of medical misconduct. Reckless experimentation would taint not only the reputation of the individual doctor who carried out the procedure but also the entire profession. Medical men like Simpson who practiced outside the South may have considered themselves disadvantaged in discovering new therapies. Slaves seemingly could be subjected to experimental treatment against their will. Surgery often occurred in a cabin in the countryside where supervision was nonexistent; there was no one to exercise oversight, as in a hospital. They may have feared that advances in medicine would come more rapidly in slave societies than in places where ethical constraints retarded experimental practices to protect the patient. But there is no evidence that access to enslaved (as opposed to free) patients assisted southern doctors in developing successful therapies. In fact medical experimentation on unwilling participants has occurred in other places even into modern times, and the antebellum South was generally regarded as lagging behind northern and European practitioners in medical innovation.[58] Indeed, the availability of patients who could not refuse treatment on their own behalf could just as well have had the opposite effect, inserting a degree of recklessness into treatment that made ultimately for second-rate medicine.

Whatever the advantages or disadvantages of an enslaved clientele, many northern doctors shared the southern view about the importance of regional difference in medicine. They were well aware that blacks constituted a large proportion of the typical southern practitioner's clientele and looked down upon the region's country doctors. Southern physicians were marginalized by practitioners in the North and in Europe. Over the course of the antebellum years, a specific southern medical literature emerged, alongside southern schools of medicine, both intended to offer southern medical men an arena in which to develop an approach to medicine uniquely southern. Neither their journals nor their educational institutions achieved the stature within the profession of their northern and European counterparts.[59] Southern doctors found themselves struggling to define their work as important to the advancement of medicine in the field of women's health.

———

Gynecological disorders caused women pain. Antebellum southern surgeons responded by attempting to alleviate misery, and they succeeded in developing techniques for repairing obstetric fistulas. Innovation came as doctors cooperated with slaveholders who wished to restore the worth of enslaved women suffering the condition. But surgeons had their own interests, which went beyond those of the slaveholder. They wanted to advance medicine and looked to enslaved woman as a means of developing and perfecting a range of gynecological treatments to be used on all women. Enslaved women, however, proved an unruly force and had ideas of their own about whether to cooperate and under what conditions. Slaveholders, too, had limits beyond which they were unwilling to make enslaved women available for treatment. Surgeons were able to develop corrective procedures for vesico- and recto-vaginal fistula, but other accomplishments eluded them. Among those conditions still awaiting cure at the end of the antebellum era were ovarian, uterine, and breast cancers.

8

Cancer and Other Tumors

THE ENSLAVED DELPHY, AGE FORTY-FOUR AND THE PROPERTY OF a Louisiana cotton planter, suffered pain in her right side for a month, accompanied by a fever. When she grew unable to work in the field, she was assigned lighter duties in the kitchen, but even those became too difficult over time. At last a doctor was called. The mistress reported the problem as "a wen in her right breast." A tumor had first appeared about a year previously, she said, and iodine (thought to deprive a tumor of nutrition) had been applied to reduce its size. This approach had failed.[1]

The doctor, identified as M. Marsh, determined that the whole breast was involved, as well as the surrounding tissue. He explained to Delphy's mistress that there was little hope for curing cancer. Either the patient would need "to pursue a palliative course or submit to its extirpation with the knife," which at best would bring only "a little respite or temporary relief." Although some antebellum doctors were attempting excision of tumors, the success rate was poor. An operation might give the woman a year or more to live, or it could hasten death, Marsh estimated. His account of the case—the only known source for learning about it—did not mention whether the patient understood her condition or how her cooperation was obtained, but other physicians were consulted who also advised extirpation. On their advice and that of Marsh, the mistress consented to a mastectomy.

The patient, who was tied to a chair with towels and "etherized," survived. She recovered enough that she was able to work in the kitchen, but when she was put in the field to plow, she experienced pain and swelling. Improvement followed her return to cooking. Marsh offered no comment on how long the patient lived following the surgery or on the woman's quality of life.

In the treatment of cancer or other serious illness among slaves, owners expected to be in charge. They not only made the decision to call the doctor and approved the treatment, but they also controlled the information physicians received about the development of disease. Case histories, considered an important diagnostic tool by physicians of the day, were usually collected from the mistress (as in this case), master, or overseer rather than from the patient or members of the patient's family. The way owners and overseers presented the case to the doctor shaped the course of what, if any, treatment the patient received.

The slaveholder had considerable discretion in deciding what to do about cancer. Physicians were unsure of the best course to pursue; no standard protocol existed. Accordingly, owners had wide latitude in suggesting treatment and responding to a doctor's recommendation. A specific action could not guarantee a person's survival, but taking none represented an acknowledgment that the situation was hopeless. Owners accustomed to taking command had difficulty yielding to fate without a fight. Certain treatments held hope for a woman's return to childbearing or other work and for relief of the patient's suffering. The latter consideration was not unimportant to slaveholders, particularly if the inflicted was a favorite slave. Expense was another significant issue. Some measures kept medical expenses to a minimum; others put the slaveholder's finances at risk. Doctors' fees could be high, or a slave's life lost. Faced with the necessity of deciding what to do with an enslaved woman for whom there was no sure cure, owners confronted ethical issues stemming from the inconsistency of claiming humans as property.

The decision of what to do in the face of incurable disease was no less daunting for physicians than for owners. When they recommended a plan of care, they worried about raising false hopes for cure. Slaveholder clients might call them to account if expensive medical treatment did not produce the desired result. On the other hand, they were reluctant to give up on a case solely because no standard protocol existed for treatment. To be sure, the slaveholders' wishes had to be respected, but doctors had their own reasons for wanting to move forward with medical care. Medicine might be furthered generally and a professional reputation secured through the development of a cure, the prolongation of life, or even effective palliative care.

Southern doctors who confronted cancer in slave patients published case histories and paid attention to what was happening with regard to cancer treatment in Europe and the North. Through their actions, they demonstrated a conviction that southerners could play an important part in advancing medical knowledge. That antebellum doctors did not succeed in their quest for a cure is no reason to dismiss their efforts as unimportant. In attempting to manage cancer in the slave quarter, southern physicians explored ethical questions in a manner that marked the increased professionalization of medicine throughout the nation. They were not modern men. The principled issues that doctors examined did not include the enslavement of people. Practicing within a slave society, they did not question the right of slaveholders to do as they wished with human chattels in life or in death. Southern doctors did, however, confront other ethical issues embodied in the treatment of cancer, and in doing so they demonstrated a desire to act out of their own interests and not merely those of slaveholders. When doctors teamed up with owners in an attempt to take command of cancer in the slave quarter, both parties had their own motives. Meanwhile slaves did the best they could to ease the end of life for terminally ill patients using time-honored methods.

Sick and in pain, cancer sufferers sought amelioration of symptoms from healers in the quarter, but they were also susceptible to claims by doctors that they could cure the disease. Some kept their condition hidden to avoid surgery and other doctoring, but others submitted to surgery as well as to other less invasive treatment. Enslaved women were most likely to cooperate with their owner's physician when the situation was dire.

––––––––

Many deemed the relationship between doctor and patient crucial to effective diagnosis and treatment. Patients were to defer to the medical authority of the doctor, but the doctor (according to the doctrine of specificity, which prevailed at the time) was expected to cultivate an intimate relationship with the afflicted person in order to tailor treatment to the latter's specific attributes.[2] The taking of a case history helped the doctor understand the patient. Yet when the patients were enslaved, owners insisted that only they could identify a problem, define it for the doctor, and approve a plan of care. Doctors did not come to know individual patients so much as to know their particular owners. Stereotyping of patients by race, class, and gender often came to stand in for a genuine knowledge of a patient's individual attributes, and the owner's desired outcome came to substitute for a genuine cure. Doctors could and usually did insist on a physical examination of the patient, which allowed them to make their own judgment about the patient's condition, but in the days before technology allowed diagnosis of patients through laboratory tests and X rays, the doctor could hardly come up with a diagnosis or treatment plan that ignored the slaveholder's assessment of the problem. Delphy's mistress defined the slave's condition in terms of her inability "to perform her duty." The doctor assumed the role of rendering her once again useful to the mistress by treating her malady.

It was the slaveholder who made the decision to go ahead with treatment after the doctor outlined a plan of care. The patient and members of her family had little to say in the matter. They were expected to go along with whatever the doctor and owner determined. Although the mastectomy performed on Delphy was considered by the majority of medical professionals to be rash and ineffective, the choice was made to go forward with it anyway. An insistence on bold action by slaveholders encouraged the practice of heroic surgery in the South. Risktaking to save a life fell in line with southern medical tradition. To declare a remedy "entirely safe, is almost equivalent to saying it is of but little value," one doctor remarked.[3] The comment reflected slaveholders' thinking as much as any doctor's.

The mistress's explanation of Delphy's condition no doubt shaped Marsh's recommendation for a risky procedure. Delphy had reached a point at which she could no longer be of service to her owner. A more cautious approach had been tried already and found wanting from the owner's perspective. Only more drastic action held out promise of recovery. Marsh's description of the hoped-for cure reveals the extent to which he shared the slaveholder's view of the situation: successful surgery would allow her to regain "the ability to render valuable service to her owner." He was not without sympathy for the patient: the procedure promised to relieve her of pain and to prolong her life as well. Presumably the owner hoped for all three outcomes.[4] The problem was that mastectomies rarely succeeded. Cancer was little understood, and surgery for removing it was far from perfected. Operations, no matter what their purpose, posed a risk of their own to the patient. Surgery to remove a cancerous growth might do more harm than good.

Marsh was not the only southern surgeon resorting to implausible treatment in an effort to restore a slave woman's usefulness. Ephraim McDowell, who pioneered the surgical removal of a diseased ovary in 1809, performed his second operation in 1813 upon an enslaved woman at the "earnest solicitation of her master." The Kentucky surgeon considered the woman's condition "hopeless" and surgery contraindicated by the rigidity of the tumor, but a regimen of mercury administered over three or four months left her "still unable to perform her usual duties." McDowell later explained his thinking: "I agreed to experiment" because of the master's entreaty and the woman's "distressful condition." Once his hand entered her abdomen, McDowell feared the extraction "would be instantly fatal; but, by way of experiment, I plunged the scalpel into the diseased part." Miraculously, the woman survived. McDowell's third ovariotomy also occurred on an enslaved woman. She, too, recovered sufficiently, in the doctor's words, to officiate "in the laborious occupation of cook to a large family."[5]

Marsh and McDowell had responded to the owner's concerns about the patient's ability to perform productive labor. But other doctors recommended treatment on the basis of an owner's concern about a woman's reproductive capacity. Virginia physician J. F. Peebles confronted an ovarian tumor in a mature black woman who had menstruated regularly but never conceived. She was of the type that intrigued doctors and slaveholders alike: married without children. The doctor described her as age thirty-eight and married since she was seventeen. The tumor had existed throughout the woman's married life. Peebles hoped to explore the connection of the tumor to the woman's infertility; at least this is what he emphasized in his write-up of the case. Like other doctors, he linked ovarian tumor and sterility and searched for cause and cure. Although the tumor apparently had produced no discomfort for two decades, Peebles devised a treatment plan that involved bleeding. "Active venesection [opening a vein] and the application of leeches over the abdomen" produced "a slight purulent discharge from the vagina," according to the doctor's account. The tumor gradually diminished and by the third month had been reduced to "about the size of a pullet's egg."[6]

Concern about childbirth encouraged John A. Cotter to team up with a colleague to remove two tumors from the vagina of a slave woman belonging to E. H. Stone in Mississippi. She was between seven and eight months pregnant at the time of the operation and subsequently delivered a healthy baby. As evidence of a successful cure, Cotter offered that she went on to bear three or four additional children without further complaint. H. J. Richards of New Orleans operated on a black woman whom he described as about forty-two years old, "married, but never impregnated." After removing a growth on an enslaved woman's cervix, R. L. Scruggs informed colleagues that the forty-eight-year-old mother of twelve children might give birth to yet more. Such cases were known to occur, he added, no doubt anticipating skepticism on the part of his colleagues. Three doctors consulted in the case involving Mary, a Georgia slave who had never conceived although she had been married for years. Mary's other symptom besides infertility—great irregularity in menstruation—suggested to the doctors the presence of a tumor. Renowned southern surgeon Paul F. Eve performed the operation to remove it.[7]

Eve later insisted that the patient wanted him to perform the operation. Mary, he said, agreed to the operation "without persuasion or influence of any kind." Marsh said the same about Delphy. Henry R. Frost, M.D., of Charleston, South Carolina, assured readers of the *Western Journal of Medicine and Surgery* that a slave mother under his care had approved his performing an embryotomy during a long and difficult labor. The purpose of an embryotomy was to dismember a fetus so that it could be removed when natural delivery proved impossible. It resulted in the death of the infant, of course, but it also posed a risk to the mother; hence the doctor's care to stipulate the consent of the mother. But everyone knew that the owner's consent was necessary, not the slave's. Surgeons or other physicians who treated slaves carried out their work, in the words of J. Marion Sims, "whether the patient is willing or not." When W. A. Brown of Georgia received criticism for administering medication thought to have caused abortions in two women, the doctor defended his position as follows: "The owners of the property were apprised of what would probably be the result, but as we regarded it as the least of two evils, the owners consented to its administration."[8]

At no time was consent for medical treatment more important than when doctors encountered cancer. Cancer, of course, affects members of both sexes, but certain malignancies fell into the category of women's diseases. Ovarian, uterine, and breast tumors each drew the attention of southern medical men. Since all were potentially deadly, doctors took particular care to inform slaveholders of the prognosis and to involve them in decisions about treatment.

Eve, Marsh, Frost, and other surgeons emphasized that they gained the express consent of black patients for proposed operations. Alban S. Payne of Virginia noted the enslaved Clary's agreement to a procedure to dissect a rectal tumor that prevented menstruation and caused the patient a lot of pain. William G. Smith, also from Virginia, maintained that the enslaved Maria consented to a caesarean after it was explained to her that both she and her baby would meet "certain death" without the operation. John Bellinger, who in 1835 removed an ovarian tumor from an enslaved woman, reported that she, too, had "fully consented" before the operation began. Aware of the controversial nature of the surgery, Bellinger addressed the issue head on. The woman complained of soreness and pain, and this fact together with the "favorable state of the patient's constitution" outweighed "in our minds" (by which he apparently meant the four or more doctors who examined her) any objections against its removal by operation. Bellinger may have been particularly sensitive on the issue of patient consent. He had performed an unsuccessful operation in 1828, and the procedure performed in 1835, before three doctors and two medical students, nearly came to a halt when the patient strenuously objected in the middle of the operation.[9] Both incidents no doubt encouraged the doctor to stipulate as to the woman's consent when he wrote later about the 1835 case for colleagues.

The outcome from the 1835 operation was positive, but Bellinger performed the procedure on another black woman in 1846 who died five days following the surgery. The patient was experiencing pain and heavy bleeding. The dangers of the operation "were distinctly explained to her, at the same time that she was encouraged to hope that it would be successful," Bellinger wrote. According to his account, she made the decision to go ahead with the operation anyway.[10]

The southern surgeon's insistence that he had obtained the consent of an enslaved patient was a response to sentiment outside the region that surgery could go forward only if the patient legally agreed to the procedure. When it came to treatment that was untested or considered especially risky or unlikely to produce the desired outcome, gaining the consent of the patient was particularly important. Because they worked with enslaved patients who were not legally capable of giving their consent, southern doctors found themselves on the defensive. In expectation that their accounts of medical practice might be publicized outside the region, doctors stipulated that they had gained their patients' consent for treatment within a system that denied its legal necessity. Although most southern medical men who wrote publicly about their cases did so for southern medical journals, nineteenth-century periodicals frequently picked up stories one from another without seeking permission from either the author or the journal in which an article first appeared. Southern doctors no doubt feared that their colleagues in the North and in Europe would be skeptical of a system in which a slave owner substituted his or her consent for that of the patient.

All the same, in discussing surgery performed on black women, the majority of southern doctors did not address the issue of consent except by implication or did so only in vague terms. When physician T. Lipscomb of Tennessee decided to examine a slave woman internally "by the touch" to ascertain the cause of hemorrhaging, he did so, he said, "by consent," without specifying exactly whose consent he had obtained. A New Orleans woman subjected to two successive surgeries to remove an ovarian tumor may have found the "constant hemorrhage and leucorrheal discharge" aggravating enough that she agreed to the surgery on both occasions. H. J. Richards, who performed both operations, simply stated later that "the patient did not complain of pain."[11] His wording, and that of other doctors who maintained that black patients endured surgical procedures quite well, may have been intended to reassure a wide audience (and perhaps themselves) that surgical operations were at least accepted if not welcomed by black women. Their cooperation was offered as evidence of consent.

At times there was an element of truth in physicians' claims to have involved slaves in decisions about medical procedures, particularly surgery. In the days before anesthesia was widely used in operations, doctors considered the cooperation of patients essential to their successful completion. Surgeons dreaded having to halt action in the middle of an operation in order to calm a hysterical patient. In the case of slaves, doctors relied on the authority of owners and their own authority as white men to command cooperation. Slaves were accustomed to adjusting behavior to suit the expectations of members of the owning class; even so, they could find surgery so painful that they became agitated. A struggling slave not only interfered with the surgeon's work but also violated the sacrosanct southern principle that slaves must obey. Moreover, doctors and slave owners discussed surgery as an extension of the owner's benevolence toward slaves. A paternalistic ethos supposedly ensured black men and women access to medical care that was frequently unavailable to poor whites. In return for treatment, the patient was supposed to be obliging and thankful, not frantic and fearful. A patient who resisted medical intervention called into question the equation between medical attention and benevolence. She also raised questions about the ability of the owning class to exercise mastery over slaves in general and black women in particular. In light of this circumstance, doctors could hardly discount entirely the wishes of slaves when it came to surgery. They sought their cooperation to ensure the success of the procedure but also the continuation of the paternalistic drama that was said to characterize the relationship between white men and their black charges.

Excision before the widespread use of anesthesia required great fortitude. No known record exists of an enslaved woman's experience of pain associated with surgical removal of a breast, but a northern white woman had this to say of the operation she endured in 1814: "My suffering was severe beyond expression, my whole being seemed absorbed in pain." Although they consented to the procedure, some free women had to be strapped down because they flailed at and struggled against the surgeon, who was expected to act boldly and swiftly in wielding his knife. A black woman, probably free, was described as "writhing and screaming with all her power" during an operation to remove "the entire mamma, as also an indurated axillary gland." Even after the successful introduction of anesthesia in surgery in 1846, doctors hesitated to put patients under its influence, especially black women, who were believed to endure pain better than white women and who were terrified of losing consciousness. Surgeons did not routinely use anesthesia on all patients until the 1890s.[12] Enslaved patients who endured surgical procedures were the ones whom owners and doctors deemed most likely to cooperate.

Whether patients were fully informed about possible risks and outcomes is a separate issue from that of cooperation. Tumors brought pain, and patients wanted a cure or at least the alleviation of symptoms. Consequently, cancer patients might have been easily swayed by the promise of a cure even when it was far from certain. Most doctors who performed surgery emphasized their successes rather than their failures. Surgeons knew no sure way to restore health. Indeed doctors were divided as to whether cancer could be cured at all. It is not clear that this message was conveyed to surgical candidates, however.

Enslaved women would have been encouraged to cooperate by the knowledge that they could practice their own healing measures alongside those of the doctor, although indigenous methods of cure would have been tried and found wanting. Both slaves and slave-holders expected that home remedies would have been exhausted before the doctor was called to help. These would have included roots, herbs, and, for those who believed in them, supernatural remedies. Cancer was rare enough among the enslaved population that healers would have had little or no experience in identifying specific curative matter and procedures; however, the symptoms would have provided clues as to what substances and spells held promise for relief.

Despite poor outcomes from surgery, southern doctors operated without much fear of reprisal for failure. This state of affairs encouraged them to innovate as long as they obtained the permission of a slave owner. Malpractice suits were rarer in the South than in the North. In both regions, courts tended to excuse a physician for the death of the patient, so long as he had obtained the patient's consent.[13] In the South, physicians were not legally obligated to obtain the consent of the slave, but they did not dare to operate on any slave without an owner's consent. Because slaves made up a major portion of the southern doctor's clientele, acts resulting in the death of a patient did not often end up in court as the subject of litigation.

The *Atlanta Medical and Surgical Journal* in the summer of 1856 weighed in on the issue of patient consent and authority by reproducing the words of a Pennsylvania judge upon the subject. Physicians could not guarantee the result of a treatment, he explained. Instead, they could only promise to exercise "a reasonable degree of skill, such as is ordinarily possessed by a profession generally, and to exercise that skill with reasonable care and diligence." The doctor could not be held responsible for a mistake in judgment. Nurses and other attendants also affected the outcome of the case.[14] In the South, attendants were often black women—midwives, nurses, family, and friends—who frequently came in for criticism by doctors and owners alike either for failing to follow physician orders or for general ineptitude.

The author of the article in the Atlanta periodical, identified as

Judge Minot, expounded on the idea of physicians' as well as patients' rights. If a physician was engaged to perform duties, he should be allowed to do his work without interference from other doctors. Consultants might be called in, a measure that was entirely proper. But the attending physician should not be criticized or discharged except in cases of "manifest gross ignorance, negligence, or moral delinquency." Only a "*bastard* doctor" would take on a client for a trial period and drop that client if the cure was not satisfactorily achieved within a given time. No respectable physician would take on another's client unless the attending physician had given up the case voluntarily. It was not uncommon, however, for patients to be handed from one doctor to another without permission from (and in some cases without even notification to) the attending doctor. All such practices should cease.[15]

The editor of the Atlanta journal pronounced Minot's opinions "common sense." Southern slave society placed a high premium on honor. There was no honor in being second-guessed, criticized, or displaced. Slaveholders understood this notion, and they frequently sought permission from the attending physician before calling for the opinion of another or for a change in treatment. Mary Jeffries' husband, for example, sought the consent of the attending physician, C. W. Ashby, before taking his wife to a second doctor in Flinthill.[16] Delphy's mistress assured Marsh upon his arrival that the previous physician had been a capable practitioner. A doctor frequently requested a consultation with another practitioner before the owner demanded that he do so, particularly in surgical cases, where the chance of something going awry was high. In this way doctors and slaveholders acknowledged a common set of interests and membership in the elite class. Slaveholders supported the physician's claim to professional status, just as doctors upheld the idea of the slaveholder's right to claim human property.

Occasionally a doctor became fascinated with a particular condition and wanted to perform surgery solely to satisfy his own curiosity and to edify his colleagues. Especially for procedures promising no benefit to the slaveholder, physicians found it necessary to win the confidence of a slave before proposing the plan to the owner. William D. Haskins, who hoped to alter the sexual identity of the man he regarded as of doubtful sex, first found it necessary to gain the slave's agreement to an examination. Haskin arranged to meet the slave "by accident," then explained his desire to help the slave, all the while promising him the "strictest secrecy." The unnamed slave agreed to the initial probe, no doubt in the hope of improving his chance for marriage. He feared initiating sexual activity in his current condition and worried that "his deformity would be discovered" by a sexual partner. However, when the slave who had lived his entire life as a man learned that the doctor proposed surgery to make him a woman, he adamantly refused. Apparently the doctor did not pursue the matter with the master, who would have worried about the possible risk posed by the procedure to his bonded property. When it came to terminal illness, slaveholders did not face the same constraints in approving medical procedures. Because the slave would die anyway, an owner might grant permission for a highly risky procedure. Power relationships in the antebellum South hindered free choice among the enslaved. A fine line separated consent and coerced cooperation. Even if patients consented to an operation, it was the slaveholder's wishes that were being carried out.[17]

The same situation did not prevail when doctors sought the consent of white women for surgery, although the issue was still complicated by the patriarchal nature of southern society. As heads of households, masters could give or withhold consent or otherwise oversee the medical treatment of their wives and daughters as well as of their slaves. When C. W. Ashby treated Mary Jeffries for a menstrual problem in Virginia, he informed her husband "that I could not promise her any permanent relief." After Mary heard that a doctor practicing in Flinthill had successfully treated a case similar to her own, it was her husband who went to see the physician to determine whether his remedy would relieve Mary's symptoms. Presumably discussions would go no further if he disliked either the doctor or his approach. Farther north, husbands also expected to approve the gynecological care wives received at the hands of doctors. When Charles A. Hentz practiced medicine in Cincinnati, he managed to build up an obstetric practice by obtaining the consent of Irish stable hands to attend their wives. Nonetheless, surgeons customarily gained the consent of their white female patients as well as of their husbands. "Mrs. H," a Kentucky native, suffered from an ovarian tumor. A written account of the case stressed the woman's participation in the decision to operate: she "was informed of the nature of her disease and of the necessity of an operation for its cure." Understanding the danger of allowing the tumor to remain, "she decided to undergo the operation." A subsequent conversation confirmed that the patient was "very desirous of having the operation."[18]

The participation by free white women in decisions about medical procedures included the right to request treatment, not simply consent to it. Despite the presence of adhesions, which other surgeons considered a contraindication for surgery, James Bolton performed an ovariotomy on a white woman whose tumors were "numerous and extensive." Doctors had tried previously to tap (drain) the tumor, but the patient's condition only worsened. Bolton justified the *"extremely hazardous operation"* on the ground that she was about to die. Under these circumstances, he maintained, "the patient has a right to demand that course which gives the best chance for his life."[19] Enslaved women of course did not have a "right" to treatment by physicians. Their bodies belonged to someone other than themselves. They had no means of requesting a doctor's care on their own behalf. Only the slave owner could command such medical treatment.

The majority of slaves did not live long enough to develop any type of cancer. In an age before antibiotics and routine immunization, most people—regardless of race—tended to die of infectious disease. But all doctors were expected to treat a cancerous condition when it occurred among their patients, slave and free. Even laypeople learned of remedies that might be employed at home. *Domestic Medicine* touted two home cures, which were sandwiched between pages discussing cures for lockjaw and treatments for scalds and burns. One involved applying a substance to the affected body part—a corrosive sublimate—that was considered especially powerful and painful to endure. *Domestic Medicine*'s author, physician John C. Gunn, cautioned that opium or laudanum would be needed to dull the patient's pain. For this reason, he thought that the best remedy in many cases was excision by a physician, but he outlined the treatment nevertheless.[20]

One difficulty for doctors in treating cancer was that they could not with any degree of certainty distinguish between benign and malignant tumors. The situation complicated the search for a cure because some reported successes involved tumors that were nonmalignant. Leading European surgeon Alfred-Armand Velpeau insisted that cancerous tumors of the breast could be identified with the aid of a microscope, but other doctors doubted whether the instrument could be used for this purpose. An 1854 issue of the *New Orleans Medical News and Hospital Gazette* quoted a European authority who maintained that malignant and nonmalignant tumors of the breast could be distinguished by the presence or absence of a discharge from the nipple. Cancerous tumors produced atrophy in the mammary gland, which in turn produced no discharge. Nonmalignant tumors, on the other hand, "are always attended with more or less discharge or oozing."[21] But again without the twentieth-century aid of biopsy, not everyone agreed.

Some benign tumors that resembled cancer were "extirpated by mistake," a circumstance that not only put patients at needless risk but also inflated the number of "successful" operations surgeons were said to have performed. One Kentucky doctor charged that benign breast and testicular tumors in particular were frequently mistaken for malignancies and removed. The phenomenon, he thought, explained the supposed success of renowned European surgeons. Even in cases in which life might appear prolonged, the surgeon had not necessarily cured the patient. Velpeau claimed to have cured many women of the disease through surgical removal of the breast and underlying chest muscles, but his critics charged that the doctor had mistaken benign for malignant tumors. At any rate, the Frenchman kept track of few patients over a period of years, so no one could speak with certainty about the outcome of his cases.[22] Meanwhile, Marsh and other doctors operated on what they thought were malignant tumors and ulcerations that could not otherwise be cured.

The fact that surgeons did not know why cancer developed further obstructed the quest for a cure and the ability to diagnose cancer. Some tumors resulted from an accumulation of fluid; others represented an unyielding growth. By the nineteenth century, physicians had ruled out contagion as a cause. They also recognized that the disease occurred most often in older adults, and some physicians thought that it had a tendency to be genetic in origin. A. G. Grinnan, M.D., of Virginia, for one, called the condition "hereditary in some families." Such observations were of little help to individual practitioners as they confronted patients in practice. A. S. Helmick, of Prince Edward County, Virginia, was called in the fall of 1854 to see an enslaved woman around the age of twenty described as athletic and never sick before in her life. The woman complained of back pain, nausea, and tenderness in the region of her uterus. Other symptoms included constipation, fever, and a rapid pulse. The women's mistress judged her situation so serious that she expected the woman to die. In a desperate effort to save the patient, Helmick tried mercurial purgatives and diuretics, cupping (a form of bleeding), opium, and calomel, along with slippery elm water (made from the bark of the tree) injected into her vagina and rectum. When she failed to improve, he raised "a blister to be constantly kept running, either upon the loins, or over the pubis." Eventually blisters were extended to cover the entire abdomen and the inside of her thighs. Although Helmick—like the woman's mistress—concluded that the patient was dying, he tried not to give up on her. He saw her every day and took over the management of her diet. Finally in desperation he added iodide of iron (a salt made through the evaporation of a mixture of iron filings, distilled water, and iodine) and spirits of turpentine to the treatment regimen. Six months after Helmick first saw the patient, she died. An autopsy revealed massive abdominal adhesions. Still uncertain what had happened, the attending physician described the case for colleagues in the pages of *The Stethoscope*. Could it have been cancer? he asked. "There has been so many different descriptions of cancer given by those writing upon the subject—and so vague, indeed, is the sense in which the term cancer is sometimes applied, that it is quite impossible to recognize the complaint from their descriptions," he remonstrated.[23] Helmick's query exposed a very real problem confronting doctors who hoped to cure cancer.

The problem of diagnosing and treating cancer prompted a search for information outside the South. When *Atlanta Medical and Surgical Journal* editor W. F. Westmoreland traveled to France in the mid-1850s to observe and report the latest in surgical techniques, he penned accounts that among other things focused on ovarian tumors. As was the case with surgery for vesico-vaginal fistula, no one method could suffice for all cases, he thought. Yet the editor and medical professor also questioned the worth of surgery generally for the condition. Whether tumors should be treated with surgery depended in his estimation upon their character with regard to the liquid they contained, their walls, and structure. Some tumors were best left alone, others punctured, still others excised. The decision about which treatment to use was complicated by the fact that the same treatment might produce different results under different circumstances.[24]

Although certain principles held true for tumors in general, doctors considered ovarian, uterine, and breast cancer separate diseases and developed treatment for each independently of the others. Ephraim McDowell performed the first recorded removal of an entire ovary on a white woman in Kentucky in 1809. He used no antisepsis or anesthetic. His next four operations were performed on black women. Three of the women recovered, and one improved temporarily but succumbed when the cancerous tumor grew back. The fifth died shortly after the operation. The second physician to experiment with the removal of an ovary was Yale Professor Nathan Smith, who performed the operation on a white woman from Vermont. Alban G. Smith of Kentucky was the third successful ovariotomist. He operated on Patient, a slave, in 1823.[25] Despite these earlier efforts, interest in ovariotomies waned until the 1840s and remained controversial into the 1870s. The mortality rate associated with them was exceedingly high, in part because of the risk of infection, which only hastened the patient's demise.

Ovarian tumors struck fear into everyone because they could claim a woman's life with seeming rapidity. Because they grew slowly and were difficult to detect, a woman might be near death before their discovery. The practice among slaves and slaveholders of trying home remedies before seeking outside help only added to the problem. Most cancer encountered by doctors in the slave quarter was in an advanced state of development. Doctor Samuel Sexton in June 1838 purchased an enslaved woman about twenty-four years of age who died from a tumor the following year. She appeared to be in good health at the time of purchase, but about three months before her death she was seized with violent pains in the abdomen accompanied by high fever. Her new owner examined her externally and internally, as did Sexton's physician friend, named in the record as Griffith. Neither could determine the character of her problem. Warm embrocations (applications of a liquid such as a liniment, especially by rubbing) appeared to help, and she performed "her usual labors until within two weeks of her death, except for a few days about her menstrual periods," which had been regular. Two days before she died she walked about and appeared to her owner and doctor to be comfortable and convalescing. She grew worse, however, and died twenty-four hours later.[26]

As Sexton's case demonstrates, sometimes ovarian tumors were discovered only through an autopsy. One victim, a Louisiana slave woman around the age of fifty-five and the mother of three children, had never complained of pain, at least to her owner. Her first symptoms were partial memory loss, followed by dementia. At the end, she fell into a complete stupor. The doctor in attendance did not suspect any disease of the reproductive system or cancer of any kind, and the two doctors who performed the postmortem examination were convinced that the cause of death would be located in the brain. The woman's owner, however, requested that the two doctors investigate the abdomen, whether out of curiosity or because he had more knowledge of the case is unknown.[27] Perhaps he knew of home remedies that she had been using at the time of her death. Because autopsies were rarely undertaken in the era, the performance of this one suggests unusual concern about the cause of death.

Uterine disorders were widespread in the antebellum South, but uterine cancer was not. It appeared infrequently, but a uterine tumor, cancerous or not, rendered an enslaved women "unsound" in the eyes of slave owners and traders because it could become "a permanent cause of abortion." The tumor's presence prevented the uterus from expanding during pregnancy. In addition, uterine tumors caused hemorrhaging, which in itself impaired a woman's constitution. One planter described the slave Seraphine as pregnant at the time of her sale, rather than afflicted with a very large tumor as was actually the case.[28] He would have had difficulty finding a buyer otherwise. Not only would her ability to bear children have been questioned, but so would her capability of working in any capacity.

As with ovarian cancer, uterine cancer was difficult to detect, eluding both vaginal and rectal examinations. Tennessee slave Grace appeared to suffer from symptoms of miscarriage at the age of thirty-five. She thought she was pregnant, and a doctor was called to treat her. Within two hours of his arrival, she lay dead. After her death, speculation began about what had caused the hemorrhaging that claimed her life. Was it a miscarriage? Or perhaps kidney problems were to blame. Some people charged that she had been poisoned. An autopsy revealed as the cause of death hemorrhage originating in a cancerous growth on her uterus. A fourteen-year-old Kentucky slave exhibited signs of pregnancy, including enlarged breasts and very dark areola. She in fact had an abdominal tumor. "Most of the Medical Faculty of Nashville University" had examined her by the time the tumor was identified. In fact it was an autopsy that finally confirmed the tumor's presence.[29] The owner who sold Seraphine may have been unscrupulous in presenting her as pregnant or merely wrong in his judgment.

Just as a cancerous tumor might be mistaken for pregnancy, so, too, a woman who appeared to have an abdominal tumor might actually be pregnant. A Louisiana doctor treated an enslaved woman for cancer without good result—the tumor continued to grow. Only when the owner in desperation consulted another physician was her condition correctly diagnosed: the pregnant woman gave birth to twins five months later. Physician James Overton operating in 1818 was surprised to observe irregular movements in the tumor he expected to extricate following an incision into the abdomen of a white woman in Tennessee. Surmising the truth—the woman was pregnant—he quickly closed the incision. Overton, who operated before a large crowd eager to observe the procedure that had heretofore brought him fame, never overcame the mistake. His medical career effectively came to an end.[30] Overton's situation was unusual. Most doctors did not operate in so public a sphere. Those who operated on slaves often did so in cabins without the scrutiny of colleagues. Any consultants on the scene shared in the attending doctor's successes and failures. Nevertheless, a mistake in diagnosis might injure a doctor's reputation. Doctors wanted to be sure that cancer had been diagnosed correctly before operating, but correct diagnosis was not easily accomplished.

The incidence of breast cancer was difficult to document, but doctors believed that it occurred more frequently than uterine or ovarian cancer. John C. Gunn's *Domestic Medicine* considered breast cancer one of the most common manifestations of the disease. Medical textbooks of the day echoed Gunn's claims. Slaveholders were interested in cures because breast complaints were common enough and seriously detracted from the worth of a female slave. J. E. Carson, a slave trader from Augusta County, Virginia, purchased a woman without examining her carefully at the time. He soon asked to renegotiate the price. A more thorough examination had revealed a "bad teet." The woman admitted to a "brest complaint"; a "blister mark on her brest"—a sure sign of medical treatment—confirmed the truth of her statement. She told the trader she had seen a doctor, presumably for a tumor. The trader's response was an attempt to recoup at least part of her purchase price.[31]

When confronted with breast, ovarian, and uterine tumors, doctors tried a variety of means to eliminate them, some bolder than others. The most timid physicians exercised faith in traditional measures intended to reduce the tumor's size. They blistered, bled, dosed, and drained. Physician S. B. Robison of Tennessee ordered "leeches to the tumor" and a dose of oil at night for an enslaved patient who was suffering from an inflammation of the right ovary. He continued to prescribe them along with medicines and poultices for at least one month. D. Warren Brickell, professor of obstetrics at the New Orleans School of Medicine, advocated draining as a treatment for ovarian tumor. In March 1858 he described his procedure, which centered upon extracting pus, applying poultices, and dosing the patient (in this case a free black woman who had sent for the doctor on her own) with narcotics. The patient died, but Brickell did not fault the procedure. Instead he blamed the patient for having waited too late to summon him. A month later Brickell tried the same therapeutic approach on an enslaved woman. She survived, and the doctor attributed the better outcome to treatment begun at an earlier stage of the tumor's development. A doctor known in the record only as Fenner lanced a tumor in the external sex organs of a black woman who had recently given birth. This, along with poultices, afforded her some relief through the oozing of accumulated blood, he reported.[32]

Solutions other than draining generally focused on preventing the tumor's growth. Techniques for achieving this outcome included the application of iodine ointment to the neck of the womb in the case of uterine cancer (which supposedly worked because it deprived the tumor of nutrition). The British medical journal *Lancet* promoted treatment of ovarian cysts with injections of iodine, following the usual tapping (draining). According to the *Lancet* article, reproduced in a Virginia medical journal, only one patient had died from the procedure in Paris, but it was so painful that it had taken the strength of four men to hold down one of the surviving women.[33]

Tumors could be excised as well as drained, although there was some disagreement among doctors about the efficacy of different methods of removing ovarian tumors, spurred by fear of hemorrhage. In the early part of the nineteenth century, gradual detachment through a "sloughing process" following the application of a ligature was favored over the tumor's immediate detachment. The editors of the *New Orleans Medical News and Hospital Gazette* ended up with a "beautiful specimen . . . nicely put up in alcohol" of a uterine tumor removed from a black woman through this method. The physician H. J. Richards intended the "polypus uteri" specimen to serve as evidence of the protocol's success. By 1856, however, the editor of a New Orleans medical journal expressed regret that many physicians clung to this older method of removal. When a tumor was excised through a speedier process, hemorrhaging seldom presented a problem, at least not to the extent of threatening life, the editor maintained. A year earlier, Moses M. Pallen, professor of obstetrics at the St. Louis Medical College, had recommended that all tumors classed as polyps be removed through surgery.[34]

Pallen's advice ran counter to traditional thinking. Surgery generally was considered the treatment of last resort for medical problems. The chances of recovery were low for gynecological surgery, as for other operations. There was danger of shock, hemorrhage, and infection. "Only acute pain, discomfort, and fear" could convince a person to submit to surgery of his or her own free will. Given the state of knowledge concerning oncology, surgery to remove tumors was at best empirical, at times experimental. *Brown, On Surgical Diseases of Women,* published in Philadelphia, laid out the circumstances under which an ovariotomy was justified. These included knowledge that the tumor was increasing in size and the expectation that the tumor would prove fatal. The doctor also had to establish that the tumor was not cancerous, something that was difficult to do. The patient had to be strong enough to withstand the operation, and there could be no adhesions present. Finally, other, less invasive treatments that appeared suitable should have been tried in advance. Individual surgeons modified the criteria in accordance with the facts of a particular case, but everyone considered timing important. One did not operate too soon (before the disease grew imminently fatal) or too late (after the disease had progressed to the point of no hope). An operation performed too late was not only of no use but also "cruel and unwise"; "no humane surgeon would attempt it," in the words of one practitioner.[35] Thus, intuition as well as knowledge factored into a decision to operate.

Most advocates of removal admitted that to be considered operable, a tumor had to be small and easily accessed in addition to fatal. Very large tumors or those located in inaccessible places were unlikely candidates for successful excision. In these cases, doctors did what they could on the basis of instinct and what they had at hand. Some tried to reduce the tumor's size in the hope of rendering it operable. Unfortunately, an increase in the tumor's size during the period when other measures were being tried compounded the problem of its removal. When other measures failed, a doctor might resort to surgery because no other course held hope for recovery. John Bellinger excised a tumor after watching it enlarge over the course of a year.[36]

In the case of cancerous tumors for which there was little hope for recovery, the only options available to the doctor (as well as to the patient) may have been experimentation or resignation to the impending death. Some prominent surgeons had been espousing the former course since the eighteenth century. Excision seemed to be the best path to many nineteenth-century surgeons despite warnings to the contrary. Hentz, who drained the abdominal tumor of the slave known as Frances, joined two colleagues in attempting to remove surgically a small, tumorlike growth (polyps uteri) from the uterus of Polly, another enslaved woman. Her disease had grown worse over time, and the operation apparently was undertaken because of the advanced state of the cancer and the doctors' assessment that the patient would probably die.[37]

Most doctors, however, assessed the individual patient and recommended less drastic treatment when feasible, and even when all else failed, many doctors did not recommend surgery. South Carolinian Charles Witsell "was called" to see an enslaved woman about forty years old who was debilitated from four years of bleeding. Examining her "per vaginam," he found a mass too large for an operation. A friend recommended injecting "perchloride of iron" into the mass, presumably in the hope that this would reduce the size of the tumor enough that surgery could be attempted. Since Witsell "happened to have none of the perchloride of iron in my office," he substituted tincture of iron and water in equal parts. "The injection caused an intense burning, which lasted about twelve hours," the doctor reported. He repeated the procedure two days later, this time doubling the strength of the solution. No pain ensued, but the patient was clearly failing. Hemorrhaging had ceased after the first injection; nevertheless, the woman's condition deteriorated, in the doctor's opinion as a result of her earlier loss of blood. The case took on "such a hopeless appearance, that I left off visiting the patient," Witsell wrote. The overseer told him later that the woman died two weeks later.[38]

Doctors dreaded encountering cancer because such outcomes were all too predictable. The cases did not fit into the heroic narratives they fashioned to explain their work. Witsell, who became so discouraged that he stopped visiting the patient altogether, defended his course of action in print. He advised other doctors "to give the iron by injection a fair trial; the perchloride being preferable to the preparation I used." He put the blame for the patient's demise on her constitution; she would have survived had she been strong enough "to stand repeated injections." Once the tumor had been reduced by means of the injections, it might have been surgically removed.[39]

Physicians who advocated surgery as a cure for cancer in the face of high mortality rates found themselves on the defensive and sometimes in denial concerning the poor outcome of an operation. J. Marion Sims performed surgery to remove a breast on three occasions from 1849 to 1853, although he did not publicly discuss his involvement until 1857. Tennessee physician John Travis observed that operations performed by others to remove a cancerous growth were not always successful. He personally knew of cases in which surgeons removed a cancerous tumor only to have the disease soon return and destroy the patient. But he rejected the idea that cancer could not be cured. In all cases, delay explained the poor outcome, he said. As with all operations performed too late (in the case of breast cancer "after the disease penetrates the ribs, or has reached the inside of the chest"), surgery did not work. Travis asserted that the key to success was early excision, before the cancer spread. In 1836 he claimed to have effected a cure of some years' standing by removing "the right breast of a negro girl, aged 26 years," who had suffered from the condition for twelve months. Her "breast was indurated and knotty" and at times quite painful. Following the plan for removal outlined by the eminent English surgeon Astley Cooper, Travis "made two semi-lunar incisions with the scalpel in the integuments," then carefully removed the whole breast, which weighed eight ounces. "I cut down to the pectoral muscle, and removed every particle of the schurrus," Travis wrote. He then closed the incision. The woman recovered within thirty days. The entire operation had taken one hour and twenty minutes, during which the woman lost one pint of blood.[40]

Doctors did not always acknowledge the recurrence of cancer. The announcement of a successful operation often meant that the patient was alive immediately after the procedure, or a few weeks longer at most. B. W. Avent of Murfreesboro, Tennessee, however, followed an enslaved woman long enough to see that the operation he performed had not produced a cure. In April 1854 he removed the right breast of a slave woman who lived only fourteen months. At first the thirty-five-year-old mother had appeared to be doing well; within a few weeks "she was able to perform the ordinary house labor of a female servant." But a year later a tumor reappeared "in the axilla." Avent lanced and drained it, and planned another operation to remove it. However, the patient died before the second operation could be performed.[41]

Researcher and physician Washington L. Atlee, who in 1852 published "A Table of All the Known Ovariotomies" in the *Transactions of the American Medical Association*, documented 222 operations. Although 146 patients purportedly recovered from the procedure, the other 76 died. Atlee himself claimed to have performed the operation on 18 women, 6 of whom did not survive.[42] Atlee did not explain his statistics clearly. His figures probably refer to patients who survived the immediate surgery or who were still alive shortly after the operation.

Eminent physician E. Randolph Peaslee, who practiced medicine in the North but who maintained an honorary membership in the Louisville Obstetrical Society, also maintained a set of statistics on ovariotomies purporting to show that 117 operations had been performed throughout the country in the first three quarters of 1863, in which 68 patients recovered and 49 died. Peaslee believed that his figures fell short by at least 200 operations, bringing the total number performed to more than 317.[43] Again, the meaning of the statistics for the long-term survival of patients is far from clear. Peaslee no doubt meant to indicate that the number of operations was increasing (it was) and that the success rate was improving (this is less certain).

Peaslee estimated that ovariotomies began to achieve acceptance by doctors only after 1855. Even then city surgeons "opposed it for some years afterward," leaving the procedure under the purview of country doctors. Statistics from northern hospitals indicate that the availability of anesthesia increased the incidence of the operation. Whereas the operation had once been limited to desperate cases to remove life-threatening tumors, after 1846 the number of operations increased, including those clearly of an experimental nature.[44] There is no reason to believe that the situation differed in the South, where a large portion of a doctor's patients would have been enslaved women.

At a meeting of the American Medical Association in 1853, a doctor identified as Yandell of Kentucky gave the following report "on the results of surgical operations for the relief of malignant diseases" in his state. Cancers, "particularly of the mammary glands, have always, with a few rare exceptions, been regarded by practitioners as incurable . . . Nature never cures a disease of the kind; nor can this be effected by any medicine or internal remedies known to the profession." Surgery in cases of "genuine cancer" was almost always followed by relapse, usually within weeks or months of the operation. Nearly all practitioners consequently opposed surgery. It not only failed to work but it "frequently destroys the patient more rapidly than when it is permitted to pursue its own course." Yandell further complained that physicians almost always provided an imperfect account of their surgical cases. For example, "the time and nature of the patient's death" or the "period of relapse" might be distorted or omitted. Although there was a high rate of relapse, most doctors performing excision preferred to operate in the early stages of the tumor's development. Yet there was no guarantee of success even then.[45]

Although Yandell intended to raise the ethical issue posed by doctors who performed surgery despite poor outcomes, his remarks also reveal a real interest on the part of southern doctors in participating in an international effort to identify cancer and its cure. Doctors performed surgery in the manner of their European counterparts and reported their experiences in the pages of medical journals and at medical society meetings. Their behavior mirrored that of physicians in Europe and in the North who sought to enhance the professional status of doctoring. Unfortunately for everyone involved, Yandell's assessment of cancer treatment reflected all too accurately the state of oncology as it existed in the antebellum era.

Surgeons in the South sought to improve knowledge and treatment of cancer and considered terminally ill slaves suitable candidates for experimentation as long as owners acknowledged in advance the possibility that the slave would die or turned over ownership of the slave to the doctor. Under either of these circumstances, doctors considered themselves to have considerable latitude to do as they wished with women's bodies. Believing the patient doomed within a few months to a year, surgeon Paul F. Eve in 1840 decided in consultation with other doctors to perform "a heroic operation" on Mary to remove her entire uterus, a procedure that Eve's former mentor, noted Philadelphia physician Charles D. Meigs, said did not hold out hope for recovery even when performed correctly. Eve's later account of the events surrounding the case emphasized that everyone involved knew the woman had only a slim chance—perhaps one in a hundred—of recovery. As expected, the tumor returned, and Mary died. She lived three months and a week following the procedure.[46]

Doctors like Eve justified surgery in the face of poor outcomes by insisting that it relieved suffering and made death from terminal disease easier. They presented themselves as professionals performing a legitimate procedure of benefit to patients and to the medical profession. J. Mason Warren in 1848 urged the American Medical Association to sanction the surgical removal of a cancerous breast solely as a palliative measure. Physicians published accounts of their cases regardless of the outcome for the edification of their colleagues, and in this way the surgeries—even if unsuccessful—could be said to advance medical knowledge. Surgeons also put diseased body parts on display for observation and study. Mary's uterus ended up in Meigs's medical museum, a curiosity. The uterus from John Bellinger's dead patient was put on display at the museum of the local medical college, along with the tumor removed from his first patient (black) and yet another from a white woman.[47] Marsh cited relief from suffering as a factor in operating on Delphy.

Although it seems unlikely that slaveholders sought surgery upon slaves solely for this purpose, they, too, wanted to alleviate suffering. But whether doctors acknowledged the fact or not, slaveholders who consented to seemingly hopeless operations on enslaved women did so because they hoped to reclaim the worth of a valuable property. They also approved experimental surgery because it promised to result in a remedy for all women, not just the individual slave. Turning over a slave woman for experimentation also relieved the planter of the cost of caring for an unproductive person. When medical men like J. Marion Sims assumed the management of disease among enslaved women like Anarcha, they often agreed to bear the cost of their care. Moreover, slaveholders expected to control all aspects of a slave's life. When a woman contracted a life-threatening disease such as cancer, the decision for an operation was an extension of this control, even to her death. The same might be said for medical men, who shared slaveholders' sense of mastery over patients. Death was to be managed according to the wishes of slaveholders but also in line with prevailing medical principles.

It is difficult to know what enslaved women wanted with regard to tumors, particularly those that were cancerous. Those in pain surely wanted relief. Almost none of hundreds of slaves who spoke about health matters when interviewed by government agents in the 1930s mentioned cancer, however. Given the difficulty of diagnosis, it is likely that some cases of cancer went undetected. Death may have been attributed to other causes. There may have been a reluctance to discuss the matter. Mattie Fritz's mother died soon after the enslaved girl's birth. The explanation given to the daughter was that her mother "died from the change of life," but Fritz suspected that her mother had a cancerous tumor.[48] It is not clear why this cause was not discussed. Perhaps slaves and former slaves shared the general reluctance of modern people to speak of the dreaded disease. Or the incidence of cancer may have been so low among a people who did not live long enough to contract the disease that the subject seldom came up.

Other health problems were of greater importance to former slaves. Issues of consent did emerge in the interviews, however. Time and again, former slaves mentioned that slave owners decided whether a slave's condition warranted a doctor's treatment and not the slave herself. This is not to say that slaves went without treatment when the owner decided against calling a doctor. Slaves had their own healing practices, which did not involve cutting.

Women who suffered from cancer or other tumors reacted differently depending on their degree of pain, their faith in orthodox or traditional methods of healing, and the degree of pressure or subterfuge owners used to coerce them into accepting the ministrations of the regulars. Although some black women no doubt sought physician assistance through owners, others had it forced upon them. Still others went to great lengths to conceal conditions and avoid the slaveholder's intervention. Enslaved women often preferred to keep serious medical conditions to themselves so as to follow their own healing customs. Doctor J. L. Jones discovered for the first time during an autopsy that a slave woman had suffered from ovarian cancer. She had never complained of pain, and the physician who had treated her during her last illness never suspected any disease of the reproductive system. Another slave woman complained a lot about a tumor until doctors were called in to decide on a cure, at which time she insisted she felt much better. Although she continued to menstruate, she said she was pregnant, probably in an attempt to ward off the operation the doctors were contemplating.[49]

Patients' concerns differed from those of owners and physicians. The women would have wanted to live out their days as free from pain and suffering as possible, but most were under no illusion that the slaveholder's doctor could consistently alleviate suffering, let alone ward off impending death. When it came to healing, they could exercise choice to a certain degree: they could turn to spiritual and herbal healers in the quarter rather than or in addition to surgeons. Especially when death seemed likely, slaves wanted to manage events according to their own customs, perhaps to say good-bye to loved ones or to engage in other rituals marking the end of life.

Consent was a troublesome matter for surgeons of the antebellum South, especially so in cases of cancer, for which there was no sure remedy. Acting as part of a larger medical community, they searched for a cure. But northern and European colleagues, who operated in a different social environment, were exploring ethical issues along with cure for disease. For some an enslaved clientele was problematic because slaves could not consent legally to treatment or refuse an owner's decision in favor of it. Certain southern surgeons who cared about their reputations beyond the South handled the matter by stipulating that they gained a slave woman's permission for specific procedures. Others publicly acknowledged the authority of the slaveholder to withhold or arrange for treatment. Still others sought cooperation by both.

Whether they stipulated that they wanted treatment or not, black women found it difficult to have a say in the unfolding of events after the fact of cancer was established by an owner. To maintain control over their own bodies, they might have to suffer in silence. Most women wanted help for debilitating conditions, however. They could fall back on traditional measures intended to ease the end of life, but suffering led some to cooperate with the doctor in the hope that they might be relieved. By the end of the antebellum era, a small number of enslaved women were submitting to treatment by the surgeon at the behest of owners. Too often they bore as burdens not only the pain of disease and surgery but also the coercion that characterized slavery.

9

Freedwomen's Health

W. C. BELLAMY, M.D., OF COLUMBUS, GEORGIA, BEGAN TO EXPER-
iment with the cotton plant in 1866. He had first read of its use to
stimulate contractions in parturient women and to bring on tardy
menstruation in the 1858 U.S. Dispensary, but Bellamy had spurned
its use then in favor of the standard treatment, ergot. The disruption
of the Civil War cut off his supply of ergot, however, and he sought a
substitute for the substance that doctors commonly used to stimulate
contractions and bring on the menses or speed labor. He turned to
cotton root. He used it first to relieve a black woman suffering from
what he termed a case of "tedious labor." She was a patient of another doctor who had called Bellamy for advice. Uncertain of the
plant's effect, Bellamy hesitated to prescribe the full dose specified in
the Dispensary, recommending instead a reduced dosage. Before
leaving the woman's bedside, he asked the attending physician to
keep him informed about her condition. The attending doctor, who
lacked faith in the plant's efficacy, administered Bellamy's recommended dosage before leaving to visit another patient. He was gone
an hour at most, but by the time he returned, the delivery was already complete; "a good-sized, healthy child" had been born "with
very little trouble."[1]

Reflecting on the wartime experiences of southern physicians,
Bellamy noted that other doctors had experimented with folk reme-
dies. The war had cut off the flow of medical supplies from the
North, where many were manufactured or imported. A northern

blockade of southern ports likewise kept exotic plants and their medicinal preparations unavailable. Isolated from the rest of the world,
physicians had to apply "whatever indigenous remedies we might
possess," Bellamy remarked. Innovation continued in the immediate
aftermath of war because access to medical supplies remained a
problem for doctors in the defeated and economically devastated
South. In 1867 Atlanta Medical College professor J. G. Westmoreland observed continued interest in local therapeutic agents. One
positive aspect of the war, he told readers of an Atlanta medical journal, was that the blockade forced doctors to seek new drugs from
nearby fields and forests.[2]

Bellamy used the cotton plant in several other cases of tedious
labor with good results and concluded that it would be effective in
treating menstrual problems (specifically amenorrhea and dysmenorrhea). One case involved a white woman who had not had her period for a year. The treatment produced only a scanty show of blood
the first month, Bellamy said, but thereafter her menses were restored to normal. He tried it on another woman—"a robust, sanguine young widow"—and again it produced the desired result. On
the basis of these experiences, Bellamy was "fully satisfied" that the
cotton plant worked as well as (if not better than) ergot "in promoting the various functions of the uterine organs."

Bellamy pronounced the cotton plant (gossypium) "sure, speedy
and safe . . . not only for difficult, painful, contracted labors, but
also to control all the irregularities of females and to alleviate their
peculiar monthly sufferings." It was powerful enough "to produce
miscarriage, if administered during pregnancy," he observed. His enthusiasm spurred him to begin making arrangements to package his
formula, under the name Tilden's Fluid Extracts, for physicians who
might like to try it. He did not plan to patent the medicine, he said,
because it should be available to everyone. Perhaps Bellamy realized
the futility of attempting to patent a prescription that was well
known throughout the South. No doubt recognizing that others

would prepare the drug for themselves, Bellamy added a helpful tip: the best time to gather the plant was during October and November, when it was mature but uninjured by frost.

By the time Bellamy reported his experiments with cotton root, its origins as a remedy for women's ailments had been obscured. It had long been used within the black community, but the 1858 Dispensary had credited Doctor Bouchelle of Mississippi with discovering the plant's usefulness. Bouchelle previously had freely acknowledged its habitual use by slaves, but when Bellamy reported his experiences in the *Atlanta Medical and Surgical Journal*, he did not mention the role of black women in identifying the curative power of the plant.[3] He was either unaware of or unwilling to admit the importance of black women in establishing the efficacy of this indigenous plant for ensuring women's well-being.

Just as black women's knowledge of healing was absent from the public discourse concerning medicine in the South, so, too, was the part played by black women as patients. The system whereby white men provided medical care to slaves began to collapse during the Civil War. An exodus of physicians from southern plantations occurred as medical men enlisted in the Confederate cause. "One day he went off," a former slave said in reference to her physician-owner; her mother said he had gone to war. Southern medical schools closed their doors because droves of students and faculty alike also enlisted in military service. Southern medical journals suspended publication as sponsoring medical schools shut their doors and editors turned to other pursuits.[4]

Medical practice shifted in emphasis to military needs. Located in Union territory, the University of Louisville's Medical Department closed its doors for the 1862–63 session. When it reopened for the 1863–64 term, its curriculum concentrated on military surgery. The *Atlanta Medical and Surgical Journal* suspended publication in 1861, but not before the war's influence was apparent in its pages. The September issue included articles on the condition of sick and

wounded Confederate troops in Virginia, the treatment of wounds,
and other war matters; the issue contained only one reference to
women's health—a brief originally published in a foreign journal
about a woman who died in an attempt to induce an abortion by taking camphor.[5]

When medical journals resumed publication after the war, case
histories involving African Americans were conspicuously diminished in number. Whereas once their cases had appeared regularly in
the descriptions southern doctors gave of their medical practices,
postwar references to blacks were infrequent either by name or by
race. In some ways, the disappearance of black names was under-
standable given the changing nature of medicine. The journals
themselves reflected a shifting idea of medical therapeutics. Before
the war, southern doctors had clung to the notion that medical treatment had to be adjusted to the individual characteristics of patients.
Now doctors were embracing a new therapeutic concept that universal treatments might be identified through clinical trials. This notion
was reflected in a new style of writing about medical practice that
subsumed the individual patient's experience in the doctor's practice
and emphasized universal, abstract theories of diagnosis and treatment often derived from clinical trials rather than extracted from
one or two cases randomly encountered in a country doctor's practice. But the new style of medical writing cannot explain entirely
why blacks in general received less attention in the postwar period
than in the antebellum era.[6]

Former slaves left largely to fend for themselves in medical matters responded differently depending on their individual assessment
of whether the slaveholder's doctor had helped more than harmed
his black patients. Some who had come to accept the ministrations
of regular doctors felt the loss keenly and looked for ways as freed
people to gain access to the services of doctors. Others were more
sanguine about the situation, particularly with regard to women's
health. Displeased with the way white men had tried to manage

black women's reproductive role in slavery, in freedom they turned to more familiar and trustworthy healers and health practices.

The withdrawal of physicians from the countryside that began during the war continued after the ceasefire. The closure of medical schools during the war limited the number of new doctors trained to replace those who died or retired, so there were fewer practicing physicians. More important and no doubt related, the end of slavery diminished the monetary rewards for doctoring. Medical schools reopened, but medicine appeared to many a less lucrative career than before the conflict, when slaveholders might be counted on to pay the costs of medical care for slaves. As one former slave observed, before the war, white doctors attended black patients at the slaveholder's request, "but not after." When the Georgia Medical College reopened in 1866, it had difficulty recruiting students. S. H. Stout, professor of surgical and pathological anatomy, in an introductory address marking the start of the college's eighth regular summer course of lectures, lamented that many worthy men had abandoned the practice of medicine since the war because "the prospects of pecuniary independence" were gloomy. An editorial in an 1867 issue of the *Atlanta Medical and Surgical Journal* bemoaned the current situation involving former slaves, which "has resulted in great embarrassment and pecuniary loss to the physician."[7]

Increased racial animosity further reduced the number of white physicians willing to see black patients. Those willing to treat freed people risked alienating white clients. In some places, vigilante groups such as the Ku Klux Klan intimidated white doctors who might otherwise have been willing to do so. A federal official stationed in Raleigh went so far as to declare a conspiracy among citizens and physicians to withhold medical care from freed people.[8]

Freed people's lack of funds was an obvious reason cited for the withdrawal of practicing physicians from black communities. Freed people who worked could barely pay for food and clothing, let alone medical attention, and the interest of former slaveholders in the medical care of workers had diminished considerably. The reluctance of many doctors to treat freed women and men placed a heavy burden on those who were willing to visit the former slaves. Medications posed a separate problem. Even if physicians visited gratis, former slaves had difficulty paying for prescriptions, and doctors could not afford to provide them for nothing.[9]

In an annual report issued in 1867, James M. Laing, an official in the Bureau of Refugees, Freedmen, and Abandoned Lands (Freedmen's Bureau), established by the U.S. Congress to aid the transition from slavery to freedom, explained the problem in Georgia. Doctors charged $2.00 for each visit, double for night visits. In addition, they charged $1.00 per mile to travel to the patient. The purchase of medicine further increased the cost: patients could expect to pay $1.00 for a dose of twenty grains of quinine, 25 cents for a small dose of castor oil. Yet freed people received only about $8.00 to $12.00 a month in wages. S. P. Anderson, a teacher at a freedman's school located in Tennessee, registered a similar concern. Doctors' bills were too high for freed people to pay. Charging from $2.50 to $3.00 for one visit, physicians asked whether the former slaves had any money before responding to a request for care.[10]

Wages were indeed too low to cover fees for doctors and medicines. Doctor J. G. Temple of Kentucky estimated that only one-quarter of former slaves could pay for short-term medical care. Long-term medical problems represented even greater financial disaster. Physicians in South Bend, Arkansas, complained of being unable to collect fees from freed people because they had no means of paying. Kentucky freedman Eli Coleman also blamed the impoverishment of the black worker for inadequate medical care in the black community. He knew firsthand its tragic consequence. When Eli's wife, Nora, became ill following the war, he waited until she was "nearly dead" and unable to speak before summoning the doctor. By then it was too late. The two arrived at the cabin only to find that Nora had died.[11]

The practice whereby individuals and families incurred medical expenses on behalf of themselves and family members could leave whole families destitute if the cost of care mounted. The Wells family in Arkansas had only twelve dollars to last them for the coming year after the family's employer deducted medical expenses from its share of the crop. Sarah and her four children had been sick much of the previous year, leaving Sarah's husband in the position of trying to ensure the welfare of his family without her help. Sarah blamed the planter's wife as much as anyone else for the situation. She was mean, the former slave said, because she did not check on Sarah or her children during their sickness. Apparently the young mother expected the practice whereby the mistress monitored the medical needs of slaves to continue after the war and emancipation.[12]

Freed black women, who were poorly reimbursed for their work and who were subject to periodic unemployment because of the demands of childbirth and childcare, were especially hard pressed to afford medical care. Temple observed that women in labor generally could not afford even the fee charged by a midwife. The assistant commissioner of the Freedmen's Bureau for Alabama in 1867 reported the usual wages of freedmen as ten to twelve dollars per month. Freedwomen, in contrast, earned six to ten dollars. And women who worked as domestic servants were particularly vulnerable to the loss of jobs, Temple said. If they became ill, they were immediately let go.[13]

Feeling keenly the loss of income previously available for treating enslaved people, many physicians looked to the federal government to restore the status quo by guaranteeing payment for medical services from former slaveholders now turned employers. After all, the former slaves remained in the South and presumably had the same need for medical care as previously. T. K. Leonard of Florida frankly acknowledged that before emancipation ("while they were property"), the medical treatment of blacks represented the greatest portion of a southern physician's practice. Leonard hoped that the Freedmen's Bureau might help doctors collect fees for treating the freed people. Through the bureau, the federal government might require planters to deduct medical expenditures from freed people's wages or to withhold a portion of the crop specifically to pay for any medical services the former slaves received. In this way the planter would be held responsible for paying the doctor's bills, as before the war. As freed people returned to work on plantations, physicians like Leonard found galling the idea that planters were pocketing the profits of their labor without distributing any to their former colleagues in the medical profession.[14] No doubt many of the doctors expressed genuine concern about the health of freed people, but they also had a monetary incentive to seek a continuation of the prewar pattern whereby planters paid the cost of medical care for workers.

Desperate, doctors in Atlanta attempted in January 1866 through collective action to secure payment for tending former slaves by publicly declaring that they would hold employers accountable for the medical care provided to plantation workers. "A notice to that effect was published in the newspaper"; however, planters would not comply. Only a few doctors collected payment. The same physicians proposed a new plan the following year: planters could stipulate that they would withhold a modest fee for medical services in labor contracts. Thus physicians would be assured of at least some funds for services rendered, unlike the previous year, when they were unable to collect any fees for the care they provided. Similar schemes had been advanced in other southern states. An Atlanta journal supported the measure and recommended an aggregate deduction, either weekly or monthly, from an employee's wages. Each employee would be free to choose his or her physician, and the doctor would base his charge on a fee bill to be developed by the city, village, or county, as appropriate. Local fee bills were thought necessary because the disease environment and character of workers varied from place to place. The Atlanta medical journal also carried a call from a petitioner for a different solution: state support. In Germany and other European nations, the government paid for medical treatment of the poor; the state of Georgia could do the same.[15]

Both bureau officials and physicians proposed schemes for reimbursing doctors for attending freed people, none of which bore fruit. John E. Tallon, who served as one of the bureau's medical directors and who was a physician himself, suggested that the government levy a tax on each planter employing freed people specifically for the purpose of hiring physicians or nurses. Bureau official James Sinclair proposed a tax of one dollar to be levied on each freed adult. The money would be used to reimburse a surgeon of the bureau's choosing. Captain W. Storer How, superintendent of Virginia's Sixth District, forwarded a few medical bills for indigent freed people directly to headquarters, asking on behalf of physicians that they be paid. Bureau officials responded by discouraging the practice. All physicians should collect fees from the freed people able to pay, but they also should expect to provide services gratis to some indigent people.[16] The Freedmen's Bureau would not act as a third-party payer.

The Freedmen's Bureau was also reluctant to act as a collection agent on behalf of physicians or to provide medical services directly to patients. Its officials encouraged individual planters to care for the sick and disabled among the workforce. Presumably when a planter did so, he or she assumed an obligation to see that the bill was paid. But the bureau stopped short of assuming any burden for the provision of health services to the former slaves or for collection of physician accounts that were in arrears. The Freedmen's Bureau had a Medical Department, which had some resources for temporarily assisting infirm and destitute freed people. The bureau took over the hospitals operated by the Union Army during the war and established dispensaries for the distribution of medical care and drugs in

those areas without hospitals. These efforts were short-lived, however, and they never reached effectively into the rural areas, where
the majority of freed people resided. At any rate, the bureau's Medical Department had all but disappeared by 1867.[17]

Despite the bureau's reluctance to assume responsibility for the
medical care of former slaves, officials confronted the issue indirectly
when they exercised oversight of freed people's conditions of labor.
Efforts by agents to ensure fair working conditions, which peaked in
1866 and 1867, achieved different results in different places because
planters were not required by law to gain bureau approval of working
conditions, and those who sought the bureau's endorsement of labor
contracts were not obliged to address the issue of medical care. In
some places agents reviewed a large proportion of labor agreements,
but in others they examined few. Bureau agent James Sinclair in
Lumberton, North Carolina, on 25 August 1856 approved twenty-
five contracts between freed people and planters, only eleven of
which guaranteed any type of medical care. In contrast, Assistant
Commissioner J. B. Kiddoo of Texas reported that "physicians of the
State manifest a commendable willingness to give medical attendance to the freedmen, and in all contacts that I have seen, there is
some promise made for medical attention to the Negroes."[18]

Although considerable variation existed, Freedmen's Bureau officials often operated under the assumption that planters would provide needed medical care for workers and their dependents. The
issue was not so much whether the care would be provided as who
would pay. Employers were expected to play a key role in fronting
the funds needed for doctors and medicines, but they were left to decide whether to absorb the cost themselves or to pass it along to the
laborer, whose wage or share of the crop would be reduced accordingly.[19] As it turned out, former slaveholders proved eager to make
freed people responsible for medical expenses.

Many of the initial contracts submitted for approval to the
Freedmen's Bureau cited conditions that differed little from slavery

days, except that medical care was specifically exempted from the employer's responsibility. A contract between planter B. C. Wyly and freed couple Ephraim and Clary on behalf of themselves and their five children spelled out the expectation that all members of the family would work as domestic servants from July through December. In exchange the family would have "board and lodging as heretofore," along with corn and pork at the end of the year. Wyly agreed to furnish everything the family might need except medical care. One former slave when asked in the 1930s about the difference between slavery and freedom noted that under freedom people paid for medical care but under slavery owners assumed responsibility for the doctor's bill. Freedwoman Josephine Tippit Comptom recalled that her Texas employer often paid the doctor's bill for workers. But this was not always the case with other planters. Indeed, Compton's boss apparently did not do so consistently, and many freed people in her community had to rely on the generosity of one doctor who provided his services to former slaves gratis.[20]

Rather than spelling out the planter's unwillingness to provide medical care, the majority of labor contracts made no mention of the matter. Thus the agreement between Pettis Smithson and Robert Harvey dated 28 December 1865 addressed neither medicine nor medical attention for Harvey, his wife, and their two children. The same was true of a contract between planter William Hamilton and the freed Miller family dated 7 January 1867. A contract between David S. Johnston and forty-two freed people in Early County, Georgia, left unstated who would pay medical costs, but the document pledged the planter to furnish clothing, food, and shelter "as heretofore." Working hands were responsible for supporting "the infirm & helpless this year," which presumably meant that they would pay for any needed medical care in addition to food and shelter.[21]

Of those planters who agreed to assume some degree of responsibility for the medical needs of their employees and dependents, many attempted to establish a nonwage labor system modeled on slavery. In 1866 William Lynn, of Henry County, Alabama, and his wife pledged "to take good care of [his former slaves] in sickness and pay all docktor bills also goods and clothing as heretofore furnished." He promised neither wages nor a share of the crop but instead access to land, every other Saturday off for cultivating it, and stock. Eight men and nine women signed on behalf of themselves and eighteen children, putting themselves in a relationship that resembled slavery in fact if not in name. Three women of Alexandria, Virginia, agreed to serve Thomas Henderson in return for room and board, clothing, and medical attendance and supplies. No wages were mentioned. Nathan, Sarah Ann, and their two eleven-year-old children (Jim and Betsy) were expected to be on "call at all times as heretofore," in exchange for, among other things, "all medical aid" needed by the family. Penelope and her fourteen-year-old daughter agreed to work (cooking, washing, ironing, and other household work) as before the Civil War in exchange for "their usual food & raiment, lodging, food & medical attention." Planter Edward H. Turner in Fauquier County, Virginia, promised no wages in a contract dated November 1865. Instead he would provide freedwoman Eliza Pinkwood with rations, clothing, "and all necessary medical attendance and supplies in case of sickness" for herself and her two children.[22]

Planters who provided medicines and doctors for workers tried to maintain control over expenses, much as they had done under slavery. Although contracts were generally secured by a lien on the crop, Turner's contract with Pinkwood was secured with twenty dollars. Consequently, the contract could be bought out for that sum should Pinkwood's medical care exceed this amount. Planter W. C. Penick of Alabama agreed in the spring of 1865 to make medical care available only to the extent that his medical training allowed. Being "formerly for many years a physician," Penick promised "the said Negroes whose names are signed to the contract . . . his own individual medical attention without charge." Neither his employees nor their families could expect him "to employ or pay for any physician to attend on them" if they became indisposed. H. R. Felder made similar promises to the eighteen freed people he employed in January 1867. Among other things, the contract obligated the planter "to furnish the freedmen and freedwomen and their children such medical attention as he or his father . . . can *themselves* give." The care would be free of charge except for quinine. McQueen McIntosh in 1865 offered several dozen freed people nurses, medicines, and a physician if they would relocate. "Medical attendance and medicine" would also be provided for their dependants, but "at the expense of the laborers," who would have the costs deducted from their wages.[23]

Women entered into contracts as part of labor gangs and family groups, and as individuals. As occurred with men, most assumed responsibility for paying for their own medical care. Again, the major difference was whether the employer agreed to absorb the cost initially and seek reimbursement later or whether the woman would pay for all medical care out of pocket. The contract signed in January 1866 by Polly Minor in Carolina County, Virginia, on behalf of herself, her three sons, and two daughters obligated the mother to pay for their medical bills. Minor was to receive fifty dollars for the year, one of her sons to receive ten dollars. The others worked in exchange for room and board. The sixty dollars acquired by the family had to cover clothing in addition to medical expenses, and might be reduced if any of the Minors—mother or children—lost time from work because of illness or for another reason.[24]

Contracts that survive from the period reveal other freedwomen contracting on their own behalf. Hetty Conquest agreed to work as a cook and washer for S. T. Lucas of Accamac County, Sallie Pettegrew contracted to work for six months in Lynchburg at unnamed tasks, and Netty Ann Webb went to work as a nurse in an undisclosed Virginia location.[25] These women were particularly vulnerable to suffering the want of life's necessities and medical attention should they become pregnant or suffer from gynecological disease, because they appear to have had no family nearby who could assist them. Many entered into contracts so vague that they failed to promise even a rudimentary wage or shelter, let alone medical attention.

Dulcena, who signed a contract with Benjamin F. Pope in Alabama, promised that she and her fourteen-year-old son Henry would serve "respectfully & politely" in exchange for food. If they stayed through the end of the year, Dulcena was to receive five dollars per month. The contract made no mention of medical care or shelter.[26] The expectation of medical care may have gone without saying. Planters were used to making decisions unilaterally about engaging a physician. The choice reflected a variety of concerns, including the perceived seriousness of the problem; the ability of the planter, worker, or family member to handle the problem through time-honored home remedies; the press of work about the plantation and household; the cost and likely effectiveness of the treatment; the availability of a physician; and the humanitarian impulse that encourages people to come to the aid of those who suffer from illness. Pope would probably have taken all these factors into account if Dulcena became incapacitated while in his employ.

Planters who reimbursed workers with wages or a share of the crop expected to deduct a portion for any time lost due to sickness. Patsy Teackle of Virginia was hired for thirty-six dollars in yearly wages, to be paid in installments every three months. "All time lost" because of sickness was to be deducted from the total. An agreement between planter Miles W. Abernathy and freedman Wesley specified that the freedman was to do farm and domestic work as before the war and to attend church. In exchange Wesley was to receive eight dollars monthly, along with shelter, fuel, and food for his family as well as "medical attention in sickness, loss of time to be deducted." A preprinted contract circulating in 1867 listed the administering of medicine as a duty of the employer, and a reduction in wages as the consequence of missing time from work "by reason of sickness." Alfred Walker and eight other heads of household signed such a contract on behalf of their families; their wives would have their pay reduced for time lost because of childbearing.[27]

Some planters tried to extend the concept of payment for lost time to recoup the cost of rations distributed to workers who lost time on the job as a result of illness. For example, two contracts negotiated between planters and freed people in Gouchland County, Virginia, called for the payment of rations consumed by anyone absent from work in excess of fifteen days on Westview Plantation or more than twenty days on Pocahontas Plantation. No exception was made for pregnancy and childbirth; consequently, the penalties would have hit young families especially hard. The existence of the policy demonstrates how planter attitudes had changed since the end of the war and emancipation: whereas once the planter might have released a new or expectant mother from productive labor or reduced her work assignment to help ensure the birth and survival of children, now the planter refused to make such concessions. Those women and men who wanted children would need to weigh their ability to pay not only the cost of caring for a young child but also the cost of sustaining the mother through the pregnancy, childbirth, and the early weeks or months of childrearing.[28]

Women of childrearing age typically made up part of a planter's workforce, some of whom might be listed as dependents for an extended period. James E. Waddy of Louisiana journeyed to Georgia in late 1866 or early 1867 to recruit hands for his plantation called Dixie. He found forty hands aged twelve or older, who were accompanied by forty children younger than twelve. The group included few dependents other than the children and one elderly couple—a mother and father—who apparently accompanied grown children to Louisiana. Age alone did not define one as a dependent, however. Lucinda Favor, who was sixty-five and listed as an "invalid," was nevertheless designated a "Class 3" hand, which apparently meant that she was capable of earning her own living. Two younger women were listed as dependents: the twenty-nine-year-old wife of Willis Austin was "unhealthy," as was the wife of Tillman Bass, her age unspecified. The use of the term "unhealthy" suggests that the women either were pregnant, had recently given birth, or suffered health problems, possibly from complications of childbirth. And the plantation owner faced the prospect of losing the work of other hands: 30 percent of the adult workforce consisted of women between fifteen and forty, the age span of childbearing.[29]

Pregnancy, childbirth, and gynecological disorders—many resulting from complications of childbirth—no doubt accounted for much of the time women lost from the field. Planters distinguished between short-term absences of a week or two, even a month, and the long-term absences typically associated with women's reproductive health. Freedman Jim Sharpe signed a contract for 1867 with H. H. Haddock pledging himself and his wife, Catherine, to work for the planter. Jim was to begin work on the first of the year, but Catherine would not begin until the first of March, presumably after she had recovered from childbirth. One Mississippi planter who signed an agreement with Georgians to work on his plantation in 1866 contracted with 161 people. Of these, only 100 were adult. Forty-four of the adults were women, but 8 of these were "unserviceable"—that is, incapable of work. None of the 56 men were listed in this category, and of the 8 "unserviceable" women, all but 2 were of childbearing age. Sarah Gomer and Kilki Frazier were ages sixty and fifty respectively; the rest were between ages seventeen and thirty-seven. Martha Anthony, age thirty-one, was on the list because she was "pregnant, feet & legs swollen so badly." Lucy Bailey, seventeen; Mary Dill, thirty-five; Francis Jones, twenty-two; Dilsie Gains, thirty-five; and Dinah Graves, thirty-seven, were listed as dependent on their husbands. All were sick or disabled, which in the terminology of the nineteenth century could mean recovering from or suffering the complications of childbearing.[30]

To assemble this workforce, Clark Anderson and Company, which represented the Mississippi planter, had promised wages, shelter, food, fuel, and "medical attendance and supplies in case of sickness." At the same time, the contract assessed penalties for missing days of work: "one dollar per day during the spring and summer months, and two dollars during cotton picking season." Further penalties applied to those who "lost time for protracted sickness." In such cases, the medical expenses and supplies would be deducted from wages.[31] The agreement protected planters from the situation in which a woman worker earning wages might lose time from the field to give birth or require medical attention because of health problems. In these instances, the cost of the care would be shifted to the husband.

Freed people devised strategies for coping with confinement and complications of childbirth. Generally these did not differ significantly from those used to cope with illness. Wages might be maintained if a woman promised to make up lost time in the future. More commonly, a family member or friend might work in the woman's place. A contract between planter John B. Morton of Cumberland County, Virginia, and five freedmen specified that "their wives & children their mules & horses" would perform work on the same basis as the men, but if any could not perform chores because of sickness or another valid excuse, they would "owe" the planter that number of days in the future. On Coffin's Point plantation of St. Helena Island, sisters and friends took over "the tasks of the lying-in women." Exchanges of labor were important because a woman might lose her allotment of the crop if she could not complete her share of the work.[32]

As slaves, blacks had grown used to helping one another. Former Texas slave Thomas Cole specifically recalled that no one wanted to help someone who was lazy, but many people would pitch in to assist when someone was ill, a condition that covered women in labor and those recovering from childbirth as well as convalescents from sickness. Freedman Campbell Armstrong also noted the tendency of former slaves to help one another out. The assistant commissioner of

the Freedmen's Bureau in Texas, General J. B. Kiddoo, reported that
freed people assisted one another, a practice that he encouraged.
Often it was a family member who came to someone's aid. Isabell
Henderson of North Carolina married following freedom at the age
of twenty-two. When pregnancy left her feeling ill, she returned to
her stepfather's house for a time.[33]

Collective action could go beyond the immediate family. In
Nashville, freed people formed a benevolent aid organization and
succeeded in establishing a hospital. Former slaves in Augusta,
Georgia, also banded together in a freedmen's aid society for the
purpose of providing medical care to the black community. They
raised enough money to support a lying-in ward and a black midwife
in addition to a hospital and physician.[34] Not all freed people benefited from such organizations, however. They took time and money
to establish. Many former slaves had instead to negotiate assistance
from family members.

Freedwoman Parthenia Oaks agreed to work for H. H. Haddock
during 1867 with the specific understanding that when she became
unable "to do good reasonable work" (presumably during confinement) her mother would take her place for a spell. Haddock drew up
the contract to make clear that he would not assume any responsibility for doctor's bills for either the workers or their dependents. "They
alone are responsible," he wrote. Oaks and her father shared a yearly
wage of $120. Haddock paid shared wages to others; Mary Rose
shared one income with her nephew Henry, for example.[35] Shared
wages ensured that women absent from work because of childbirth
or the need to nurse an infant could survive through another's labors
during periods when they could not work.

Freed people expected a woman to withdraw temporarily from
contract work for childbirth, but planters sometimes expected
women to complete reduced work throughout the pregnancy and
soon after confinement, much as they had done under slavery. In
Georgia the different expectations became obvious in a dispute in-

volving planter Phocion Ramsey and freedman Anderson Garret. Garret expected to work for Ramsey in exchange for five dollars each month along with food and shelter for his family. Ramsey considered that the whole family was obligated to work for the sum. In an affidavit filed with the Freedmen's Bureau, Garret explained that his wife was never part of the contract because she was pregnant and nearing confinement. She required "the usual time for child bearing" both before and after the birth. Ramsey argued that the family had failed to fulfill its obligations. Not only did the wife refuse to help in the field, but also the three children proved incapable of performing work there. A Freedmen's Bureau official decided the case in the planter's favor, and the Garret family found themselves turned off the Columbus County plantation.[36]

Another dispute over the work of a new mother flared elsewhere in Georgia and came before the Freedmen's Bureau for resolution. In this 1866 case, Isham Crowell complained that he had been charged for items he did not receive, including medical attendance for his wife's confinement. She had given birth without assistance, Crowell stipulated. "A negrowoman Patience" had been called, but because the child arrived before she did, Patience declined to charge for her visit. "No Doctor stepped in." The husband also complained that his wife's pay had been reduced for the loss of ninety-seven days of work because of her confinement. She "lost four weeks by confinement," and she also suffered from chills and fever on occasion, but she had not been so many days out of work.[37]

Crowell further complained that his wife's pay had been reduced on the assumption that she had cared for her child. The child died one day after birth, Crowell stated, and the mother had "lost no time out of the field" either for care or for mourning. Yet she still suffered a reduction in wages. Customary pay in the region was $100 a year for able-bodied hands, $75 for women who had a child to tend. The lower pay reflected the time lost from work for confinement and care of the child. Crowell apparently believed that his wife was entitled to

$100 a year, minus an amount equal to about a month's wages.[38] This calculation reflected the practice under slavery in which a parturient woman might be given up to four weeks to recover from childbirth before returning to fulltime work. Less labor also might be expected from women with infants than from those without because the women needed time for breastfeeding and other chores related to a newborn's care. The outcome of the Crowell case is unknown.

Eventually the system of contract labor gave way to family sharecropping in which planters furnished land, seeds, and supplies to kin groups in return for a portion of the crop, usually 50 percent. This arrangement allowed the members of a household to determine who would do specific types of work. Family members could substitute for new mothers as they wished. Former slaves preferred the system in part because it gave them a degree of independence; it allowed women (at least those with able-bodied husbands or other family members to work the crop) to allocate their labor more directly for the support of the family.[39]

As for medical attendance, freed people varied in their response to the withdrawal of regular physicians from the black community following the war. Even before the end of the war, one was grumbling about the lack of access to regulars occasioned by their service to the Confederacy. Former slave Mary Thompson blamed the absence of medical treatment by trained physicians for much of the sickness and many of the deaths experienced by slaves in the postwar period. So did Pauline Howell, who was turned off an Arkansas plantation after slavery ended. Boston Blackwell lodged a similar complaint. Texas freedman William Byrd considered the loss of medical attention a negative aspect of freedom. Under slavery, workers were too valuable to let die, so owners paid doctors' bills, he explained. After emancipation, they were not as valuable in the employer's eyes. When a laborer became ill, the boss could find a replacement without incurring any cost. Frances Fluker, who had been enslaved in Arkansas, said simply that she never thought about being sick after the war because she knew she could not afford the doctor's bill.[40]

Former slaves not only found the refusal of employers to pay medical expenses troubling; they also found their lack of interest in the freed person's troubles scandalous. Henry Murray and others on the Murray plantation in Dallas County, Alabama, must have been shocked when the master burned the plantation hospital after the war. Henry explained later that as slaves they had been used to proper medical attention when they became ill. Freedwoman Alice Cole lamented the loss of good medical care in freedom, although she had in mind the "old-time remedies" as much as the pills white doctors gave to their patients. Former Texas slave Hattie Cole also regretted the lack of medical attention that freedom brought. Interviewed in the 1930s by government agents, Cole said that as a freedwoman she sometimes received needed medicine, at other times not. In slavery days she had always obtained something, even if only herbal remedies provided by her master.[41]

Other freed people appeared content to dispense with a doctor's care in favor of folk remedies or expressed a desire to consult a doctor of their own choosing. Former Alabama slave Joe Hawkins apparently did not regret the loss of doctors, who would "bleed you for most any sickness." For the most part, slaves had maintained a pragmatic attitude toward the provision of medical care by owners. Unable to control when doctors were called in, they nevertheless observed treatment and cooperated more or less depending on their assessment of outcomes. Former slaves sought help from regulars when they perceived the treatment efficacious, affordable, under their control, and after home remedies had proven wanting.[42]

A group of freed men working for planter John Strain in Perry County, Alabama, arranged with a local physician to attend all the hands on the plantation. The arrangement came to Strain's attention only when the physician approached the planter for payment out of the freed people's wages. Strain was incredulous and wrote the

Freedmen's Bureau to learn how it should be handled. The hands are already "in my *debt*, from $20 to $90 each," Strain complained; yet "the physician thinks I am bound to pay." One reason Strain found the situation galling was that he had promised the freed people "such medical attention as my superintendent and self could give." Clearly, the former slaves judged their services lacking. In Grooverville, Georgia, freed people hired physician W. R. Joiner under a contract that called for the workers to pay for his services out of their annual wages. The contract between McQueen McIntosh and his workers explicitly stated that the "laborers are entitled to select a plantation physician, who will be sent for by the said proprietor when necessary." The underlining of this clause in the original suggests that this was a particularly sore point with the workers.[43]

When it came to women's reproductive health, doctors provided few services that resulted in positive outcomes for women; thus they generally preferred to rely on one another rather than on a physician. Subjected to invasive procedures, inexperienced doctors, and experimental intervention under slavery, black women were wary of a white doctor's services. Freedmen and women regularly sought other types of medical care from installations of the Freedmen's Bureau, but few approached the bureau to ask for assistance with managing pregnancy, childbirth, or other reproductive health problems. Laing advised his superiors that "uterine disease from abortion and miscarriage" prevailed "to an alarming extent." Still, few women sought assistance. When in June 1868 bureau doctor J. G. Temple of Kentucky reported the cases he had treated, he listed only 2 involving complications of childbirth out of a total of 432. Eighty-eight involved measles, and 52 acute diarrhea. He described his cases for the month as typical.[44]

Yet gynecological and obstetric problems were prevalent among former slaves, as physician John E. Tallon found when in 1863 he visited the Louisiana plantation known as Hickory Place. Of the twenty-four people who were laid up there, thirteen were women.

Four of them suffered from general debility, sometimes accompanied by diarrhea. Five, however, suffered from suppressed menstruation (amenorrhea), two others from vaginal discharges (leukorrhea, or the "whites"). The conditions of two women were unclear. In contrast, eleven men and children suffered mostly from worms, although two had diarrhea, one displayed general debility, and another had croup along with fever.[45]

The distrust that freed people had of white doctors reflected in part their knowledge of the racist attitudes held by regular physicians. After the war, former slaves in one Arkansas community recognized the white doctor who used to attend slaves on their plantation among the members of the Ku Klux Klan who shot at freed blacks attending a political meeting. A North Carolina doctor who said he attended "many *she niggers* during their accouchement" described his patients as "unfaithful, profligate, unprincipled, thievish, tyrannical, usurping, overbearing, and insulting." Bureau medical director John E. Tallon reported to superiors that when freed people asked for medical care, "the planter sends for a rebel physician who attends the planter's family and who always feels largely for the planter, but for the negro contempt and disdain." Tallon reported a conversation with one doctor who expressed the hope that all freed people would die. Gideon Lincecum, who had retired from medical practice in the antebellum years, obtained a license from the federal government to practice in Texas after the war. His racist attitude—termed "harsh and strident" by the editors of his correspondence—led him to describe slavery as "natural," contend that blacks could not "be elevated to a level with the white race" by any means, and advocate as a means of improving society the enslavement of free black northerners and castration of rebellious slaves. Onnie Lee Logan, who served as midwife to a black clientele in the mid-twentieth century, maintained that poor treatment of black women by white doctors encouraged them to rely on midwives.[46]

Freed people in Kentucky stayed away from Louisville in part because the medical director of the University of Louisville's Medical Department, Joseph W. Benson, was rumored to have seized and sold the corpses of black infants to the medical school for study and even to have murdered some of the children to ensure the availability of cadavers. Benson was convicted and imprisoned for fraud in connection with a government contract and later charged with tampering in the affairs of the local Freedmen's Bureau hospital, circumstances that did nothing to inspire the freed people's confidence. In addition, he was a well-known southern sympathizer. Providing further evidence of its sympathies, the Medical Department after the war also reemployed doctor David W. Yandell, who had left Kentucky to serve as a surgeon in the Confederate military. Freed people in other parts of the South shared a similar distrust of white doctors who had fought for the Confederacy and against emancipation.[47]

There was another reason for black women to avoid medical men. Doctors had cooperated with slaveholders in their attempts to manage women's sexuality and childbearing in the slave quarter. When they had intervened in conception, childbirth, complications of childbirth, and women's diseases, they had done so at the owners' behest and for the owners' purposes. This fact was not lost on black women and men, who spurned their services when slavery ended.

Men have traditionally exerted control over subordinate groups through regulation of sexual relationships.[48] Slaveholders in the antebellum South were no exception. Elite white men assumed that it was their prerogative to interfere with sexuality in the slave quarter, going so far as to demand access to the bodies of enslaved women for their own sexual pleasure and to insist that certain slaves mate in an effort to ensure the birth of strong and healthy children in bondage. Much of this sexual exploitation occurred out of public view. Particularly when it came to liaisons between elite white men and enslaved black women, powerful slaveholding families would not stand for the public flouting of legal and social conventions that confined acceptable sexual relationships to members of the same race and class.

But in the antebellum South, sexual dominance could be expressed publicly under the guise of medical treatment. Medical men and slave owners cooperated in subjecting the most intimate of human acts to outside scrutiny so that the goal—conception and the birth of a slave—would be achieved to the slaveholders' satisfaction.

The withdrawal of physicians from service to the black community offered black women an opportunity to gain control over their bodies. To be sure, atrocities continued in the postwar period as some white men forcibly violated black women. However, medical men might be kept at a distance, and this circumstance would allow women to handle pregnancy, childbirth, and other health concerns according to their own notions of propriety.

For those suspicious of white doctors, home remedies passed down from older generations inspired confidence that freed people could treat health problems on their own, an important consideration among a people largely too poor to afford white medicine anyhow. Harriet Collins, born a slave in Texas, learned home cures from her mother, who in turn had learned them from a member of the previous generation. The origin of certain of her cures stretched all the way back to Africa, and some had their genesis in the cultural practices of Amerindians who had once inhabited the southern landscape. Some remedies consisted of the popular herbal and root teas made from such substances as sassafras, mullein, or various flowers. Others were made from whatever else was at hand. Bleeding could be stopped with soot and cobwebs but also by letting a dog lick the injury. Some substances acted magically, protecting the person from present or future ills. For example, a nutmeg worn on a string around the head could cure headache; a dime strung around an ankle prevented leg cramps. A sack half filled with salt and containing nine grains of red pepper and four buckeyes worn around the neck warded off chills. No doubt, European and European-American practices also influenced Collins' approach to healing. Jim Allen, who as a boy learned to gather the herbs used by the mistress and a physician, explained in the 1930s that he could still identify the plants. Collins and other former slaves continued to gather and use whatever remedies they considered efficacious, no matter who had originally advocated them.[49]

Harriet Barrett of Texas practiced medicine before and after the war using much the same remedies. Charcoal, onion, and honey were especially good for a little baby; camphor tied in a sack around a child's neck worked against chills, fever, and problems associated with teething. A rabbit's foot worn around the neck also warded off chills and fever as well as other diseases. Louisa Adams, formerly enslaved in North Carolina, kept herbs in her kitchen—the same ones used by slaves decades earlier. One Louisiana woman maintained faith in the cami weed, red oak bark, and peach tree leaves, which she continued to gather in the woods, until her death in the late 1920s. A former Georgia slave assured an interviewer in the 1930s that the herb used by slaves to treat fever was "good now . . . if you can get it." Former slave Fred Forbes, who lived in Nebraska after the war, made a cure for a cold in much the same way as his mother. The concoction not only provided a "sure cure" but also served as a powerful link to the past and the customary practices that no doubt provided comfort as much as cure. For problems that did not respond to folk cures, freed people could take preventive action or consult spiritual healers as before the war. Former slave Rachel Santee continued in the 1930s to throw salt on the fire or place a broom across the door when she heard an owl and to carry a rabbit's foot and buckeye in her pocket. The existence of "preacher faith" doctors such as Lewis Hill suggests that a link between spirituality and medicine continued in some communities beyond the Civil War. One factor encouraging the retention of folk healing was the inability of physicians to cure illnesses resulting from social factors. These required spells. Therefore, conjurers continued to hold out hope for people beyond the pale of regularly trained doctors, although as before the war not everyone accepted the need for them.[50]

The majority of former slaves relied on traditional root and herbal remedies to treat women's health problems. Teshan Young, who in Texas gathered herbs and other plants to treat children and adults, boiled red shank into a juice for "female trouble." Teas made of birthroot, squaw weed, horsemint, and cotton speeded labor, eased the discomfort of menstruation, ensured recovery from childbirth, and brought on menstruation when it appeared tardy. Even today such herbal remedies remain popular and are sometimes incorporated into nurse-midwifery practice.[51]

Former slaves thus returned to the practice whereby women managed pregnancy and childbirth without the help of medical men. Before the war, physicians were available on many plantations and farms for those cases in which enslaved women experienced complications of birth. Following the collapse of slavery, former slaves who lacked the cash to pay could not count on a doctor's assistance with childbirth or for any other ailment. Physician Robert Wright thought that it was "a rare thing in this section of the country for a Physician to attend at the birth of a child particularly among the coloured people." Children were born at home with the aid of a midwife even when complications developed.[52]

Traditional birth attendants did not have the skills to ward off tragic outcomes in all cases of complicated birth. Midwife Margaret Thornton estimated that she oversaw the births of 2,000 infants in North Carolina and "closed as many eyes" as did other midwives.[53] But doctors had not always saved mother and child either. Midwives did what they could to avoid tragedy, but they also aided parents in understanding any unavoidable and unfortunate outcome, including the stillbirth of a child or the death of the mother. They helped loved ones cope with loss by guiding them through traditional responses that invested the moment with meaning.

Some of the midwives who practiced in the postwar period were the same ones who had done so in slavery. Mariah Bell became a midwife in slavery and continued to tend women after the war, serving altogether for forty-five years. Jennie Butler assisted with cases of childbirth until 1912, quitting only when traveling around the countryside became difficult and the pay too low. Granny Pernell in Mississippi also continued the practice of midwifery after the war. The only difference was that she had to visit her clients on foot; before the war, she had access to her owner's horse. Lucretia Brown, who apparently became a midwife under the tutelage of her mistress, continued to practice after the war. She employed traditional herbs, including "sassafras bark and black root . . . boneset, St. John Weed, and smartweed," all of which she gathered herself. Katy Elmore in Louisiana also worked before and after the war as a midwife serving black and white women and children.[54]

As occurred under slavery, some midwives worked under the supervision of physicians. Cyntha Jones's old slave master had been a doctor. Following the war, when Jones was just twenty-one years old, her former owner helped her get started as a midwife. She apprenticed with "old Dr. Clark." He and others—including presumably her former owner, Simpson Dabney—read medical texts to Jones until she understood enough to obtain a medical license. Jones practiced in Arkansas for about fifteen years under the supervision of five different doctors, assisting altogether in the delivery of 299 babies. Jennie Butler, who attended childbirth cases in Arkansas through 1912, termed herself a physician's assistant rather than a midwife because she worked under the direction of a doctor. "We women did all the work," she later maintained. The doctor visited in the parlor; at times he did not even enter the birthing room, according to Butler's testimony. Dicey Thomas became a nurse after the war and worked with all the prominent white doctors in Little Rock. Bell Williams followed a somewhat different path into midwifery. At first the local doctors sent for her to act as a nurse, but she soon became known in the neighborhood, and people began calling her to serve as midwife on her own.[55]

States (Montreal: Eden Press
-Floyd and Carolyn F. Sargent,
Cultural Perspectives (Berkeley:
ol P. MacCormack, "Adaptation
of Fertility and Birth, ed. Mac-

frican American culture in the
body of literature. See esp. Ira
turies of Slavery in North Amer-
rd University Press, 1998) and
-American Slaves (Cambridge,
s, 2003); John W. Blassingame,
ntebellum South, rev. ed. (New
Dusinberre, *Them Dark Days:*
rk: Oxford University Press,
merican Institutional and Intel-
go Press, 1976); Drew Gilpin
: A Design for Mastery (Baton
Robert W. Fogel and Stanley
cs of American Negro Slavery
enovese, *Within the Plantation*
th (Chapel Hill: University of
ing, *Prelude to Civil War: The*
1836 (New York: Harper and
oll: The World the Slaves Made
omy of Slavery: Studies in the
Vintage, 1967); Herbert G.
1750–1925 (New York: Pan-
nd Patriarchy: Charleston,
45–72; Walter Johnson, *Soul*
Cambridge, Mass.: Harvard
e Riverside: A South Carolina
Press, 1984); Lawrence W.
-American Folk Thought from
Press, 1977); James Oakes,
s (New York: Knopf, 1982);
tic Slavery," in *Slavery and*
ord University Press, 1982);
: Slavery in the Antebellum

By World War II, obstetricians had replaced midwives in most routine cases of childbirth throughout most of the country. Only among southern blacks did the tradition of home births linger. Maria Jackson kept up a midwifery practice well into the twentieth century. Liddie Boechus, who bore twelve children in as many years and became a midwife following the Civil War, practiced for decades. By the time Boechus spoke about her experience in the 1930s, the number of births attended by lay midwives had fallen to less than 15 percent in the nation as a whole. Most women preferred attendance by a physician. Eighty percent of practicing midwives lived in the South, however, where they assisted in the delivery of 50 percent of black infants.[56] For almost 100 years after the end of slavery, the midwife continued to serve the black community, and childbirth remained the work of women. For a people without means and distrustful of the white physician, this was how children were born.

in *Yucatan, Holland, Sweden, and the Unite*
Women's Publications, 1980); Robbie E. Davi
Childbirth and Authoritative Knowledge: Cross
University of California Press, 1997); and Car
in Human Fertility and Birth," in *Ethnography*
Cormack (New York: Academic, 1982).

4. The debate over the nature of slavery and *A*
antebellum South has produced a vast and rich
Berlin, *Many Thousands Gone: The First Two Cer*
ica (Cambridge, Mass.: Belknap Press of Harva
Generations of Captivity: A History of African
Mass.: Belknap Press of Harvard University Pres
The Slave Community: Plantation Life in the A
York: Oxford University Press, 1979); William
Slavery in the American Rice Swamps (New Y
1996); Stanley M. Elkins, *Slavery: A Problem in A*
lectual Life, 3d ed. (Chicago: University of Chic
Faust, *James Henry Hammond and the Old South*
Rouge: Louisiana State University Press, 1982);
L. Engerman, *Time on the Cross: The Econom*
(Boston: Little, Brown, 1974); Elizabeth Fox-G
Household: Black and White Women of the Old Sou
North Carolina Press, 1988); William W. Freehl
Nullification Controversy in South Carolina, 1816–
Row, 1966); Eugene D. Genovese, *Roll, Jordan, R*
(New York: Vintage, 1976) and *The Political Eco*
Economy and Society of the Slave South (New York
Gutman, *The Black Family in Slavery and Freedom,*
theon, 1976); Michael P. Johnson, "Planters
1800–1860," *Journal of Southern History* 46 (1980)
by Soul: Life Inside the Antebellum Slave Market (
University Press, 1999); Charles Joyner, *Down by t*
Slave Community (Urbana: University of Illinois
Levine, *Black Culture and Black Consciousness: Afro*
Slavery to Freedom (New York: Oxford University
The Ruling Race: A History of American Slaveholder
Willie Lee Rose, "The Domestication of Domes
Freedom, ed. William W. Freehling (New York: Ox
and Kenneth M. Stampp, *The Peculiar Institution*
South (New York: Vintage, 1956).

5. Histories of slavery and medicine pay little attention to black women's health. See Diane Price Herndl, "The Invisible (Invalid) Woman: African-American Women, Illness, and Nineteenth-Century Narrative," in *Women and Health in America: Historical Readings,* ed. Judith Walzer Leavitt, 2d ed. (Madison: University of Wisconsin Press, 1999), pp. 131–132; Loretta J. Ross, "African-American Women and Abortion: A Neglected History," *Journal of Health Care for the Poor and Underserved* 3 (fall 1992): 275.

6. Steven M. Stowe, *Doctoring the South: Southern Physicians and Everyday Medicine in the Mid-Nineteenth Century* (Chapel Hill: University of North Carolina Press, 2004), pp. 30, 281n29.

7. On medical journals of the antebellum era, see Steven M. Stowe, "Seeing Themselves at Work: Physicians and the Case Narrative in the Mid-Nineteenth-Century American South," *American Historical Review* 101 (February 1996): 41–42; Myrl Ebert, "The Rise and Development of the American Medical Periodical, 1797–1850," *Bulletin of the Medical Library Association* 40 (1952): 243–276; Walter Fisher, "Physicians and Slavery in the Antebellum Southern Medical Journal," *Journal of the History of Medicine and Allied Sciences* 23 (January 1968): 36–49.

1. Procreation

1. Details of Lulu Wilson's life are extracted from George P. Rawick, ed., *The American Slave: A Composite Autobiography* (Westport, Conn.: Greenwood, 1972–1979), SS2, vol. 10: Tex., pt. 9, pp. 4191–98. Hereafter this collection of slave narratives is cited by series, supplement (if any), and volume.

2. The idea that medical practice reflects the setting in which it occurs is discussed by Judith Walzer Leavitt, "'A Worrying Profession': The Domestic Environment of Medical Practice in Mid-Nineteenth-Century America," *Bulletin of the History of Medicine* 69 (1995): 1–29, esp. p. 3; Charles Rosenberg, "The Practice of Medicine in New York a Century Ago," ibid., 41 (1967), esp. p. 253.

3. On the work of enslaved children and its importance for family, see Marie Jenkins Schwartz, *Born in Bondage: Growing Up Enslaved in the Antebellum South* (Cambridge, Mass.: Harvard University Press, 2000), pp. 9, 123, 132–134; idem, "Family Life in the Slave Quarter," *Magazine of History* 15 (summer 2001): 36–41; idem, "One Thing, Then Another: Slave Children's Labor in Alabama," *Labor's Heritage* 7 (winter 1996): 22–33, 56.

4. S2, vol. 8: Ark., pt. 1, p. 168, and vol. 14: N.C., pt. 1, p. 360, and vol. 15: N.C., pt. 2, pp. 131, 229, 417; SS1, vol. 9: Miss., pt. 4, p. 1817; SS2, vol. 10: Tex., pt. 9, p. 4111; T. Lindsay Baker and Julie P. Baker, eds., *The WPA Oklahoma Slave Narratives* (Norman: University of Oklahoma Press, 1996), p. 488; W. Michael

Byrd and Linda A. Clayton, *An American Health Dilemma*, vol. 1: *A Medical History of African Americans and the Problem of Race* (New York: Routledge, 2000), p. 282.

5. Melanie Pavich-Lindsay, ed., *Anna: The Letters of a St. Simons Island Plantation Mistress, 1817–1859* (Athens: University of Georgia Press, 2002), p. 301; Erika L. Murr, ed., *A Rebel Wife in Texas: The Diary and Letters of Elizabeth Scott Neblett, 1852–1864* (Baton Rouge: Louisiana State University Press, 2001), p. 275. Jennifer L. Morgan discusses the importance placed on enslaved women's reproductive capacity for future generations of slaveholders during the colonial years in *Laboring Women: Reproduction and Gender in New World Slavery* (Philadelphia: University of Pennsylvania Press, 2004), chap. 3.

6. The slave population in the United States, in contrast to that of Cuba and other American nations, had been growing through human reproduction since the early eighteenth century. Only in the United States did the rate of slave births so exceed the rate of slave deaths that the slave population can be said to have grown through "natural means." The U.S. slave population became the largest in the Americas even though the country imported a much smaller number of slaves than many other nations. See Philip D. Curtin, *The Atlantic Slave Trade: A Census* (Madison: University of Wisconsin Press, 1969), pp. 88–89, 92; Paul E. Lovejoy, "The Volume of the Atlantic Slave Trade: A Synthesis," *Journal of African History* 23 (1982): 473–501; Joseph E. Inkori and Stanley L. Engerman, "Introduction: Gainers and Losers in the Atlantic Slave Trade," in *The Atlantic Slave Trade: Effects on Economies, Societies, and Peoples in Africa, the Americas, and Europe*, ed. Inkori and Engerman (Durham, N.C.: Duke University Press, 1992), pp. 5–6; David Eltis and David Richardson, "The 'Numbers Game' and Routes to Slavery," *Slavery and Abolition* 18 (April 1997): 2; Philip D. Curtin, *The Rise and Fall of the Plantation Complex: Essays in Atlantic History* (New York: Cambridge University Press, 1990), pp. 173–174; Rebecca J. Scott, *Slave Emancipation in Cuba: The Transition to Free Labor, 1860–1899* (Princeton: Princeton University Press, 1985), p. 10. On Louisiana's sugar-producing plantations, the slave population decreased rather than increased in the nineteenth century. See Richard Follett, "Heat, Sex, and Sugar: Pregnancy and Childbearing in the Slave Quarter," *Journal of Family History* 28 (October 2003): 510–539.

7. Thomas Affleck, "On the Hygiene of Cotton Plantations and the Management of Negro Slaves," *Southern Medical Reports* 2 (1850): 434; S2, vol. 11: Mo., p. 215. On fertility rates among slaves, see Richard Sutch, "The Breeding of Slaves for Sale and the Westward Expansion of Slavery, 1850–1860," in *Race and Slavery in the Western Hemisphere: Quantitative Studies*, ed. Stanley L.

Engerman and Eugene D. Genovese (Princeton: Princeton University Press, 1975), pp. 173–210.

8. S2, vol. 8: Ark., pt. 1, p. 47, and vol. 11: Ark., pt. 7, p. 245, and vol. 15: N.C., pt. 2, p. 274, and vol. 17: Fla., pp. 55, 223; SS1, vol. 7: Miss., pt. 2, pp. 600–601, and vol. 9: Miss., pt. 4, pp. 1453–54; SS2, vol. 1: Ala., Ariz., Ark., and Other Narratives, p. 255, and vol. 6: Tex., pt. 6, p. 2081; "Management of Slaves," *DeBow's Review* 13 (August 1852), in *Advice among Masters: The Ideal in Slave Management in the Old South*, ed. James O. Breeden (Westport, Conn.: Greenwood, 1980), p. 242.

9. Although slaves could not marry legally, most owners recognized certain slave unions as such and granted privileges for married couples, including in some cases a promise not to separate the couple through sale. I have discussed this issue at length in *Born in Bondage*, chap. 7.

10. S2, vol. 15: N.C., pt. 2, p. 350; SS2, vol. 2: Tex., pt. 1, p. 168; Charles L. Perdue Jr., Thomas E. Barden, and Robert K. Phillips, eds., *Weevils in the Wheat: Interviews with Virginia Ex-Slaves* (Charlottesville: University Press of Virginia, 1976), p. 105; A. M. French (Mrs.), *Slavery in South Carolina and the Ex-Slaves; or, The Port Royal Mission* (New York: Negro Universities Press, 1969), p. 93. See also Kate E. R. Pickard, *The Kidnapped and the Ransomed: The Narrative of Peter and Vina Still after Forty Years of Slavery* (Philadelphia: Jewish Publication Society of America, 1970), p. 153.

11. S2, vol. 10: Ark., pt. 5, p. 277; SS1, vol. 1: Ala., p. 432, and vol. 7: Miss., pt. 2, p. 511; Southron, "The Policy of the Southern Planter,"*American Cotton Planter and Soil of the South,* n.s., 1 (October 1857), in Breeden, *Advice among Masters,* p. 146; John Spencer Bassett, *The Southern Plantation Overseer as Revealed in His Letters* (New York: Negro Universities Press, 1968), p. 32.

12. P. C. Weston, "Management of a Southern Plantation," *DeBow's Review* 22 (January 1859), in Breeden, *Advice among Masters,* p. 260. See also Bassett, *Southern Plantation Overseer,* p. 32; S2, vol. 8: Ark., pt. 2, p. 132, and vol. 17: Fla., pp. 242, 257, 342; SS1, vol. 7: Miss., pt. 2, pp. 440–441, 611.

13. S2, vol. 8: Ark., pt. 1, p. 311.

14. S2, vol. 8: Ark., pt. 1, pp. 42, 157; 8 May 1845, Diary, George Augustus Beverly Walker Papers, ADAH.

15. S2, vol. 14: N.C., pt. 1, p. 124; SS2, vol. 3: Tex., pt. 2, p. 587.

16. S2, vol. 8: Ark., pt. 1, p. 105; Baker and Baker, *WPA Oklahoma Slave Narratives,* pp. 126, 172. Grayson eventually married and gave birth to ten children.

17. Perdue, Barden, and Phillips, *Weevils in the Wheat,* pp. 33, 71, 128.

18. S2, vol. 8: Ark., pt. 1, pp. 128–129, 299, and vol. 11: Mo., pp. 303–304.

19. Baker and Baker, *WPA Oklahoma Slave Narratives*, pp. 19, 22n2. The classic study of the slaveholder's conception of honor is Bertram Wyatt-Brown, *Southern Honor: Ethics and Behavior in the Old South* (New York: Oxford University Press, 1982). See also Drew Gilpin Faust, *James Henry Hammond and the Old South: A Design for Mastery* (Baton Rouge: Louisiana State University Press, 1982); Walter Johnson, *Soul by Soul: Life Inside the Antebellum Slave Market* (Cambridge, Mass.: Harvard University Press, 1999); and Ariela J. Gross, *Double Character: Slavery and Mastery in the Antebellum Southern Courtroom* (Princeton: Princeton University Press, 2000).

20. SS2, vol. 2: Tex., pt. 1, p. 26; Schwartz, *Born in Bondage*, chap. 7.

21. S1, vol. 2: S.C., pt. 2, p. 23; S2, vol. 8: Ark., pt. 1, pp. 122–123, and pt. 2, p. 132, and vol. 15: N.C., pt. 2, pp. 78, 98, and vol. 17: Fla., pp. 101, 127, 168; SS2, vol. 2: Tex., pt. 1, p. 26; Schwartz, *Born in Bondage*, chap. 7.

22. James Trussell and Richard Steckel, "The Age of Slaves at Menarche and Their First Birth," *Journal of Interdisciplinary Studies* 8 (winter 1978): 492.

23. S2, vol. 8: Ark., pt. 1, p. 211, and vol. 15: N.C., pt. 2, p. 434, and vol. 17: Fla., pp. 127–128, 167, 185; SS2, vol. 3: Tex., pt. 2, p. 555, and vol. 10: Tex., pt. 7, pp. 4121–23.

24. S2, vol. 8: Ark., pt. 1, p. 119, and vol. 10: Ark., pt. 6, p. 223; SS2, vol. 10: Tex., pt. 9, p. 4158.

25. SS2, vol. 2: Tex., pt. 1, pp. 105–106.

26. S2, vol. 17: Fla., p. 110; SS1, vol. 9: Miss., pt. 4, p. 1801; SS2, vol. 10: Tex., pt. 9, pp. 3985, 3998, 4065, 4110, 4158.

27. S2, vol. 14: N.C., pt. 1, pp. 30–31; SS2, vol. 10: Tex., pt. 9, p. 4362. For an example of a slave woman who believed she had been born of a forced pairing, see Baker and Baker, *WPA Oklahoma Slave Narratives*, pp. 140–141.

28. SS2, vol. 10: Tex., pt. 9, pp. 4295–96. On trickster tales, see Lawrence W. Levine, *Black Culture and Black Consciousness: Afro-American Folk Thought from Slavery to Freedom* (New York: Oxford University Press, 1977), chap. 2.

29. S1, vol. 3: S.C., pt. 4, p. 243; S2, vol. 16: Kans., Ky., Md., Ohio, Va., and Tenn., pt. 8, p. 33; SS2, vol. 2: Tex., pt. 1, pp. 303, 305, 309–310, 317, 322; Perdue, Barden, and Phillips, *Weevils in the Wheat*, p. 198; Virginia Pound Brown and Laurella Owens, eds., *Toting the Lead Row: Ruby Pickens Tartt, Alabama Folklorist* (University: University of Alabama Press, 1981), p. 148.

30. William G. Craghead, "Case of Catamenial Retention from Imperforated Hyman," *The Stethoscope* 5 (April 1855): 193; Steven M. Stowe, ed., *A Southern Practice: The Diary and Autobiography of Charles A. Hentz, M.D.* (Charlottesville: University Press of Virginia, 2000), p. 541; Ronald L. Baker, comp., *Homeless,*

Friendless, and Penniless: The WPA Interviews with Former Slaves Living in Indiana (Bloomington: Indiana University Press, 2000), pp. 117, 245; Perdue, Barden, and Phillips, *Weevils in the Wheat,* pp. 84, 117, 257; Baker and Baker, *WPA Oklahoma Slave Narratives,* p. 506; S2, vol. 8: Ark., pt. 1, pp. 51, 250, and pt. 2, p. 35, and vol. 9: Ark., pt. 3, pp. 25, 218, 340; Thelma Jennings, "'Us Colored Women Had to Go Though a Plenty'": Sexual Exploitation of African-American Slave Women," *Journal of Women's History* 1 (winter 1990): 60–66; Frederick Douglass, *Narrative of Frederick Douglass* (New York: Dover, 1995), p. 2.

31. Howard A. Kelly and Walter L. Burrage, *Dictionary of American Medical Biography* (Boston: Milford House, 1971), pp. 142, 932; Warren Stone, "Observations upon Diseases of the Uterus," *New Orleans Medical News and Hospital Gazette* 1 (1 November 1854): 341, also p. 350.

32. John R. Turner, "Plantation Hygiene," *Southern Cultivator* 15 (May–June 1857), in Breeden, *Advice among Masters,* p. 195; "Sterility among Negroes: A Case from a Country Practitioner," *New Orleans Medical News and Hospital Gazette* 3 (1 September 1856): 391–392.

33. "Bibliographical," *Atlanta Journal of Medicine and Surgery* 2 (November 1856): 185; W. Tyler Smith, "A Course of Lectures on the Theory and Practice of Obstetrics," *New Orleans Medical News and Hospital Gazette* 3 (April 1856): 112.

34. Deborah Gray White, *Ar'n't I a Woman? Female Slaves in the Plantation South* (New York: Norton, 1985), p. 31.

35. Steven M. Stowe, "Seeing Themselves at Work: Physicians and the Case Narrative in the Mid-Nineteenth-Century American South," *American Historical Review* 101 (February 1996): 41. See also Lamar Riley Murphy, *Enter the Physician: The Transformation of Domestic Medicine, 1760–1860* (Tuscaloosa: University of Alabama Press, 1991); John Duffy, *From Humors to Medical Science: A History of American Medicine,* 2d ed. (Urbana: University of Illinois Press, 1993), p. 23.

36. Ira Berlin has discussed the growing paternalistic attitudes of planters in *Generations of Captivity: A History of African-American Slaves* (Cambridge, Mass.: Belknap Press of Harvard University Press, 2003), chap. 2.

2. Healers

1. J. Y. Bassett, "Report on the Topography, Climate, and Diseases of the Parish of Madison Co., Ala.," *Southern Medical Reports* 1 (1849): 264.

2. John Harley Warner, *The Therapeutic Perspective: Medical Practice, Knowledge, and Identity in America, 1820–1885* (Princeton: Princeton University Press, 1997), p. 12; James O. Breeden, "States-Rights Medicine in the Old South,"

Bulletin of the New York Academy of Medicine 52 (March–April 1976): 3481; John Duffy, ed., *The Rudolph Matas History of Medicine in Louisiana,* vol. 1 ([Baton Rouge]: Louisiana State University Press, 1958), pp. 269–270; Sally G. McMillen, *Motherhood in the Old South: Pregnancy, Childbirth, and Infant Rearing* (Baton Rouge: Louisiana State University Press, 1990), pp. 9–15. This approach to healing, which was characteristic of American colonial physicians, was falling out of favor by the 1830s in the North. See John Duffy, *From Humors to Medical Science: A History of American Medicine,* 2d ed. (Urbana: University of Illinois Press, 1993), p. 14.

3. Those scholars who note differences in black and white medical practice in the Old South include Todd L. Savitt, "Black Health on the Plantation: Masters, Slaves, and Physicians," in *Science and Medicine in the Old South,* ed. Ronald L. Numbers and Todd L. Savitt (Baton Rouge: Louisiana State University Press, 1989), pp. 351–354; idem, *Medicine and Slavery: The Diseases and Health Care of Blacks in Antebellum Virginia* (Urbana: University of Illinois Press, 1978); Sharla M. Fett, *Working Cures: Healing, Health, and Power on Southern Slave Plantations* (Chapel Hill: University of North Carolina Press, 2002); Lawrence W. Levine, *Black Culture and Black Consciousness: Afro-American Folk Thought from Slavery to Freedom* (New York: Oxford University Press, 1977), pp. 63–66; William Dosite Postell, *The Health of Slaves on Southern Plantations* (Gloucester, Mass.: Peter Smith, 1970), p. 108; Richard H. Shryock, "Medical Practice in the Old South," *South Atlantic Quarterly* 29 (1930): 172. See also S2, vol. 8: Ark., pt. 1, p. 124; T. Lindsay Baker and Julie P. Baker, eds., *The WPA Oklahoma Slave Narratives* (Norman: University of Oklahoma Press, 1996), pp. 206–207, 289. The idea that sickness can originate in either the physical or the supernatural has been found to exist among many people throughout history. See Roy Porter, *The Greatest Benefit to Mankind: A Medical History of Humanity* (New York: Norton, 1997), pp. 33–34.

4. *New Orleans Medical News and Hospital Gazette* 1 (15 April 1854): 54; Duffy, *From Humors to Medical Science,* p. 31; Charles E. Rosenberg, "The Therapeutic Revolution: Medicine, Meaning, and Social Change in Nineteenth-Century America," in *The Therapeutic Revolution: Essays in the Social History of American Medicine,* ed. Morris J. Vogel and Charles E. Rosenberg ([Philadelphia]: University of Pennsylvania Press, 1979), p. 10; Fett, *Working Cures,* pp. 38, 43.

5. On alternative medicine in the mid-nineteenth century, see Alex Berman and Michael A. Flannery, *America's Botanico-Medical Movements: Vox Populi* (New York: Pharmaceutical Products Press, 2001); John S. Haller Jr., *Medical Protestants: The Eclectics in American Medicine, 1825–1939* (Carbondale: Southern Illinois University Press, 1994); James C. Whorton, *Nature Cures: The History of Alternative Medicine in America* (New York: Oxford University Press, 2002);

William G. Rothstein, *American Physicians in the Nineteenth Century: From Sects to Science* (Baltimore: Johns Hopkins University Press, 1972), chaps. 7 and 8.

6. Duffy, *From Humors to Medical Science,* pp. 130, 144, 203; Dwayne D. Cox and William J. Morison, *The University of Louisville* (Lexington: University Press of Kentucky, 2000), p. 25.

7. Steven M. Stowe, *Doctoring the South: Southern Physicians and Everyday Medicine in the Mid-Nineteenth Century* (Chapel Hill: University of North Carolina Press, 2004), pp. 24, 69.

8. J. Marion Sims, *The Story of My Life* (New York: Da Capo, 1968), p. 150.

9. Stowe, *Doctoring the South,* pp. 55, 281n29; Rothstein, *American Physicians in the Nineteenth Century,* p. 92; Judith Walzer Leavitt, *Brought to Bed: Childbearing in America, 1750–1950* (New York: Oxford University Press, 1986), p. 40.

10. This description applies to physicians throughout the nation; Duffy, *From Humors to Medical Science,* pp. 141, 182; Lamar Riley Murphy, *Enter the Physician: The Transformation of Domestic Medicine, 1760–1860* (Tuscaloosa: University of Alabama Press, 1991), pp. 107–108. By the 1840s the tendency of the public to judge practitioners by genteel criteria was breaking down, according to Martin S. Pernick, *A Calculus of Suffering: Pain, Professionalism, and Anesthesia in Nineteenth-Century America* (New York: Columbia University Press, 1985), p. 68. I contend that this trend obtained much less in the South than in the North.

11. Wilma King, ed., *A Northern Woman in the Plantation South: Letters of Tryphena Blanche Holder Fox, 1856–1876* (Columbia: University of South Carolina Press, 1993), p. 52; Jean V. Berlin, ed., *A Confederate Nurse: The Diary of Ada W. Bacot, 1860–1863* (Columbia: University of South Carolina Press, 1994), p. 40; Sims, *The Story of My Life,* pp. 153, 154, 159.

12. Herbert M. Morais, *The History of the Afro-American in Medicine* (Cornwells Heights, Pa.: Publisher's Agency, 1978), p. 17; T. K. Leonard, M.D., Miccosukie, Fla., 2 February 1866, LR, June 1865–June 1869, Series 586, RG 105; Steven M. Stowe, "Obstetrics and the Work of Doctoring in the Mid-Nineteenth-Century American South," *Bulletin of the History of Medicine* 64 (winter 1990): 547; "Negro Hospital," *Charleston Medical Journal and Review* 15 (November 1860): 851.

13. Stowe, *Doctoring the South,* pp. 8–9; William Dosite Postell, "The Doctor in the Old South," *South Atlantic Quarterly* 51 (1952): 397; Arnold [to Dr. Herber Chase, Philadelphia], 13 October 1836, in *Letters of Richard D. Arnold, M.D., 1808–1876,* ed. Richard H. Shryock (New York: AMS, 1970), p. 13; Steven M. Stowe, ed., *A Southern Practice: The Diary and Autobiography of Charles A. Hentz, M.D.* (Charlottesville: University Press of Virginia, 2000), pp. 530, 531, 536;

Donald P. McNeilly, *The Old South Frontier: Cotton Plantations and the Forma-tion of Arkansas Society, 1819–1861* (Fayetteville: University of Arkansas Press, 2000), p. 56; S2, vol. 15: N.C., pt. 2, p. 77. When one retiring physician offered his practice in southwestern Virginia for sale in 1854, he estimated the projected income at between $2,500 and $3,000 annually; advertisement, *The Stethoscope* 4 (September 1854): n.p. Not everyone agreed that doctors moving to the South could reap great profits. See George Rosen, *Fees and Fee Bills: Some Economic Aspects of Medical Practice in Nineteenth Century America* (Baltimore: Johns Hop-kins Press, 1946), p. 18. On the relative financial well-being of antebellum and postwar medical practitioners, see S. H. Stout, "An Address, Introductory of the Eighth Regular Summer Course of Lectures in the Atlanta Medical College," *Atlanta Medical and Surgical Journal* 7B (July 1866): 206. Particular places in the South came to have a superabundance of physicians from the viewpoint of doc-tors trying to make a living. See Stowe, *A Southern Practice*, p. 66; idem, *Doctor-ing the South*, p. 276n12.

14. Arney R. Childs, ed., *Rice Planter and Sportsman: The Recollections of J. Motte Alston, 1821–1909* (Columbia: University of South Carolina Press, 1999), p. 47; Rosen, *Fees and Fee Bills*, pp. 29, 43; S2, vol. 15: N.C., pt. 2, p. 58; Celsus, "Year Practice—Hireling Doctors," *The Stethoscope and Virginia Medical Gazette* 3 (April 1853): 238; "Tariff of Fees, Etc.," *The Stethoscope* 4 (January 1854): 99; King, *Northern Woman in Plantation South*, pp. 35, 48. Many former slaves recalled a plantation physician when they were interviewed by representatives of the federal Works Progress Administration in the 1930s. See for example Baker and Baker, *WPA Oklahoma Slave Narratives*, pp. 26, 271, 333.

15. Bennett H. Wall, "Medical Care of Ebenezer Pettigrew's Slaves," *Mississippi Valley Historical Review* 37 (1950): 460–461; Stowe, *Doctoring the South*, p. 81. Tryphena Blanche Holder Fox's behavior suggests that physicians' wives played a role in pleasing paying customers. This physician's wife tried her best "to keep on the right side" of the mistresses in the neighborhood, even those she disliked, so as not to harm her husband's practice; King, *Northern Woman in Plantation South*, p. 46. Judith Walzer Leavitt demonstrates that physicians whose practice took them to the homes of patients might alter medical practices to suit family and friends. See "'A Worrying Profession': The Domestic Environment of Med-ical Practice in Mid-Nineteenth-Century America," *Bulletin of the History of Medicine* 69 (1995): 26, 28.

16. Charlotte Ann Allston to Robert F. W. Allston, 19 April 1820, in J. S. East-erby, ed., *The South Carolina Rice Plantation as Revealed in the Papers of Robert F. W. Allston* (Chicago: University of Chicago Press, 1946), p. 54; S2, vol. 15: N.C., pt. 2, p. 58; SS2, vol. 3: Tex., pt. 2, p. 930; Jan Furman, ed., *Slavery in the Clover Bottoms: John McCline's Narrative of His Life during Slavery and the Civil*

War (Knoxville: University of Tennessee Press, 1998), p. 12. See also S2, vol. 9: Ark., pt. 3, p. 2, and vol. 14: N.C., pt. 1, pp. 170, 273, and vol. 17: Fla., pp. 196–197, 242; SS1, vol. 9: Miss., pt. 4, p. 1472; SS2, vol. 10: Tex., pt. 9, pp. 3950, 4068, 4281; Sims, *The Story of My Life,* pp. 148, 190, 201; James Oakes, *The Ruling Race: A History of American Slaveholders* (New York: Knopf, 1982), p. 40; Stowe, *Doctoring the South,* p. 78.

17. Claudia L. Bushman, *In Old Virginia: Slavery, Farming, and Society in the Journal of John Walker* (Baltimore: Johns Hopkins University Press, 2002), 213; Oakes, *The Ruling Race,* p. 63; Duffy, *Rudolph Matas History of Medicine,* pp. 290–307; Rosen, *Fees and Fee Bills,* p. 19; William K. Scarborough, "Science on the Plantation," in Numbers and Savitt, *Science and Medicine in the Old South,* pp. 88–90; McNeilly, *The Old South Frontier,* pp. 72–77. Some northern physicians also found it difficult to support their families with income from a medical practice, and many turned to farming. See Leavitt, "'A Worrying Profession,'" p. 9. Former slaves recalled numerous owners who both planted and practiced medicine; see Baker and Baker, *WPA Oklahoma Slave Narratives,* pp. 132, 184, 200, 208, 214, 265, 365, 406; S2, vol. 8: Ark., pt. 2, p. 232, and vol. 15: N.C., pt. 2, pp. 287, 433.

18. McNeilly, *The Old South Frontier,* pp. 72–77; Ira Berlin et al., eds., *Free at Last: A Documentary History of Slavery, Freedom, and the Civil War* (New York: New Press, 1992), pp. 356–357; S2, vol. 10: Ark., pt. 6, pp. 111, 216; SS2, vol. 3: Tex., pt. 2, p. 880.

19. Elizabeth Barnaby Keeney, "Unless Powerful Sick: Domestic Medicine in the Old South," in Numbers and Savitt, *Science and Medicine in the Old South,* pp. 280–281; advertisements, *Atlanta Medical and Surgical Journal* 7A (October 1861): n.p.; Murphy, *Enter the Physician,* pp. 18–19, 28, 61; Stowe, *Doctoring the South,* pp. 28–29.

20. Murphy, *Enter the Physician,* pp. 63–67, 78–80, 93.

21. Neblett's father-in-law was a physician, which may explain why she came to have a copy of Beach in her possession. Erika L. Murr, ed., *A Rebel Wife in Texas: The Diary and Letters of Elizabeth Scott Neblett, 1852–1864* (Baton Rouge: Louisiana State University Press, 2001), p. 251. On Beach, see Duffy, *From Humors to Medical Science,* p. 83.

22. Melanie Pavich-Lindsay, ed., *Anna: The Letters of a St. Simons Island Plantation Mistress, 1817–1859* (Athens: University of Georgia Press, 2002), p. 321; Wall, "Medical Care of Ebenezer Pettigrew's Slaves," pp. 453, 470.

23. C. R. Harris, "The Epidemic of Puerperal Fever of Mount Solon and Vicinity," *The Stethoscope and Virginia Medical Gazette* 2 (July 1852): 379. On home care of slaves by slaveholders, see Savitt, *Medicine and Slavery,* pp. 153–161. On

home care among southern whites, see Kay K. Moss, *Southern Folk Medicine, 1750–1820* (Columbia: University of South Carolina Press, 1999). See also Keeney, "Unless Powerful Sick," pp. 276–277, 281–285.

24. E. M. Pendleton, "Reports from Georgia: General Report on the Topography, Climate, and Diseases of Middle Georgia," *Southern Medical Reports* 1 (1849): 336–337; Todd L. Savitt, "Patient Letters to an Early Nineteenth Century Virginia Physician," *Journal of the Florida Medical Association* 69 (1982): 690–691; James Douglass to Charles Brown, Charles Brown Papers, Manuscripts and Rare Books Department, Swem Library, College of William and Mary; S2, vol. 8: Ark., pt. 2, p. 294; SS2, vol. 3: Tex., pt. 2, p. 646, also p. 710; A. S. Helmick, "An Interesting Case in Practice," *The Stethoscope* 5 (December 1855): 717.

25. James Douglass to Charles Brown, Charles Brown Papers; letters from Charles R. Battaile, 16 November 1827; John W. Selden, 17 February [18—]; Elizabeth Gordon, 17 October [18—]; Polly Fox, [18—]; William Jones, 4 March [18—]; all in Letters to Doctor James Carmichael and Son, Historical Collections at the Claude Moore Health Sciences Library, University of Virginia, http://etext.lib.virginia.edu/healthsci/carmichael/collection. Vitriol (sulfuric acid) was sometimes used to stem hemorrhaging; see Moss, *Southern Folk Medicine*, p. 210. The bark referred to was no doubt Peruvian bark (also known as cinchona), which was used for a variety of ailments. Laudanum was prepared from opium. Charles E. Rosenberg has observed that home remedies and the therapies associated with orthodox physicians were based on similar assumptions generally within the United States; "The Therapeutic Revolution," p. 13.

26. Letters from William Jones, 4 March [18—]; Charles R. Battaile, 30 May 1826; N. Seddon, [18—]; William Richardson, 4 August 1828; Lucy Alexander, 2 November 1826; George W. B. Spooner, [18–]; Ann G. Patton, 23 January 1820; William Payne, 17 August 1828; Brodie S. Hull, 24 September 1821; E. Herndon, 13 May [18—]; all in Letters to Doctor James Carmichael and Son; Pavich-Lindsay, *Anna*, p. 333.

27. Ray Mathis, *John Horry Dent: South Carolina Aristocrat on the Alabama Frontier* (University: University of Alabama Press, 1979), p. 84.

28. Advertisement, *Atlanta Medical and Surgical Journal* 4 (June 1859): n.p.; advertisement, *The Stethoscope and Virginia Medical Gazette* 3 (February 1853): n.p.; advertisement, ibid., 1 (February 1851): n.p.; advertisement, *Atlanta Medical and Surgical Journal* 7A (October 1861): n.p.; SS2, vol. 1: Ala., Ariz., Ark., and Other Narratives, p. 54, and vol. 3: Tex., pt. 2, p. 513.

29. Robert Collins, "Essay on the Treatment and Management of Slaves," *Southern Cultivator* 12 (July 1854), in *Advice among Masters: The Ideal in Slave*

Management in the Old South, ed. James O. Breeden (Westport, Conn.: Greenwood, 1980), p. 23; S2, vol. 14: N.C., pt. 1, p. 290; letter from N. Seddon, 2 May 1828, Letters to Doctor James Carmichael and Son; Pavich-Lindsay, *Anna,* p. 394; Wall, "Medical Care of Ebenezer Pettigrew's Slaves," pp. 454–455; Bushman, *In Old Virginia,* p. 168; G. W. Cocke, letter to the editor, *The Stethoscope and Virginia Medical Gazette* 3 (April 1853): 220–221. See also Childs, *Rice Planter and Sportsman,* p. 57; Charles E. Rosenberg, "Introduction to the New Edition," in *Gunn's Domestic Medicine: A Facsimile of the First Edition,* Tennesseeana ed. (Knoxville: University of Tennessee Press, 1986), p. xvi.

30. Pendleton, "Reports from Georgia," p. 336; Ariela J. Gross, *Double Character: Slavery and Mastery in the Antebellum Southern Courtroom* (Princeton: Princeton University Press, 2000), p. 104; William Hampton Adams, "Health and Medical Care on Antebellum Southern Plantations," *Plantation Society* 2 (May 1989): 266; Keeney, "Unless Powerful Sick," p. 291; Morais, *The Afro-American in Medicine,* p. 17; Franklin, "Overseers," *Carolina Planter* 1 (August 1844), in Breeden, *Advice among Masters,* p. 297; Collins, "Treatment and Management of Slaves," p. 23; Savitt, *Medicine and Slavery,* pp. 156–159.

31. Brickell quoted in Felice Swados, "Negro Health on the Ante Bellum Plantations," *Bulletin of the History of Medicine* 10 (1941): 460–472; J. B. Garden, "Pneumonia," *The Stethoscope* 5 (January 1855): 3; Harris, "The Epidemic of Puerperal Fever," p. 380; Gross, *Double Character,* p. 104. The award by the Alabama court was limited to the value of the contract for hire, rather than to the worth of her person sold on the market.

32. SS2, vol. 10: Tex., pt. 9, p. 3911; Mrs. N. B. DeSaussure, *Old Plantation Days: Being Recollections of Southern Life before the Civil War* (New York: Duffield, 1909), pp. 17, 36–37, 63; T. L. Ogier, "Amenorrhea Treated Successfully with the Water Pepper," *Southern Journal of Medicine and Pharmacy* 1 (May 1846): 298.

33. Thomas H. Todd, "On the Use of Cathartics in Retention of the Placenta," *Western Journal of Medicine and Surgery* 7 (May 1843): 350; A. T. Noe, "Treatment of Dysmenorrhea by Mechanical Dilation," *Nashville Journal of Medicine and Surgery* 3, no. 4 (1852): 347; R. L. Scruggs, "Medical and Obstetric Cases," *Western Journal of Medicine and Surgery,* 2d ser., 7 (March 1847): 199; Walter Fisher, "Physicians and Slavery in the Antebellum Southern Medical Journal," *Journal of the History of Medicine and Allied Sciences* 23 (January 1968): 42; Savitt, *Medicine and Slavery,* pp. 160–161; Catherine Clinton, *The Plantation Mistress: Woman's World in the Old South* (New York: Pantheon, 1982), pp. 28, 143–147.

34. Postell, *Health of Slaves on Southern Plantations,* p. 105.

35. SS2, vol. 3: Tex., pt. 2, p. 803; Fett, *Working Cures*, pp. 147–158; Eugene D. Genovese, *Roll, Jordan, Roll: The World the Slaves Made* (New York: Vintage, 1976), pp. 225–226; Levine, *Black Culture and Black Consciousness*, pp. 63–65; Savitt, *Medicine and Slavery*, p. 149. Doctors were known to castrate slaves at the behest of the state. See Petition of Samuel Kerfott, in *The Southern Debate over Slavery*, ed. Loren Schweninger, vol. 1: *Petitions to Southern Legislatures, 1778–1864* (Urbana: University of Illinois Press, 2001), pp. 38–39; Clarence L. Mohr, *On the Threshold of Freedom: Masters and Slaves in Civil War Georgia* (Athens: University of Georgia Press, 1986), p. 220.

36. SS2, vol. 1: Ala., Ariz., Ark., and Other Narratives, p. 136.

37. Baker and Baker, *WPA Oklahoma Slave Narratives*, p. 323; letters from William Herndon Jr., 27 January and 15 February 1820, Letters to Doctor James Carmichael and Son; Savitt, "Black Health on the Plantation," p. 351.

38. Frances Webster to Frances Kirby Smith, 10 August 1851, in *The Websters: Letters of an American Army Family in Peace and War, 1836–1853*, ed. Van R. Baker (Kent, Ohio: Kent State University Press, 2000), pp. 262–263; S2, vol. 15: N.C., pt. 2, pp. 373–374. See also vol. 14: N.C., pt. 1, p. 108; S1, vol. 2: S.C., pt. 1, p. 125; letters from George Banks, 10 August 1826, and William Jackson Jr., 25 July 1823, Letters to Doctor James Carmichael and Son. Wormseed is also known as Jerusalem oak.

39. SS2, vol. 3: Tex., pt. 2, pp. 849–850.

40. Baker and Baker, *WPA Oklahoma Slave Narratives*, p. 121; Helmick, "An Interesting Case in Practice," p. 719; Bushman, *In Old Virginia*, p. 156; DeSaussure, *Old Plantation Days*, pp. 36–37; Fett, *Working Cures*, pp. 176, 120–122; Savitt, *Medicine and Slavery*, p. 162.

41. Morais, *The Afro-American in Medicine*, pp. 16–17; Childs, *Rice Planter and Sportsman*, p. 57; Sims, *The Story of My Life*, p. 116; Duffy, *From Humors to Medical Science*, p. 102.

42. Bassett, "Topography, Climate, and Diseases of Madison Co., Ala.," p. 264; Edwin Adams Davis, ed., *Plantation Life in the Florida Parishes of Louisiana, 1836–1846, as Reflected in the Diary of Bennet H. Barrow* (New York: Columbia University Press, 1943), pp. 265, 266, 299–300, 365.

43. Davis, *Plantation Life in Louisiana*, pp. 198, 269.

44. Rosenberg, "The Therapeutic Revolution," p. 14; Drew Gilpin Faust, *James Henry Hammond and the Old South: A Design for Mastery* (Baton Rouge: Louisiana State University Press, 1982), pp. 77–82, 132; Plantation Manual of James H. Hammond of Beach Island, South Carolina, ca. 1834, Joseph I. Waring Research Files, Waring Historical Library, Medical University of South Carolina, Charleston.

45. Murphy, *Enter the Physician*, pp. 92–93; Walker quoted in Bushman, *In Old Virginia*, p. 72; see also pp. 7, 81, 152–153, 156–157.

46. S2, vol. 9: Ark., pt. 3, p. 333, and vol. 11: Mo., p. 1, and vol. 15: N.C., pt. 2, pp. 394, 435; SS1, vol. 6: Miss., pt. 1, p. 267, and vol. 9: Miss., pt. 4, p. 1480; SS2, vol. 3: Tex., pt. 2, pp. 734, 914; Baker and Baker, *WPA Oklahoma Slave Narratives*, p. 72.

47. J. Douglass, "Ergot in Placenta Previa—Abortion at Three Months, Delivery of Another Child Six Months After," *Charleston Medical Journal and Review* 15 (March 1860): 328; Moses Roper, *A Narrative of the Adventures and Escape of Moses Roper, from American Slavery*, 4th ed. (London: Harvey and Darton, 1840), p. 5; Baker and Baker, *WPA Oklahoma Slave Narratives*, p. 209; Harriet A. Jacobs, *Incidents in the Life of a Slave Girl*, ed. Jean Fagin Yellin (Cambridge, Mass.: Harvard University Press, 1987), p. 61; S2, vol. 8: Ark., pt. 2, p. 84, and vol. 9: Ark., pt. 3, p. 329, and vol. 10: Ark., pt. 5, p. 310; Deborah Kuhn McGregor, *From Midwives to Medicine: The Birth of American Gynecology* (New Brunswick, N.J.: Rutgers University Press, 1998), p. 32.

48. Bushman, *In Old Virginia*, pp. 5, 66, 152–153; William Ed Grimé, *Ethno-Botany of the Black Americans* (Algonac, Mich.: Reference Publications, 1979), p. 67; Petition of Residents of Maury, Bedford, Giles, Hickman, Williamson, and Lincoln Counties, in Schweninger, *The Southern Debate over Slavery*, pp. 137–139; Fett, *Working Cures*, p. 47; Morais, *The Afro-American in Medicine*, pp. 12–14.

49. John R. Hicks, "African Consumption," *The Stethoscope* 4 (November 1854): 628; "Medico-Chirurgical Society of the City of Richmond—First March Meeting," *The Stethoscope and Virginia Medical Gazette* 3 (April 1853): 231. For an earlier case in Virginia (1777) see Petition of Archer Payne, in Schweninger, *The Southern Debate over Slavery*, p. 3. Medicine was not the only area in which slaves learned more about their owners' practices than vice versa. See for example Sidney W. Mintz and Richard Price, *The Birth of African-American Culture: An Anthropological Perspective* (Boston: Beacon, 1992), p. 28.

50. John Thornton discusses the idea that enslaved people might select aspects of European, Euroamerican, or Amerindian culture for incorporation into their own understanding of aesthetics; *Africa and Africans in the Making of the Atlantic World, 1400–1680* (New York: Cambridge University Press, 1992), p. 224. See also Mintz and Price, *The Birth of African-American Culture*, p. 45.

51. Baker and Baker, *WPA Oklahoma Slave Narratives*, pp. 328–331, 333; S2, vol. 17: Fla., p. 136; SS2, vol. 1: Ala., Ariz., Ark., and Other Narratives, pp. 181, 185, 196–198; Yvonne Chireau, "The Uses of the Supernatural: Toward a History of Black Women's Magical Powers," in *A Mighty Baptism: Race, Gender, and*

the Creation of American Protestantism, ed. Susan Juster and Lisa MacFarlane (Ithaca: Cornell University Press, 1996), p. 177; David H. Brown, "Conjure/ Doctors: An Exploration of a Black Discourse in America, Antebellum to 1940," *Folklore Forum* 23 (1990): 8; Elliott J. Gorn, "Black Magic: Folk Beliefs of the Slave Community," in Numbers and Savitt, *Science and Medicine in the Old South*, pp. 295–326.

52. S2, vol. 14: N.C., pt. 2, pp. 128–129; SS1, vol. 7: Miss., pt. 2, pp. 722, 723, 724, and vol. 9: Miss., pt. 4, p. 1888; Fett, *Working Cures*, p. 101. White conjurers were not unknown. See S2, vol. 15: N.C., pt. 2, p. 361.

53. SS1, vol. 7: Miss., pt. 2, pp. 722–724.

54. Fett, *Working Cures*, p. 107.

55. S2, vol. 9: Ark., pt. 3, p. 114; SS2, vol. 10: Tex., pt. 9, pp. 4024–25, 4027; A. G. Grinnan, "Remarks on the Topography and Diseases of Madison County, Virginia," *The Stethoscope and Virginia Medical Gazette* 3 (March 1853): 131; Stowe, *Doctoring the South*, p. 51.

56. SS2, vol. 1: Ala., Ariz., Ark., and Other Narratives, p. 118, and vol. 3: Tex., pt. 2, p. 513, and vol. 10: Tex., pt. 9, p. 3916. Slaves from Surinam used hot peppers to restore health; Grimé, *Ethno-Botany of the Black Americans*, p. 88.

57. S2, vol. 10: Ark., pt. 6, p. 266; SS1, vol. 9: Miss., pt. 4, p. 1842; SS2, vol. 3: Tex., pt. 2, p. 550.

58. S2, vol. 14: N.C., pt. 1, p. 170, and vol. 15: N.C., pt. 2, p. 346; SS1, vol. 7: Miss., pt. 2, p. 697, and vol. 9: Miss., pt. 4, pp. 1716, 1872. For a former slave who did not believe in charms, see SS1, vol. 9: Miss., pt. 4, p. 1492.

59. S2, vol. 8: Ark., pt. 2, p. 39; SS2, vol. 1: Ala., Ariz., Ark., and Other Narratives, p. 199; Postell, *Health of Slaves on Southern Plantations*, p. 108.

60. Not all slaves believed in signs, but many former slaves interviewed in the 1930s by WPA workers expressed such beliefs. See for example S2, vol. 9: Ark., pt. 3, p. 251, and vol. 10: Ark., pt. 6, p. 267, and vol. 11: Ark., pt. 7, pp. 182, 188; SS1, vol. 7: Miss., pt. 2, pp. 515, 639, and vol. 9: Miss., pt. 4, p. 1674; SS2, vol. 1: Ala., Ariz., Ark., and Other Narratives, pp. 93, 98.

61. S2, vol. 9: Ark., pt. 3, p. 234, and vol. 17: Fla., p. 188; SS2, vol. 1: Ala., Ariz., Ark., and Other Narratives, pp. 127, 130.

62. SS2, vol. 10: Tex., pt. 9, p. 3980; Pavich-Lindsay, *Anna*, p. 333; Bushman, *In Old Virginia*, p. 160; Davis, *Plantation Life in Louisiana*, pp. 185, 201, 269, 297, 320; Tidyman quoted in Fett, *Working Cures*, p. 139.

63. E. M. Pendleton, "On the Comparative Fecundity of the Caucasian and African Races," *Charleston Medical Journal and Review* 6 (1851): 351.

3. Fertility

1. William N. Morgan, "A Case of Rupture of the Uterus, with Artificial Anus at the Point of Rupture," *Western Journal of Medicine and Surgery,* 2d ser., 2 (December 1844): 498–501. See also Robert Battey, "Cinchona in Menorrhagia—Case," *Atlanta Medical and Surgical Journal* 4 (August 1859): 734–735.

2. Southron, "The Policy of the Southern Planter," *American Cotton Planter and Soil of the South,* n.s., 1 (October 1857), in *Advice among Masters: The Ideal in Slave Management in the Old South,* ed. James O. Breeden (Westport, Conn.: Greenwood, 1980), p. 47; James Oakes, *The Ruling Race: A History of American Slaveholders* (New York: Knopf, 1982), p. 74; "Judge Daniels Estimate of the Value of James River Low Grounds and Slave Labor—(Unique)," Cocke Family Papers, University of Virginia Library, Charlottesville; Rusticus, "Plantation Management and Practice," *Cotton Planter and Soil* 1 (December 1857): 375; Edwin Morris Betts, ed., *Thomas Jefferson's Farm Book* (Princeton: Princeton University Press, 1953), p. 46; Henry Wiencek, *An Imperfect God: George Washington, His Slaves, and the Creation of America* (New York: Farrar, Straus and Giroux, 2003), p. 46; S2, vol. 11: Mo., p. 314, and vol. 15: N.C., pt. 2, p. 77.

3. S2, vol. 8: Ark., pt. 1, p. 105, and vol. 11: Mo., pp. 214, 314 (on the work of a blind slave woman, see vol. 17: Fla., p. 214); T. Lindsay Baker and Julie P. Baker, eds., *The WPA Oklahoma Slave Narratives* (Norman: University of Oklahoma Press, 1996), pp. 126, 172; W. Michael Byrd and Linda A. Clayton, *An American Health Dilemma,* vol. 1: *A Medical History of African Americans and the Problem of Race* (New York: Routledge, 2000), p. 282; Marie Jenkins Schwartz, *Born in Bondage: Growing Up Enslaved in the Antebellum South* (Cambridge, Mass.: Harvard University Press, 2000), pp. 187–192; Deborah Gray White, *Ar'n't I a Woman? Female Slaves in the Plantation South* (New York: Norton, 1985), pp. 101–102, 109–110.

4. John R. Turner, "Plantation Hygiene," *Southern Cultivator* 15 (May–June 1857), in Breeden, *Advice among Masters,* pp. 195, 203.

5. Deborah Kuhn McGregor, *From Midwives to Medicine: The Birth of American Gynecology* (New Brunswick, N.J.: Rutgers University Press, 1998), p. 153; Margaret Marsh and Wanda Ronner, *The Empty Cradle: Infertility in America from Colonial Times to the Present* (Baltimore: Johns Hopkins University Press, 1996), pp. 38–40, 48, 58; W. Tyler Smith, "A Course of Lectures on the Theory and Practice of Obstetrics," *New Orleans Medical News and Hospital Gazette* 3 (April 1856): 112; Walter Johnson, *Soul by Soul: Life Inside the Antebellum Slave Market* (Cambridge, Mass.: Harvard University Press, 1999), p. 149; Steven Weisenburger, *Modern Medea: A Family Story of Slavery and Child Murder from the Old*

South (New York: Hill and Wang, 1998), pp. 265–266, 325n58; Reginald Horsman, *Josiah Nott of Mobile: Southerner, Physician, and Racial Theorist* (Baton Rouge: Louisiana State University Press, 1987), pp. 86–88, 91, 97; Juriah Harriss, "What Constitutes Unsoundness in a Negro?" *Savannah Journal of Medicine* 1 (September 1858): 145–147 and (January 1859): 293–294 (published in two parts).

6. Brenda E. Stevenson, *Life in Black and White: Family and Community in the Slave South* (New York: Oxford University Press, 1996), p. 179.

7. Ronald L. Baker, comp., *Homeless, Friendless, and Penniless: The WPA Interviews with Former Slaves Living in Indiana* (Bloomington: Indiana University Press, 2000), pp. 129, 242; SS2, vol. 10: Tex., pt. 9, pp. 3905–06, 4119, 4124, 4241; Betsy's auctioneer quoted in White, *Ar'n't I a Woman?* p. 32.

8. Harriss, "What Constitutes Unsoundness in a Negro?" Laws varied with regard to guarantees of "soundness" in a slave. Georgia required purchasers to obtain a warranty from the seller; otherwise the purchaser forfeited the right to bring suit. South Carolina law presumed that all slaves were warranted as sound unless a special certificate stated the contrary. See Sharla M. Fett, *Working Cures: Healing, Health, and Power on Southern Slave Plantations* (Chapel Hill: University of North Carolina Press, 2002), p. 22. For a schedule of physician fees listing as a service "opinion for life insurance," see George Rosen, *Fees and Fee Bills: Some Economic Aspects of Medical Practice in Nineteenth Century America* (Baltimore: Johns Hopkins Press, 1946), p. 39.

9. W. Tyler Smith, "Tyler Smith's Lectures on Obstetrics," *New Orleans Medical News and Hospital Gazette* 3 (May 1856): 164–165.

10. Johnson, *Soul by Soul*, p. 137; "Medicine in Texas," *Nashville Medical Journal* 7 (November 1854): 422; James A. Tillman and John Norwood Ledgers, vol. 2: 1859–1868, Records of Ante-Bellum Southern Plantations from the Revolution through the Civil War, ed. Kenneth M. Stampp, University Publications of America, Series J: Selections from the Manuscripts Department, SHC.

11. Ariela J. Gross, *Double Character: Slavery and Mastery in the Antebellum Southern Courtroom* (Princeton: Princeton University Press, 2000), pp. 123, 127. For fee bills listing legal testimony as a service provided by doctors, see Rosen, *Fees and Fee Bills*, pp. 20, 39.

12. Gross, *Double Character*, pp. 33, 76–77. This was true for work skills as well. A purchaser could not recover the entire cost of a slave on the basis that he or she lacked a particular skill, even though the slave had been represented at the time of the sale as having the skill. However, the shortcoming could be considered alongside other factors. Any amount awarded would be the difference in the value of a slave with and without that particular skill.

13. Quoted in Johnson, *Soul by Soul,* p. 184.

14. Walter Fisher, "Physicians and Slavery in the Antebellum Southern Medical Journal," *Journal of the History of Medicine and Allied Sciences* 23 (January 1968): 40–41. Suits pertaining to reproductive health were not disproportionate to their incidence relative to other diseases; Gross, *Double Character,* pp. 128–129.

15. White, *Ar'n't I a Woman?* p. 101.

16. John H. Morgan, "An Essay on the Causes of the Production of Abortion among Our Negro Population," *Nashville Journal of Medicine and Surgery* 19 (August 1860): 123. There was growing faith among nineteenth-century physicians generally in the healing power of nature; John Harley Warner, *The Therapeutic Perspective: Medical Practice, Knowledge, and Identity in America, 1820–1885* (Princeton: Princeton University Press, 1997), p. 4. On knowledge of and treatments for infertility among the free population of the United States, see Marsh and Ronner, *The Empty Cradle.*

17. A. A. P., "Patterson's Cases," *Transylvania Medical Journal* 1 (February 1850): 325; J. F. Peebles, "Spontaneous Recovery from an Ovarian Tumor of Twenty Years Duration," *The Stethoscope and Virginia Medical Gazette* 1 (December 1851): 668; H. W. Caffey, "Case of Catalepsy, with Remarks," *Atlanta Medical and Surgical Journal* 2 (September 1856): 9–10; letter from Uril. Taliaferro, 23 December 1819, Letters to Doctor James Carmichael and Son, Historical Collections at the Claude Moore Health Sciences Library, University of Virginia, http://etext.lib.virginia.edu/healthsci/carmichael/collection; Samuel Sexton, "A Case of Extra-Uterine Pregnancy, with an Account of the Appearances on Dissection," *Western Journal of Medicine and Surgery* 1 (February 1840): 207–208. Sexton's slave died within three months of the initial examination; Gross, *Double Character,* pp. 136–137.

18. Charles E. Rosenberg, "The Therapeutic Revolution: Medicine, Meaning, and Social Change in Nineteenth-Century America," in *The Therapeutic Revolution: Essays in the Social History of American Medicine,* ed. Morris J. Vogel and Charles E. Rosenberg ([Philadelphia]: University of Pennsylvania Press, 1979), p. 6; J. Boring, "Vicarious Menstruation," *Atlanta Medical and Surgical Journal* 1 (December 1855): 211; John Overton, "A Case of Labour Attended by Some Unusual Appearances," *Western Journal of Medicine and Surgery* 5 (January 1842): 19. On the tendency of mid-nineteenth-century physicians to link a woman's physical and mental health to the functioning of her womb and its associated organs, see McGregor, *From Midwives to Medicine,* p. 71.

19. Robert E. Campbell, "Observations upon Menstruation—Its Cause, Character and Effects upon the Female Economy," *Atlanta Medical and Surgical Journal* 2 (September 1856): 10; "Annual Commencement of the Medical

Department of Hampden-Sidney College," *The Stethoscope and Virginia Medical Gazette* 3 (April 1853): 223–224; "Announcement of Dissertation Topics," *Atlanta Medical and Surgical Journal* 7A (October 1861): 114; "Annual Announcement of Lectures in the Atlanta Medical College for the Session of 1857 with a Catalogue of the Students and Graduates of 1856," ibid., 2 (August 1857), apps.; D. Warren Bricfell [Brickell], "Obstetric Notes and Reflections," *Atlanta Surgical and Medical Journal* 2 (May 1857): 540–541; "Menstruation," *New Orleans Medical News and Hospital Gazette* 3 (1 August 1856): 367–368; D. Warren Brickell, "Obstetric Notes and Reflections," ibid. (1 February 1857): 708–712; Steven M. Stowe, ed., *A Southern Practice: The Diary and Autobiography of Charles A. Hentz, M.D.* (Charlottesville: University Press of Virginia, 2000), p. 541n79.

20. E. M. Pendleton, "On the Comparative Fecundity of the Caucasian and African Races," *Charleston Medical Journal and Review* 6 (1851): 353.

21. C. Morrill, *The Physiology of Woman, and Her Diseases from Infancy to Old Age* (New York: C. Morrill, 1848), p. 47; Joseph Warrington, *The Obstetric Catechism* (Philadelphia: J. G. Auner, 1842), p. 40; J. Henry Bennett, "Amenorrhea," *The Stethoscope and Virginia Medical Gazette* 2 (August 1852): 465; "Tyler Smith's Lectures on Obstetrics," *New Orleans Medical News and Hospital Gazette* 3 (1 June 1856): 229.

22. Bennett, "Amenorrhea," p. 465; Campbell, "Observations upon Menstruation," pp. 11–12. Joseph Warrington maintained in his medical text that "females of tropical climate" were capable of having children at age ten; *The Obstetric Cathchism*, p. 41.

23. Campbell, "Observations upon Menstruation," p. 14; Bricfell [Brickell], "Obstetric Notes and Reflections," pp. 540–541; F. H. Ramsbotham, "On the Final Cause of Menstruation," *The Stethoscope and Virginia Medical Gazette* 3 (February 1853): 115.

24. Letters from William Bernard, [18—]; M. Strachan, 29 September 1821; J. A. Banks, 18 March 1827; all in Letters to Doctor James Carmichael and Son; A. S. Helmick, "An Interesting Case in Practice," *The Stethoscope* 5 (December 1855): 717; *Thomas Jefferson's Farm Book*, quoted in Todd L. Savitt, "Slave Health and Southern Distinctiveness," in *Disease and Distinctiveness in the American South*, ed. Todd L. Savitt and James Harvey Young (Knoxville: University of Tennessee Press, 1988), p. 139; Fitzgerald quoted in Stevenson, *Life in Black and White*, p. 193. Society at large tended to hold the same assumptions about medicine and health as did physicians. See Rosenberg, "The Therapeutic Revolution," p. 13.

25. Frances Anne Kemble, *Journal of a Residence on a Georgian Plantation in 1838–1839* (Athens: University of Georgia Press, 1984), p. 214; E. M. M., "Duties of Overseers," *Soil of the South* 6 (May 1856), in Breeden, *Advice among Masters*, p. 314; Peter Pie, "Overseers," *Soil of the South* 6 (June 1856), in ibid., p. 315.

26. "Electivity in Amenorrhea," *New Orleans Medical News and Hospital Gazette* 4 (1 April 1857): 117–118; Thomas M. Matthews, "Chloroform as an Emmenagogue," *The Stethoscope and Virginia Medical Gazette* 2 (December 1852): 680–681.

27. Thomas E. Massey, "Observations upon Diseases of the Uterus," *The Stethoscope* 5 (February 1855): 166, reprinted from the *New Orleans Medical and Surgical Journal,* 15 December 1854.

28. Ramsbotham, "Final Cause of Menstruation," p. 115; E. D. Fenner, "Some Additional Remarks on the Tinctura Antacrida, a Remedy for Dysmenorrhea, and Consequent Sterility," *New Orleans Medical News and Hospital Gazette* 5 (August 1858)" 370–371; "Proceedings of the Medical Association of the State of Alabama," *Southern Medical Reports* 2 (1850): 325–326; Harriss, "What Constitutes Unsoundness in the Negro?" p. 147; William G. Smith, "Case of Caesarean Operation," *Virginia Medical Journal* 7 (September 1856): 204.

29. Fenner, "Remarks on the Tinctura Antacrida," pp. 370–371; "Proceedings of Medical Association of Alabama," pp. 325–326; Harriss, "What Constitutes Unsoundness in the Negro?" p. 147. On Mackintosh, see McGregor, *From Midwives to Medicine,* p. 141.

30. C. W. Ashby, "Stramonium, as a Remedy in Dysmenorrhea," *Atlanta Journal of Medicine and Surgery* 1 (March 1856): 392–398; J. V. Withers, "Chloroform in Dysmenorrhea," *Western Journal of Medicine and Surgery,* 3d ser., 3 (February 1849): 113–116; "Physico-Medical Society," *New Orleans Medical News and Hospital Gazette* 1 (1 May 1854): 117. Although today chloroform is used in medicine primarily as a solvent, it was formerly used principally as an anesthetic. Stramonium is the dried leaves and flowering parts of a plant popularly known as jimsonweed. Dewees recommended camphor or opium to relieve pain immediately and guaiacum (the resin of a large evergreen tree from South America and the West Indies) to cure the condition. See William P. Dewees, *A Compendious System of Midwifery,* 2d ed. (Philadelphia: H. C. Carey and I. Lea, 1826), pp. 158–159.

31. H. A. Bignon, "Treatment of Dysmenorrhea, by Quinine and Pressiate of Iron," *Western Journal of Medicine and Surgery,* 3d ser., 6 (August 1850): 148–149. See also "Miscellaneous," ibid., 1 (1 May 1854): 117.

32. Bennett, "Amenorrhea," p. 464; "Case of Conception before the Appearance of the Menses," *The Stethoscope and Virginia Medical Gazette* 3 (January 1853): 65; McGregor, *From Midwives to Medicine*, p. 155.

33. Ogier tried the treatment on other women, including two who were white; T. L. Ogier, "Amenorrhea Treated Successfully with the Water Pepper," *Southern Journal of Medicine and Pharmacy* 1 (May 1846): 298–300. See also "Electivity in Amenorrhea." One cause of sterility, venereal disease, received little attention, because many people considered it the result of divine retribution for bad behavior. Even if this had not been the case, however, physicians could not have done much more than let nature run its course, since the inefficacy of treatments was widely acknowledged. The absence of effective treatment for venereal disease left slave women vulnerable to treatment by quacks, who claimed miraculous cures from potions of various kinds. Of course, it also encouraged owners to leave slaves on their own in fashioning cures of their own design.

34. Bennett, "Amenorrhea," pp. 467, 469–472; Morrill, *The Physiology of Woman*, p. 93; "Sterility among Negroes: A Case from a Country Practitioner," *New Orleans Medical News and Hospital Gazette* 3 (1 September 1856): 392–394; William G. Craghead, "Case of Catamenial Retention from Imperforated Hymen," *The Stethoscope* 5 (April 1855): 192. Infertility generally was addressed in medical journals. See for example Dr. Kuchenmeister, "On Sterility in Relation to the Vaginal Secretions," *New Orleans Medical News and Hospital Gazette* 3 (1 November 1856): 636–638; also Fenner, "Remarks on the Tinctura Antacrida," pp. 370–371.

35. "Sterility among Negroes," pp. 392–394.

36. Craghead, "Catamenial Retention from Imperforated Hymen," p. 193.

37. Ogier, "Amenorrhea Treated Successfully," p. 298; T. F. Craig, "Ovariotomy Successfully Performed by Dr. John Craig, of Stanford, Kentucky," *New Orleans Medical News and Hospital Gazette* 1 (1 December 1854): 417; Bennett, "Amenorrhea," p. 467; "Electivity in Amenorrhea"; William R. Smith, "Case of Menorrhagia, with Complications," *Nashville Journal of Medicine and Surgery* 16 (May 1859): 393.

38. Bennett, "Amenorrhea," pp. 469–472.

39. Warner discusses the "principle of specificity" in chap. 3 of *The Therapeutic Perspective*.

40. Campbell, "Observations upon Menstruation," pp. 13, 14; Boring, "Vicarious Menstruation," p. 214. Such beliefs were found in the North as well. See McGregor, *From Midwives to Medicine*, p. 137; Bennett, "Amenorrhea," p. 468. For a Canadian example, see Hector Peltier, "Retention of the Menses Simulating Pregnancy," *The Stethoscope* 4 (February–March 1854): 111.

41. E. W. Faulcon, "Oxide of Silver in Menorrhagia," *The Stethoscope* 4 (June 1854): 333; Charles B. Dew, *Bond of Iron: Master and Slave at Buffalo Forge* (New York: Norton, 1994), p. 214.

42. Battey, "Cinchona in Menorrhagia," pp. 734–735. See also Robert G. Jennings, "Remarks on the Use of the Tampon in Uterine Hemorrhage, with a Report of Two Cases," *The Stethoscope and Virginia Medical Gazette* 2 (April 1853): 206, 209.

43. Napoleon B. Anderson, "Remarks on the Use of the Nitrate of Silver in Leucorrhea," *Western Journal of Medicine and Surgery*, 3d ser., 8 (October 1851): 295, 297.

44. Russell, "Iodine Injections in Leucorrhea," *The Stethoscope* 5 (January 1855): 31–34.

45. Bedford Brown, "Chlorate of Potash Injections in Leucorrhea and Ulceration of the Os Uteri," *New Orleans Medical News and Hospital Gazette* 4 (2 November 1857): 573–574.

46. John P. Little, "Useless Remedies," *The Stethoscope and Virginia Medical Gazette* 3 (November 1853): 638–639. See also W. L. Sutton, "Cases of Retained Placenta," *Western Journal of Medicine and Surgery*, 3d ser., 1 (January 1848): 66.

47. "Close of Vol. III—Personal," *The Stethoscope and Virginia Medical Gazette* 3 (December 1853): 722–726.

48. Quoted in William Dosite Postell, *The Health of Slaves on Southern Plantations* (Gloucester: Mass.: Peter Smith, 1970), pp. 118–119.

49. On the importance of motherhood within slave communities, see White, *Ar'n't I a Woman?* p. 159. On the importance of children within slave families, see Schwartz, *Born in Bondage.*

50. S2, vol. 10: Ark., pt. 5, p. 310, and vol. 11: Mo., pp. 129–130, 135; SS2, vol. 5: Tex., pt. 4, p. 1453; William Craft, *Running a Thousand Miles for Freedom: The Escape of William and Ellen Craft from Slavery* (Baton Rouge: Louisiana State University Press, 1999), p. 20; Lucile F. Newman, "Context Variables in Fertility Regulation," in *Women's Medicine: A Cross-Cultural Study of Indigenous Fertility Regulation*, ed. Newman with James M. Nyce (New Brunswick, N.J.: Rutgers University Press, 1995), p. 184.

51. Before the nineteenth century, most white Americans attributed barrenness to providence. People prayed about it, but women also consulted midwives, followed medicinal recipes and folk rituals concocted or handed down from family members or friends, and—if family funds allowed—occasionally visited mineral springs, all in an effort to become pregnant. On knowledge of and treatments

for infertility among the free population of the United States, see Marsh and Ronner, *The Empty Cradle.*

52. On weaning, see Schwartz, *Born in Bondage,* pp. 14, 67–69, 74; S2, vol. 17: Fla., p. 213; Tattler, "Management of Negroes," *Southern Planter* 11 (February 1851): 41.

53. T. Lipscomb, "Blighted or False Conception," *Nashville Journal of Medicine and Surgery* 8 (June 1855): 468–471; "Rules of the Plantation," *Southern Cultivator* 7 (June 1849) and "The Duties of an Overseer," *Farmer and Planter* 8 (June 1857), both in Breeden, *Advice among Masters,* pp. 205, 168; SS1, vol. 1: Ala., p. 449; Virginia Clay-Clopton, *A Belle of the Fifties: Memoirs of Mrs. Clay, of Alabama,* ed. Ada Sterling (New York: Da Capo, 1969), p. 7; Robert William Fogel and Stanley L. Engerman, *Time on the Cross: The Economics of American Negro Slavery* (New York: Norton, 1974), pp. 136–137.

54. S2, vol. 17: Fla., p. 273; Gertrude Jacinta Fraser, *African American Midwifery in the South: Dialogues of Birth, Race, and Memory* (Cambridge, Mass.: Harvard University Press, 1998), p. 215. Although Fraser discusses African American women in the twentieth century, their folk practices were handed down from an earlier era.

55. William Ed Grimé, *Ethno-Botany of the Black Americans* (Algonac, Mich.: Reference Publications, 1979), p. 122.

56. SS2, vol. 3: Tex., pt. 2, p. 568.

57. Ibid., p. 875.

58. Thos. J. Shaw, "Remarks and Observations on Gossypium Herbaceum, or 'Cotton Plant,'" *Nashville Journal of Medicine and Surgery* 9 (July 1855): 7–9; "Gossypium Herbaccum (Cotton)," *Atlanta Medical and Surgical Journal* 6 (March 1861): 481–482; John Travis, "A New Remedy for Amenorrhea," *Nashville Journal of Medicine and Surgery* 3, no. 4 (1852): 207–208.

59. Pendleton, "Comparative Fecundity of Caucasian and African Races," p. 355.

60. SS2, vol. 6: Tex., pt. 5, p. 2265. Anthropological research suggests that women do not always communicate with partners concerning fertility regulation. See Lucile F. Newman, "An Introduction to Population Anthropology," in *Women's Medicine,* p. 13.

61. Newbell Niles Puckett, *Folk Beliefs of the Southern Negro* (New York: Negro Universities Press, 1968), p. 332; Fett, *Working Cures,* p. 220n54; Grimé, *Ethno-Botany of the Black Americans,* p. 144. Other substances reportedly used by slaves to regulate menstruation include okra in South America, Barbados pride and bitter ash in Jamaica, and dracontium polyphillum in the French Antilles.

62. John Morgan, "Causes of the Production of Abortion," pp. 118–120; SS2, vol. 10: Tex., pt. 9, pp. 3959, 3961, 3981; Fett, *Working Cures*, p. 79.

63. D. E. Cadwallader and J. F. Wilson, "Folklore Medicine among Georgia's Piedmont Negroes after the Civil War," *Georgia Historical Quarterly* 49 (1965): 220, 226n75; John Morgan, "Causes of the Production of Abortion," p. 118; Kay K. Moss, *Southern Folk Medicine, 1750–1820* (Columbia: University of South Carolina Press, 1999), pp. 170, 182, 195.

64. Puckett, *Folk Beliefs of the Southern Negro*, p. 331.

65. Ibid., pp. 331–332.

66. Tom W. Shick, "Healing and Race in the South Carolina Low Country," in *Africans in Bondage: Studies in Slavery and the Slave Trade*, ed. Paul E. Lovejoy (Madison: University of Wisconsin Press, 1986), p. 111; SS2, vol. 2: Tex., pt. 1, p. 445, and vol. 5: Tex., pt. 4, p. 1830; Cadwallader and Wilson, "Folklore Medicine among Georgia's Piedmont Negroes," p. 223.

67. S2, vol. 8: Ark., pt. 1, pp. 138–139; Horsman, *Josiah Nott of Mobile*, pp. 86–88, 91, 97.

68. Fluker entered puberty after emancipation, but her reference to secrecy surrounding puberty suggests customary practice stemming from slavery days; S2, vol. 8: Ark., pt. 2, p. 319, and vol. 11: Mo., pp. 124–125, and vol. 17: Fla., pp. 136, 268–271; Charles L. Perdue Jr., Thomas E. Barden, and Robert K. Phillips, eds., *Weevils in the Wheat: Interviews with Virginia Ex-Slaves* (Charlottesville: University Press of Virginia, 1976), pp. 95–96; Anthony S. Parent Jr. and Susan Brown Wallace, "Childhood and Sexual Identity under Slavery," in *American Sexual Politics: Sex, Gender, and Race since the Civil War*, ed. John C. Fout and Maura Shaw Tantillo (Chicago: University of Chicago Press, 1993), pp. 24–26.

69. SS2, vol. 5: Tex., pt. 4, p. 1830. This is a pattern observed among modern Jamaicans; Eugene B. Brody, "Everyday Knowledge of Jamaican Women," in Newman, *Women's Medicine*, p. 176.

70. "Sterility among Negroes," pp. 391–392.

71. Modern scientific studies have demonstrated that some methods of regulating fertility used by indigenous people throughout the world are efficacious, although among the many plants and other substances employed only a small number have been tested; Newman, "Introduction to Population Anthropology," pp. 10–11; and idem, "Preface to 1985 Edition," ibid., p. xii. Certain European countries as well as the World Health Organization today consider traditional use evidence of the efficacy and safety of an herbal remedy. See Cindy Belew, "Herbs and the Childbearing Woman," *Journal of Nurse-Midwifery* 44

(May–June 1999): 232. I am influenced in my thinking about the importance of female solidarity by the work of Lucile F. Newman. See her "Context Variables in Fertility Regulation" and "Preface to 1985 Edition," p. xi.

72. White goes so far as to say that becoming a mother was more important than becoming a wife for enslaved women; *Ar'n't I a Woman?* p. 159.

73. Stevenson, *Life in Black and White,* p. 246; Deborah Gray White, "Female Slaves in the Plantation South," in *Before Freedom Came: African-American Life in the Antebellum South,* ed. Edward D. C. Campbell Jr. with Kym S. Rice (Charlottesville: Museum of the Confederacy and University Press of Virginia, 1991), p. 117. White discusses the findings of various historians on age at first birth, which range from seventeen to twenty-two and a half; p. 186n85.

74. Stevenson, *Life in Black and White,* pp. 246–248. The spacing between live births fell even more drastically from the Revolutionary era, when enslaved women gave birth on average every thirty-eight months, according to Stevenson. On the other hand, Richard H. Steckel has found the enslaved population growing through the births of enslaved children throughout the antebellum years, but he has also argued that declining fertility caused the rate of population growth to decline after 1830. He notes that enslaved women had more difficulty finding suitable mates as plantations grew in size. See "The African American Population of the United States, 1790–1920," in *A Population History of North America,* ed. Michael R. Haines and Richard H. Steckel (New York: Cambridge University Press, 2000), pp. 434, 443, 445–446.

4. Pregnancy

1. W. W. Harbert, "A Case of Extra-Uterine Pregnancy," *Western Journal of Medicine and Surgery,* 3d ser., 3 (February 1849): 110–112.

2. The mother had not felt the baby move for three weeks, so Spann might have believed the baby already dead. J. W. H. Spann, "Placenta Previa Accompanied with Uterine Hemorrhage," *Nashville Journal of Medicine and Surgery* 12 (April 1857): 289; Jos. P. Logan, "Obstinate Vomiting in Pregnancy, with Abortion," *Atlanta Medical and Surgical Journal* 1 (October 1855): 75–76. Although European and American doctors generally accepted abortion as a medical procedure to save the life of the mother, some expressed the belief that more than one doctor should be consulted. See "Is the Physician Authorized to Provoke Premature Artificial Abortion to Save the Mother?" *The Stethoscope and Virginia Medical Gazette* 3 (January 1853): 67. Most southern whites in the antebellum era opposed abortion except to save the life of the mother. See Catherine Clinton, *The Plantation Mistress: Woman's World in the Old South* (New York: Pantheon, 1982), pp. 205–207; Sally G. McMillen, *Motherhood in the Old South: Pregnancy,*

Childbirth, and Infant Rearing (Baton Rouge: Louisiana State University Press, 1990), p. 108. Abortions were relatively easy to obtain in the North; it was only in the 1850s that opposition to abortion began to grow there. James C. Mohr, *Abortion in America: The Origins and Evolution of National Policy, 1800–1900* (New York: Oxford University Press, 1978); Roger Lane, *Violent Death in the City: Suicide, Accident, and Murder in Nineteenth-Century Philadelphia* (Cambridge, Mass.: Harvard University Press, 1979); Carroll Smith-Rosenberg, "The Abortion Movement and the AMA, 1850–1880," in *Disorderly Conduct: Visions of Gender in Victorian America* (New York: Oxford University Press, 1985), pp. 217–244; Suzanne Poirier, "Women's Reproductive Health," in *Women, Health, and Medicine in America: A Historical Handbook*, ed. Rima D. Apple (New Brunswick, N.J.: Rutgers University Press, 1992), pp. 232–233. On controversy within the medical community, see J. Boring, "Feticide," *Atlanta Medical and Surgical Journal* 2 (December 1856): 257–259; "Criminal Abortion or Feticide," ibid. (August 1857): 760.

3. "Bibliographic Notices," *The Stethoscope* 5 (February 1855): 141.

4. Boring, "Feticide," pp. 257–259.

5. "Criminal Abortion or Feticide," p. 760; Charles D. Meigs, *Obstetrics: The Science and the Art* (Philadelphia: Blanchard and Lea, 1863), p. 195. See also Wooster Beach, *An Improved System of Midwifery: Adapted to the Reformed Practice of Medicine* (New York: Charles Scribner, 1854), p. 82. Beach acknowledged that it would be difficult to prove criminal intent if cases of abortion were prosecuted.

6. Witness quoted in Ariela J. Gross, *Double Character: Slavery and Mastery in the Antebellum Southern Courtroom* (Princeton: Princeton University Press, 2000), p. 68; letter to the editor and editorial comment, *Nashville Journal of Medicine and Surgery* 13 (November 1857): 387–388. See also Brenda E. Stevenson, *Life in Black and White: Family and Community in the Slave South* (New York: Oxford University Press, 1996), p. 245.

7. "Sterility among Negroes: A Case from a Country Practitioner," *New Orleans Medical News and Hospital Gazette* 3 (1 September 1856): 391–392; John H. Morgan, "An Essay on the Causes of the Production of Abortion among Our Negro Population," *Nashville Journal of Medicine and Surgery* 19 (August 1860): 122–123; John Travis, "A New Remedy for Amenorrhea," ibid., 3, no. 4 (1852): 207–208; E. M. Pendleton, "Reports from Georgia: General Report on the Topography, Climate, and Diseases of Middle Georgia," *Southern Medical Reports* 1 (1849): 338.

8. "Sterility among Negroes," p. 392; Arent's opinion discussed in Morgan, "Causes of the Production of Abortion," pp. 120–121; Pendleton, "Reports from

Georgia," p. 338. Beach discussed the ineffectiveness of many approaches to abortion in *An Improved System of Midwifery*, pp. 85–87.

9. E. M. Pendleton, "On the Comparative Fecundity of the Caucasian and African Races," *Charleston Medical Journal and Review* 6 (1851): 354.

10. Ibid., p. 355.

11. Hector Peltier, "Retention of the Menses Simulating Pregnancy," *The Stethoscope* 4 (February–March 1854): 109–111. The "problem" of diagnosing unmarried ladies as pregnant continued to plague doctors after the Civil War. See D. W. Cathell, "The Physician Himself and What He Should Add to the Strictly Scientific," in *Major Problems in the History of American Medicine and Public Health*, ed. John Harley Warner and Janet A. Tighe (Boston: Houghton Mifflin, 2001), p. 209.

12. W. H. Gantt, "Post-Mortem Revelations of Case of Supposed Ascites or Pregnancy," *The Stethoscope* 6 (June 1854): 336–337.

13. Jo. Shelby, "A Case of Abortion," *Nashville Journal of Medicine and Surgery* 14 (March 1858): 211–212.

14. "Miscarriage," ibid., 13 (November 1857): 388; "Hamamelis Virginica," *Atlanta Medical and Surgical Journal*, n.s., 8 (July 1867): 239.

15. Bezaleel Brown to Charles Brown, 4 July 1816, Charles Brown Papers, Manuscripts and Rare Books Department, Swem Library, College of William and Mary; S2, vol. 11: Mo., p. 255; Plantation Manual of James H. Hammond of Beach Island, South Carolina, about 1834, p. 3, typescript copy, Joseph I. Waring Research Files, Waring Historical Library, Medical University of South Carolina.

16. John Campbell, "Work, Pregnancy, and Infant Mortality among Southern Slaves," *Journal of Interdisciplinary Studies* 14 (spring 1984): 808; entries for 20 and 21 May 1817, 26 and 28 February 1818, Medical Daybook (1816–1834), Henry Ravenel, Henry Ravenel Family Papers, 1731–1867, South Carolina Historical Society, Charleston. In 1816 Ravenel assessed a fee of twenty-five dollars for an "Instrumental Delivery" of a slave child born at night; see entry for 28 January. Doctors routinely charged more for night deliveries and those requiring instruments; entry for 30 May 1857, Jones Family Business Accounts, Virginia State Library, Richmond.

17. W. H. Robert, "Observations on the Use of Veratrum Viride," *Nashville Journal of Medicine and Surgery* 3, no. 3 (1852): 177.

18. Hammond quoted in Drew Gilpin Faust, *James Henry Hammond and the Old South: A Design for Mastery* (Baton Rouge: Louisiana State University Press, 1982), p. 79; Dent quoted in Ray Mathis, *John Horry Dent: South Carolina Aris-*

tocrat on the Alabama Frontier (University: University of Alabama Press, 1979), p. 84. See also Deborah Gray White, *Ar'n't I a Woman? Female Slaves in the Plantation South* (New York: Norton, 1985), pp. 84–85; Todd L. Savitt, *Medicine and Slavery: The Diseases and Health Care of Blacks in Antebellum Virginia* (Urbana: University of Illinois Press, 1978), p. 33; Jacqueline Jones, *Labor of Love, Labor of Sorrow: Black Women, Work, and the Family, from Slavery to the Present* (New York: Basic Books, 1985), p. 18; Thelma Jennings, "'Us Colored Women Had to Go Through a Plenty': Sexual Exploitation of African-American Slave Women," *Journal of Women's History* 1 (winter 1990): 54; Reynolds Farley, *Growth of the Black Population: A Study of Demographic Trends* (Chicago: Markham, 1970), p. 40.

19. "Dr. Thompson's Paper," *Nashville Journal of Medicine and Surgery* 5 (November 1853): 311–316.

20. B. S. Hopkins, "Excerpts from My Case Book," ibid., 9 (August 1855): 101–102; W. L. Sutton, "Cases of Retained Placenta," *Western Journal of Medicine and Surgery*, 3d ser., 1 (January 1848): 61; Jos. J. West, "Quinine in Pregnancy," *Savannah Journal of Medicine* 1 (May 1858): 26; "Transactions of the East Tennessee Medical Society," *Nashville Journal of Medicine and Surgery* 12 (June 1857): 494.

21. Kenneth Allen De Ville, *Medical Malpractice in Nineteenth-Century America: Origins and Legacy* (New York: New York University Press, 1990), pp. 4, 5, 26–31, 65, 69, 131–132.

22. A. R. Nelson, "A Case of Abortion and Retention of the Placenta," *Western Journal of Medicine and Surgery*, 2d ser., 5 (January 1846): 9–11.

23. "Annual Commencement of the Medical Department of Hampden-Sidney College," *The Stethoscope and Virginia Medical Gazette* 3 (April 1853): 224; D. Warren Brickell, "Placenta Previa, Etc.," *New Orleans Medical News and Hospital Gazette* 3 (1 June 1856): 218. See also "New Method of Inducing Premature Delivery," *The Stethoscope* 5 (May 1855): 268–269.

24. E. F. Knott, "A Case of Parturition, with Its Complications," *Atlanta Medical and Surgical Journal* 1 (September 1855): 11–12; Brickell, "Placenta Previa, Etc.," pp. 216–218; M. J. Greene, "A Case of Partial Placenta Previa, Complicated with Transverse Presentation and Rigidity of the Os Uteri," *Atlanta Medical and Surgical Journal* 1 (June 1856): 591–592.

25. John Butts, "A Case of Labor Complicated with Eclampsia," *New Orleans Medical News and Hospital Gazette* 1 (1 July 1854): 212–213. For a reference to a pregnant slave afflicted with rheumatism, see letter from Laurence Battaile, 28 March 1820, Letters to Doctor James Carmichael and Son, Historical Collections at the Claude Moore Health Sciences Library, University of Virginia, http://etext.lib.virginia.edu/healthsci/carmichael/collection.

26. Butts, "Case of Labor with Eclampsia," p. 213.

27. "Prize Questions," *Atlanta Medical and Surgical Journal* 1 (December 1855): 248; "Selections," ibid. (January 1856): 294–295.

28. V. H. Taliaferro, "Remarks upon the Medical Properties and Therapeutical Applications of Veratrum Viride," ibid., 2 (March 1857): 399–406; W. A. Brown, "Veratrum Viride," *Nashville Journal of Medicine and Surgery* 11 (October 1856): 307–312; Robert, "Observations on Use of Veratrum Viride," pp. 176–177; B. F. Newsom, "Veratrum Viride—Has It Any Abortive Properties?" *Nashville Journal of Medicine and Surgery* 12 (January 1857): 9–19. Doctors considered the drug dangerous in general. See J. C. Nott, "A Word about Norwood's Tincture of Veratrum Viride," *The Stethoscope and Virginia Medical Gazette* 3 (March 1853): 170–171; John Harley Warner, *The Therapeutic Perspective: Medical Practice, Knowledge, and Identity in America, 1820–1885* (Princeton: Princeton University Press, 1997), pp. 130, 207, 227–231.

29. Taliaferro, "Remarks upon Properties and Applications of Veratrum Viride."

30. W. H. Gantt, "A Few Remarks on Veratrum Viride as a Therapeutical Agent," *The Stethoscope* 4 (February–March 1854): 74.

31. "To Correspondents," *The Stethoscope and Virginia Medical Gazette* 2 (September 1852): 504.

32. West, "Quinine in Pregnancy," pp. 19, 26–28; J. S. Rich, "Quinine in Uterine and Other Quasi-Periodic Hemorrhages," *Charleston Medical Journal and Review* 15 (March 1860): 179; "South Carolina Medical Association," ibid., p. 271. The debate in the medical journals over the role of quinine in inducing abortion was interrupted by the Civil War, when southern medical journals suspended publication, but it resumed after the conflict. See D. L. Phares, "Is Quinine a Partus Accelerator?" *Atlanta Medical and Surgical Journal*, n.s., 7B (October 1866): 340–343. About 25 percent of U.S. women today experience some bleeding in the early months of pregnancy, which can be a sign of impending miscarriage; James R. Scott, Philip J. Di Saia, Charles B. Hammond, and William N. Spellacy, eds., *Danforth's Obstetrics and Gynecology*, 8th ed. (Philadelphia: Lippincott Williams and Wilkins, 1999), p. 144.

33. South Carolina planter quoted in Sharla M. Fett, *Working Cures: Healing, Health, and Power on Southern Slave Plantations* (Chapel Hill: University of North Carolina Press, 2002), p. 185; Memorandum Book for Birdfield Plantation, 1850–1857, pp. 29–30, 66, James Ritchie Sparkman Papers, Records of Ante-Bellum Southern Plantations from the Revolution through the Civil War, ed. Kenneth M. Stampp, University Publications of America, Series A, Part 2: Miscellaneous Collections; Berkeley's overseer quoted in Stevenson, *Life in Black and White*, p. 193. For a reference to women who pretended to be sick in

order to catch up on their washing and ironing, see S2, vol. 15: N.C., pt. 2, p. 57. See also Frances Anne Kemble, *Journal of a Residence on a Georgian Plantation in 1838–1839* (Athens: University of Georgia Press, 1984), pp. 276–277, 170, 210; Robynne Rogers Healey, "Meanings of Motherhood: Maternal Experiences and Perceptions on Low Country South Carolina Plantations," p. 20, Paper presented at the Berkshire Conference on the History of Women, Chapel Hill, N.C., 7 June 1996 (made available by the author); White, *Ar'n't I a Woman?* pp. 79–84. Internal exams may have added to the women's problems, since they introduced the possibility of infection from physicians' unclean hands and instruments. On antebellum medical knowledge of pregnancy and gestation, see McMillen, *Motherhood in the Old South,* pp. 28–31. F. H. Ramsbotham posited that the amount of time between conception and the start of labor varied, depending in part on the location of impregnation within the fallopian tube; "On the Final Cause of Menstruation," *The Stethoscope and Virginia Medical Gazette* 3 (February 1853): 115.

34. R. King Jr., "On the Management of the Butler Estate, and the Cultivation of Sugar Cane," *Southern Agriculturist* 1 (December 1828), in *Advice among Masters: The Ideal in Slave Management in the Old South,* ed. James O. Breeden (Westport, Conn.: Greenwood, 1980), p. 164; John R. Turner, "Plantation Hygiene," *Southern Cultivator* 15 (May–June 1857), in ibid., pp. 204–205; S2, vol. 10: Ark., pt. 5, p. 157; Mathis, *John Horry Dent.*

35. Raymond Bauer and Alice Bauer, "Day to Day Resistance to Slavery," in *The Slavery Experience in the United States,* ed. Irwin Unger and David Reimers (New York: Holt, Rinehart and Winston, 1970), p. 186.

36. J. Junius Newsome, "Thesis, on the Signs of Pregnancy," *Atlanta Medical and Surgical Journal* 1 (February 1856): 333–341. See also H. Letheby, "Kiesteine as an Evidence of Pregnancy," and "M. Dubois on the Auscultatory Signs of Pregnancy," both in *Western Journal of Medicine and Surgery* 5 (April 1842): 299–230, 301–302; and Elisha K. Kane, "Experiments on Kiesteine, with Observations on Its Application to the Diagnosis of Pregnancy," ibid., 6 (September 1842): 206–215.

37. Newsome, "Signs of Pregnancy," p. 335. On the shift, see Stanley Joel Reiser, *Medicine and the Reign of Technology* (New York: Cambridge University Press, 1978), esp. pp. 2–8.

38. "Statistics of Midwifery," *Western Journal of Medicine and Surgery,* 2d ser., 1 (May 1844): 454; William P. Dewees, *A Compendious System of Midwifery,* 2d ed. (Philadelphia: H. C. Carey and I. Lea, 1826), p. 168; J. S. Chisolm, "Prolonged Gestation," *The Stethoscope* 5 (February 1855): 120; Beach, *An Improved System of Midwifery,* p. 66; Meigs, *Obstetrics,* pp. 224–233.

39. John A. Cunningham, "Case of Extra Uterine Foetus, Retained Forty Years," *Virginia Medical and Surgical Journal* 4 (February 1855): 94–95; George M. Wharton, "A Complicated Case," *Nashville Journal of Medicine and Surgery* 1 (August 1851): 209–214.

40. "Superfoetation," *Nashville Medical Journal* 17 (July 1859): 65, 66. The article first appeared as a letter to the editor from W. C. Sanckford in the *Medical Journal of North Carolina*.

41. W. K. Bowling, "An Extensive Abdominal Tumor," *Nashville Journal of Medicine and Surgery* 8 (February 1855): 103–104; Andrew Askew, "A Case of Uterine Hydatids," ibid., 2, no. 3 (1852): 134–135; J. O. Sharber, "Death from Exterior Uterine Hemorrhage," ibid., 4, no. 5 (1853): 259–261.

42. William R. Smith, "Case of Menorrhagia, with Complications," ibid., 16 (May 1859): 392–397.

43. "Fatal Case of Tetanus Supervening on Abortion," *The Stethoscope and Virginia Medical Gazette* 1 (December 1851): 672–674.

44. S2, vol. 8: Ark., pt. 2, pp. 215–216, 333, and vol. 10: Ark., pt. 5, p. 239; SS2, vol. 1: Ala., Ariz., Ark., and Other Narratives, p. 59.

45. "A Question of Legitimacy," *Western Journal of Medicine and Surgery*, 2d ser., 5 (May 1845): 457; J. W. B. Garrett, "Singular Case of Monstrosity," ibid., 3d ser., 6 (July 1850): 6; T. G. Underwood, "Influence of the Mother's Mind on the Fetus," *Nashville Journal of Medicine and Surgery* 11 (August 1856): 118–122; "Monstrosities," *Western Journal of Medicine and Surgery*, 3d ser., 11 (April 1853): 369; A. O. Kellogg, "Considerations on the Reciprocal Influence of the Physical Organization and Mental Manifestations," *Atlanta Medical and Surgical Journal* 1 (May 1856): 537; Edward Warren, "Uterine Sympathy," *The Stethoscope* 4 (June 1854): 361–363. Reform physician Wooster Beach recommended indulging the longings of women (he presumably had in mind white women) lest they suffer miscarriage caused by anxiety or mark the child; *An Improved System of Midwifery*, p. 190.

46. W. P. Moore, "Influence of the Mother upon the Fetus in Utero," *Nashville Journal of Medicine and Surgery* 13 (July 1857): 34–37; John M. Watson, "On the Influence of the Mother's Mind on the Fetus in Utero," ibid., 18 (February 1860): 97–109.

47. S2, vol. 8: Ark., pt. 2, p. 333; SS2, vol. 1: Ala., Ariz., Ark., and Other Narratives, p. 131.

48. Plantation Manual of James H. Hammond of Beach Island, South Carolina, p. 1, typescript copy, Joseph I. Waring Research Files.

49. T. Lindsay Baker and Julie P. Baker, eds., *The WPA Oklahoma Slave Narra-*

tives (Norman: University of Oklahoma Press, 1996), p. 142; S2, vol. 9: Ark., pt. 4, p. 87.

50. Letter to the editor and editorial comment, *Nashville Journal of Medicine and Surgery* 13 (November 1857): 387–388; S2, vol. 9: Ark., pt. 4, p. 216; SS1, vol. 7: Miss., pt. 2, pp. 441–442. On the role of heavy work regimens in undermining pregnancy in Louisiana, see Richard Follett, "Heat, Sex, and Sugar: Pregnancy and Childbearing in the Slave Quarters," *Journal of Family History* 28 (October 2003): 510–539, esp. p. 513.

51. Ronald L. Baker, comp., *Homeless, Friendless, and Penniless: The WPA Interviews with Former Slaves Living in Indiana* (Bloomington: Indiana University Press, 2000), p. 257; SS1, vol. 7: Miss., pt. 2, pp. 441–442. See also vol. 17: Fla., p. 67.

52. Baker, *Homeless, Friendless, and Penniless,* pp. 209, 257; S2, vol. 8: Ark., pt. 1, p. 42, and vol. 9: Ark., pt. 3, pp. 9, 231, and vol. 11: Ark., pt. 7, p. 16, and vol. 14: N.C., pt. 1, pp. 312–313; SS2, vol. 3: Tex., pt. 3, pp. 536, 736; Charles L. Perdue Jr., Thomas E. Barden, and Robert K. Phillips, eds., *Weevils in the Wheat: Interviews with Virginia Ex-Slaves* (Charlottesville: University Press of Virginia, 1976), p. 63. I am grateful to nurse-midwife Debra Erickson-Owens for offering insight into the beating of pregnant women (conversation 8 March 2005).

53. Entries for 8 and 16 March 1861, in Steven M. Stowe, ed., *A Southern Practice: The Diary and Autobiography of Charles A. Hentz, M.D.* (Charlottesville: University Press of Virginia, 2000), p. 366.

54. Robert William Fogel, *Without Consent or Contract: The Rise and Fall of American Slavery* (New York: Norton, 1989), p. 153; SS2, vol. 1: Ala., Ariz., Ark., and Other Narratives, p. 347.

55. Morgan, "Causes of the Production of Abortion," with comments by Dr. Smith and Dr. Baskette, pp. 117–123.

56. James M. Larkins, "A Case of Rupture of the Uterus with the Escape of the Foetus into the Abdomen," *Western Journal of Medicine and Surgery,* 3d ser., 1 (February 1848): 110–112. Doctors were particularly fond of saving the fetuses or bodies of aborted or stillborn infants with physical deformities. See for example Garrett, "Singular Case of Monstrosity," p. 6. On the tendency of twentieth-century African American women to avoid speaking openly of pregnancy, see Gertrude Jacinta Fraser, *African American Midwifery in the South: Dialogues of Birth, Race, and Memory* (Cambridge, Mass.: Harvard University Press, 1998), p. 218.

57. Shelby, "A Case of Abortion," pp. 211–212; W. L. Sutton, "A Case of Infanticide," *Western Journal of Medicine and Surgery,* 3d ser., 11 (January 1853):

26–30; undated letter from James Old, reprinted in Todd L. Savitt, "Patient Letters to an Early Nineteenth Century Virginia Physician," *Journal of the Florida Medical Association* 69 (1982): 693; Patteson quoted in Fett, *Working Cures*, p. 176; Chisolm, "Prolonged Gestation," p. 120. See also Stevenson, *Life in Black and White*, p. 193.

5. Childbirth

1. John Overton, "A Case of Labour Attended by Some Unusual Appearances," *Western Journal of Medicine and Surgery* 5 (January 1842): 15–19.

2. Donald Caton, *What a Blessing She Had Chloroform: The Medical and Social Response to the Pain of Childbirth from 1800 to the Present* (New Haven: Yale University Press, 1999), pp. 21, 107. Numerous medical texts, domestic medical manuals, and medical journals provide details about the ability of physicians and surgeons to manage childbirth and complications of childbirth. On medical textbooks, see Lamar Riley Murphy, *Enter the Physician: The Transformation of Domestic Medicine, 1760–1860* (Tuscaloosa: University of Alabama Press, 1991), chap. 5. On domestic manuals that circulated in the South, see Elizabeth Barnaby Keeney, "Unless Powerful Sick: Domestic Medicine in the Old South," in *Science and Medicine in the Old South*, ed. Ronald L. Numbers and Todd L. Savitt (Baton Rouge: Louisiana State University Press, 1989), pp. 276–294. See also Sally G. McMillen, *Motherhood in the Old South: Pregnancy, Childbirth, and Infant Rearing* (Baton Rouge: Louisiana State University Press, 1990), pp. 96–100.

3. Steven M. Stowe, *Doctoring the South: Southern Physicians and Everyday Medicine in the Mid-Nineteenth Century* (Chapel Hill: University of North Carolina Press, 2004), pp. 30, 281n29; Judith Walzer Leavitt, "'Science' Enters the Birthing Room: Obstetrics in America since the 18th Century," in *Sickness and Health in America: Readings in the History and Medicine and Public Health*, ed. Judith Walzer Leavitt and Ronald L. Numbers, 2d ed. (Madison: University of Wisconsin Press, 1985), pp. 84–87, 93.

4. Steven M. Stowe, "Obstetrics and the Work of Doctoring in the Mid-Nineteenth-Century American South," *Bulletin of the History of Medicine* 64 (winter 1990): 554; J. V. Withers, "A Case of Eclampsia," *Western Journal of Medicine and Surgery*, 4th ser., 2 (August 1854): 103–104; S1, vol. 7: Okla. and Miss., p. 24; SS1, vol. 3: Ga., pt. 1, pp. 204–205; entry for 5 August 1845, Plantation Diary, vol. 2, Sturdivant Collection (microfilm), SHC; entry for 10 July 1858, David Gavin Diary, SHC.

5. John A. Wragg, "Case of Rupture of the Uterus," *Southern Journal of Medicine and Pharmacy* 2 (March 1847): 146; N. Bozeman, "Vesico-Vaginal Fistula, with Laceration of the Anterior Lip of the Cervix Uteri of Nearly Six Years

Standing—Cured in Two Weeks," *Western Journal of Medicine and Surgery,* 4th ser., 4 (September 1855): 234; Ronald L. Baker, comp., *Homeless, Friendless, and Penniless: The WPA Interviews with Former Slaves Living in Indiana* (Blooming-ton: Indiana University Press, 2000), pp. 101, 103, 106–107; S2, vol. 17: Fla., p. 273; SS2, vol. 3: Tex., pt. 2, p. 709.

6. S2, vol. 8: Ark., pt. 1, p. 57, and pt. 2, p. 263, and vol. 9: Ark., pt. 3, pp. 17–18, and vol. 11: Ark., pt. 7, pp. 19–22; SS1, vol. 9: Miss., pt. 4, p. 1368; Beverly Greene Bond, "'The Extent of the Law': Free Women of Color in Antebellum Memphis, Tennessee," in *Negotiating Boundaries of Southern Womanhood,* ed. Janet L. Coryell, Thomas H. Appleton Jr., Anastasia Sims, and Sandra Gioia Treadway (Columbia: University of Missouri Press, 2000), pp. 21–22. In the twentieth century black midwives also performed other jobs. See Valerie Lee, *Granny Midwives and Black Women Writers* (New York: Routledge, 1996), p. 125.

7. S2, vol. 10: Ark., pt. 5, p. 33; SS2, vol. 1: Ala., Ariz., Ark., and Other Narra-tives, p. 317; Melanie Pavich-Lindsay, ed., *Anna: The Letters of a St. Simons Island Plantation Mistress, 1817–1859* (Athens: University of Georgia Press, 2002), pp. 30, 32n1, 92, 101, 155, 298, 331, 360–361.

8. S2, vol. 9: Ark., pt. 4, pp. 138–139, and vol. 10: Ark., pt. 6, p. 163, and vol. 11: Ark., pt. 7, p. 232; SS1, vol. 9: Miss., pt. 4, pp. 1429, 1883; J. Douglass, "Ergot in Placenta Previa—Abortion at Three Months, Delivery of Another Child Six Months After," *Charleston Medical Journal and Review* 15 (March 1860): 328–329.

9. Sharla M. Fett, *Working Cures: Healing, Health, and Power on Southern Slave Plantations* (Chapel Hill: University of North Carolina Press, 2002), p. 55.

10. David H. Brown, "Conjure/Doctors: An Exploration of a Black Discourse in America, Antebellum to 1940," *Folklore Forum* 23 (1990): 8.

11. S2, vol. 11: Ark., pt. 7, pp. 19–22. See also S1, vol. 2: S.C., pt. 1, pp. 137–138.

12. S2, vol. 11: Ark., pt. 7, pp. 21–22; Bennett H. Wall, "Medical Care of Ebenezer Pettigrew's Slaves," *Mississippi Valley Historical Review* 37 (1950): 451, 469.

13. S2, vol. 8: Ark., pt. 1, pp. 57, 239, and pt. 2, p. 282, and vol. 9: Ark., pt. 3, p. 294, and vol. 10: Ark., pt. 5, p. 354; SS2, vol. 10: Tex., pt. 9, p. 4165; Pavich-Lindsay, *Anna,* pp. 8, 78. It was not unusual for black women to attend white women at childbirth.

14. William Ed Grimé, *Ethno-Botany of the Black Americans* (Algonac, Mich.: Reference Publications, 1979), p. 122; D. E. Cadwallader and J. F. Wilson, "Folklore Medicine among Georgia's Piedmont Negroes after the Civil War," *Georgia Historical Quarterly* 49 (1965): 220–221, 223, 224n5; S2, vol. 8: Ark., pt.

2, p. 283; SS1, vol. 9: Miss., pt. 4, p. 1429; Fett, *Working Cures,* p. 98. Historians of nineteenth-century childbirth have been struck by the dread of confinement among white women, in part because of the danger posed to the life and health of the mother. Among southern whites, one in twenty-five women died in childbirth; more were disabled as the result of complications. Diaries and letters addressed the matter. See for example Erika L. Murr, ed., *A Rebel Wife in Texas: The Diary and Letters of Elizabeth Scott Neblett, 1852–1864* (Baton Rouge: Louisiana State University Press, 2001), pp. 9, 65–66, 68, 75.

15. S2, vol. 11: Ark., pt. 7, p. 151, 181; SS1, vol. 11, N.C. and S.C., pp. 85–86. See also S1, vol. 17: Fla., pp. 4–5; Georgia Writers' Project, *Drums and Shadows: Survival Studies among the Georgia Coastal Negroes* (Athens: University of Georgia Press, 1986), p. 69. On the importance of folk beliefs among slaves, see Lawrence W. Levine, *Black Culture and Black Consciousness: Afro-American Folk Thought from Slavery to Freedom* (New York: Oxford University Press, 1977), pp. 55–80. On midwifery practices among blacks in twentieth-century Alabama, see Linda Janet Holmes, "African American Midwives in the South," in *The American Way of Birth,* ed. Pamela S. Eakins (Philadelphia: Temple University Press, 1986). On the existence in the early twentieth century of the belief that children born with a caul could exert special powers, including foretelling the future, see Lee, *Granny Midwives and Black Women Writers,* p. 121.

16. S2, vol. 10: Ark., pt. 5, pp. 59, 238.

17. Quotation in William H. Philpot, "A Case of Hypertrophy of the Spleen and Post Mortem Examination," *Atlanta Medical and Surgical Journal* 2 (August 1857): 707–708. See also Lee, *Granny Midwives and Black Women Writers,* p. 123.

18. S2, vol. 15: N.C., pt. 2, pp. 66–68, 71.

19. Isabelle practiced midwifery following the Civil War, but by her own declaration she approached her role much as she had in the prewar period; S2, vol. 11: Mo., p. 204.

20. "Prof. Cenas' Cases of Difficult Labor," *The Stethoscope and Virginia Medical Gazette* 1 (December 1851): 696; letters from Samuel Alsop, 29 September 1824, and D. Gatewood, 19 January 1825, both in Letters to Doctor James Carmichael and Son, Historical Collections at the Claude Moore Health Sciences Library, University of Virginia, http://etext.lib.virginia.edu/healthsci/carmichael/collection. See also Market Book, Mrs. W. G. Jones Papers, ADAH; entries for 28 July 1851, 21 and 23 July 1860, Diary and Account Book, 1850–1853, vol. 1, Philip Henry Pitts Papers, SHC; S1, vol. 4: Tex., pt. 2, p. 18; Stowe, "Obstetrics and Doctoring," p. 549. For an example of a midwife who

summoned a physician, see Henry R. Frost, "Expulsion of a Mass of Hair from the Uterus," *Western Journal of Medicine and Surgery* 6 (September 1842): 217.

21. Brown reported treating eight blacks for every six whites; W. A. Brown, "Midwifery in a Country Practice," *Nashville Journal of Medicine and Surgery* 7 (December 1854): 460. Wooster Beach, *An Improved System of Midwifery Adapted to the Reformed Practice of Medicine* (New York: Charles Scribner, 1853), p. 19. See also Daniel Drake, "Diseases of the Negro Population," *Western Journal of Medicine and Surgery*, 2d ser., 3 (February 1845): 166.

22. Entry for 5 November 1857, in Steven M. Stowe, ed., *A Southern Practice: The Diary and Autobiography of Charles A. Hentz, M.D.* (Charlottesville: University Press of Virginia, 2000), pp. 321–322. See also S2, vol. 8: Ark., pt. 1, p. 344.

23. "Tariff of Fees, Etc.," *The Stethoscope* 4 (January 1854): 99; George Rosen, *Fees and Fee Bills: Some Economic Aspects of Medical Practice in Nineteenth Century America* (Baltimore: Johns Hopkins Press, 1946), pp. 31, 39.

24. John Duffy, ed., *The Rudolph Matas History of Medicine in Louisiana*, 2 vols. ([Baton Rouge]: Louisiana State University Press, 1958, 1962), 1: 294–295; "Medicine in Texas," *Nashville Journal of Medicine and Surgery* 7 (November 1854): 423; advertisement, *The Stethoscope* 4 (June 1854), n.p.; Beach, *An Improved System of Midwifery*, pp. 97–98; Joseph I. Waring, *A History of Medicine in South Carolina, 1620–1825*, vol. 1 (Charleston: South Carolina Medical Association, 1964), p. 380; Stowe, "Obstetrics and Doctoring," p. 548; "To the Inhabitants of Louisiana and Mississippi," *Asylum*, 7 February 1824, reproduced in Duffy, *Rudolph Matas History of Medicine*, 1: n.p. Enslaved children weighed less than 5.5 pounds at birth; modern infants weigh about 7.5. Smaller size may have made for an easier birth. See Richard H. Steckel, "Birth Weights and Infant Mortality among American Slaves," *Explorations in Economic History* 23 (1986): 173–198.

25. Wall, "Medical Care of Ebenezer Pettigrew's Slaves," p. 462; entries for Col. H. Waddell and H. G. Jones and Dr. John A. Green, guardian for Miss Harris, James A. Tillman and John Norwood Ledgers, vol. 1, Records of Ante-Bellum Southern Plantations from the Revolution through the Civil War, ed. Kenneth M. Stampp, University Publications of America, Part 7: Alabama, Series J: Selections from the Manuscripts Department, SHC; Rosen, *Fees and Fee Bills*, pp. 2, 32.

26. Rosen, *Fees and Fee Bills*, p. 27; entries for Col. H. Waddell and William Bellamy, Esq., and Dr. John A. Green, guardian for Miss Harris, Tillman and Norwood Ledgers, vol. 1; and B. H. Edwards, ibid., vol. 2: 1859–1868; Wall, "Medical Care of Ebenezer Pettigrew's Slaves," p. 462.

27. "The Physician a Hireling," *New Orleans Medical News and Hospital Gazette* 4 (January 1858): 692. On such practices, see Wilma King, ed., *A Northern Woman in the Plantation South: Letters of Tryphena Blanche Holder Fox, 1856–1876* (Columbia: University of South Carolina Press, 1993), pp. 37, 40; Arney R. Childs, ed., *Rice Planter and Sportsman: The Recollections of J. Motte Alston, 1821–1909* (Columbia: University of South Carolina Press, 1999), p. 47; Martha Carolyn Mitchell, "Health and the Medical Profession in the Lower South, 1845–1860," *Journal of Southern History* 10 (1944): 435; Duffy, *Rudolph Matas History of Medicine*, 2: 101; Todd L. Savitt, *Medicine and Slavery: The Diseases and Health Care of Blacks in Antebellum Virginia* (Urbana: University of Illinois Press, 1978), pp. 198–201. The contracts were attractive, particularly to physicians just starting out; landing even one yearly contract could ensure financial stability. In 1841 Doctor J. S. earned $150 for treating the slaves on Argyle Island, a sum greater than that paid the overseer; Weymouth T. Jordan, "Plantation Medicine in the Old South," *Alabama Review* 3 (1950): 120. Richard H. Shryock argues that the practice of charging by the year was generally restricted to beginning practitioners; "Medical Practice in the Old South," *South Atlantic Quarterly* 29 (1930): 172.

28. T. Lindsay Baker and Julie P. Baker, eds., *The WPA Oklahoma Slave Narratives* (Norman: University of Oklahoma Press, 1996), p. 104; SS1, vol. 9: Miss., pt. 4, p. 1610; SS2, vol. 1: Ala., Ariz., Ark., and Other Narratives, p. 85. For examples of fees paid to midwives, see Claudia L. Bushman, *In Old Virginia: Slavery, Farming, and Society in the Journal of John Walker* (Baltimore: Johns Hopkins University Press, 2002), p. 66; Drew Gilpin Faust, *James Henry Hammond and the Old South: A Design for Mastery* (Baton Rouge: Louisiana State University Press, 1982), p. 90; Charles B. Dew, *Bond of Iron: Master and Slave at Buffalo Forge* (New York: Norton, 1994), pp. 321, 325; Wall, "Medical Care of Ebenezer Pettigrew's Slaves," p. 468; Savitt, *Medicine and Slavery*, p. 182n59.

29. Stowe, "Obstetrics and Doctoring," p. 548; Wall, "Medical Care of Ebenezer Pettigrew's Slaves," pp. 459, 470; "An Obstetric Letter," *New Orleans Medical News and Hospital Gazette* 6 (February 1860): 931; Walter Fisher, "Physicians and Slavery in the Antebellum Southern Medical Journal," *Journal of the History of Medicine and Allied Sciences* 23 (January 1968): 44.

30. Letters to Doctor James Carmichael and Son, esp. letter from Judah Dobson, 26 February 1825.

31. Douglass, "Ergot in Placenta Previa," pp. 328–329.

32. Ibid.

33. R. D. Arnold, "Separation and Delivery of Placenta, in a Case of Placenta Previa," *Savannah Journal of Medicine* 2 (January 1860): 298–299.

34. James W. Fair, "A Case of Placenta Previa," *New Orleans Medical News and Hospital Gazette* 4 (February 1861): 905–906; M. J. Greene, "A Case of Partial Placenta Previa, Complicated with Transverse Presentation and Rigidity of the Os Uteri," *Atlanta Medical and Surgical Journal* 1 (June 1856): 592–594. See also entry for 5 November 1857, in Stowe, *A Southern Practice*, pp. 321–322; D. Warren Brickell, "Placenta Previa, Etc.," *New Orleans Medical News and Hospital Gazette* 3 (1 June 1856): 216–218.

35. Douglass, "Ergot in Placenta Previa," p. 328.

36. John Harley Warner, *The Therapeutic Perspective: Medical Practice, Knowledge, and Identity in America, 1820–1885* (Princeton: Princeton University Press, 1997), p. 23; Eben Hillyer, "Extracts from the Records of the Atlanta Medical Society," *Atlanta Medical and Surgical Journal* 1 (April 1856): 460–462; D. Warren Brickell, "Rigidity of the Os Uteri, Etc.," *New Orleans Medical News and Hospital Gazette* 3 (1 July 1856): 274.

37. W. L. Sutton, "Cases of Retained Placenta," *Western Journal of Medicine and Surgery*, 3d ser., 1 (January 1848): 67–68; William E. Brickell, "Craniotomy," *New Orleans Medical News and Hospital Gazette* 3 (1 August 1856): 328–329.

38. Frost, "Expulsion of Mass of Hair from Uterus," pp. 217–218.

39. J. Y. Bassett, "Report on the Topography, Climate, and Diseases of the Parish of Madison Co., Ala.," *Southern Medical Reports* 1 (1849): 276.

40. Samuel Hogg, "Miscellaneous Cases," *Western Journal of Medicine and Surgery* 6 (October 1842): 255.

41. Carthon Archer, "Spirits of Turpentine as an Excitant of Uterine Contractions," *The Stethoscope and Virginia Medical Gazette* 3 (October 1853): 564–566.

42. W. Tyler Smith, "The Caesarian Section," *New Orleans Medical News and Hospital Gazette* 4 (1 July 1857): 279.

43. Hillyer, "Extracts from Records of Atlanta Medical Society," pp. 460–462. See also Brickell, "Craniotomy," p. 329.

44. F. E. H. Steger, "Obstetrical Case," *Nashville Journal of Medicine and Surgery* 9 (August 1855): 104–107.

45. I am grateful to nurse-midwife Debra Erickson-Owens for her insight into the problems posed by caesarean sections.

46. The first title was reprinted from the *New York Scalpel* and published in *Nashville Journal of Medicine and Surgery* 3, no. 6 (1852): 354–359; the second appeared first in the *New Orleans Medical and Surgical Journal*. The Nashville journal published the article in 7 (October 1854): 344. Herbert M. Morais maintains that black midwives may have brought from Africa a knowledge of caesarean section, but I have been unable to confirm this claim. See *The History*

of the Afro-American in Medicine (Cornwells Heights, Pa.: Publisher's Agency, 1978), p. 12.

47. Duffy, *Rudolph Matas History of Medicine*, 2: 68, 72–74, 296–297. Caesareans were performed even earlier in various places in desperate cases. For reference to one performed in Virginia on a white woman, see Joseph L. Miller, "Cesarean Section in Virginia in the Pre-Aseptic Era," *Annals of Medical History*, n.s., 10 (January 1938): 23–25, cited in Kay K. Moss, *Southern Folk Medicine, 1750–1820* (Columbia: University of South Carolina Press, 1999), p. 151.

48. Duffy, *Rudolph Matas History of Medicine*, 2: 72–74.

49. William G. Smith, "Case of Caesarean Operation," *Virginia Medical Journal* 7 (1856): 205–208; Rosen, *Fees and Fee Bills*, p. 39. Because of the difficulty of controlling bleeding and managing the patient's pain, operations in the antebellum era had to be performed as quickly as possible.

50. Eben Hillyer, "Extract from the Records of the Atlanta Medical Society," *Atlanta Medical and Surgical Journal* 1 (March 1856): 400–403.

51. Savitt, *Medicine and Slavery*, pp. 12–14; Stowe, *Doctoring the South*, pp. 49–50; C. Morrill, *The Physiology of Woman, and Her Diseases from Infancy to Old Age* (New York: C. Morrill, 1848), p. 353; William P. Dewees, *An Essay on the Means of Lessening Pain and Facilitating Certain Cases of Difficult Parturition* (Philadelphia: John Oswald, 1806), p. 7; Samuel K. Jennings, *The Married Lady's Companion, or Poor Man's Friend* (1808; reprint, New York: Arno, 1972), p. 78. The poor generally were thought to stand depletion less well than the rich; Martin S. Pernick, *A Calculus of Suffering: Pain, Professionalism, and Anesthesia in Nineteenth-Century America* (New York: Columbia University Press, 1985), pp. 134, 153.

52. Caton, *What a Blessing She Had Chloroform*, p. 16; W. L. C. Du Hamel, "Anesthetic Agents," *The Stethoscope* 5 (February 1855): 63–67; "Medico-Chirurgical Society of Richmond—First March Meeting," ibid., 4 (April 1854): 238–241.

53. Withers, "A Case of Eclampsia," pp. 103–105; Bassett, "Topography, Climate, and Diseases of Madison Co., Ala.," p. 276; "Miscellaneous: Physico-Medical Society," *New Orleans Medical News and Hospital Gazette* 1 (1 May 1854): 117. Chloroform also could be used on white women for purposes other than pain relief. See Andrew Bolton, "Morphia and Chloroform in Puerperal Convulsions," *The Stethoscope and Virginia Medical Gazette* 4 (April 1853): 255.

54. John Butts, "A Case of Labor Complicated with Eclampsia," *New Orleans Medical News and Hospital Gazette* 1 (1 July 1854): 212–213.

55. Withers, "A Case of Eclampsia," pp. 102–105. See also S2, vol. 17: Fla., p. 175; Jacqueline Jones, *Labor of Love, Labor of Sorrow: Black Women, Work, and*

the Family from Slavery to the Present (New York: Basic Books, 1985), pp. 29–30. For a case in which former slaves continued long after emancipation to blame a doctor for a poor outcome from pregnancy, see S2, vol. 9: Ark., pt. 3, p. 340.

56. Wall, "Medical Care of Ebenezer Pettigrew's Slaves," p. 461.

57. Unfortunately Harriet's fears were justified, and the birth proved difficult for mother and child; J. E. Manlove, "Remarkable Case of Monstrosity," *Nashville Journal of Medicine and Surgery* 16 (June 1859): 481–483; Withers, "A Case of Eclampsia," p. 102. For an example of a white woman who preferred a midwife, see Murr, *A Rebel Wife in Texas*, pp. 65, 102–103. Former slave Hannah Allen, who lived to be at least 107 and who was interviewed in the 1930s, attributed her longevity in part to having remained childless; S2, vol. 11: Mo., p. 8.

58. Manlove, "Remarkable Case of Monstrosity," p. 482; entry for 5 November 1857, in Stowe, *A Southern Practice*, pp. 321–322; S2, vol. 8: Ark., pt. 1, p. 344, and vol. 10: Ark., pt. 6, p. 255.

59. Dew, *Bond of Iron*, pp. 274, 279; James E. Bagwell, *Rice Gold: James Hamilton Couper and Plantation Life on the Georgia Coast* (Macon, Ga.: Mercer University Press, 2000), p. 127. See also Withers, "A Case of Eclampsia," pp. 102–105.

60. S2, vol. 8: Ark., pt. 1, p. 311, and pt. 2, pp. 42, 283; SS1, vol. 6: Miss., pt. 1, p. 20, and vol. 9: Miss., pt. 4, p. 1892; Philpot, "A Case of Hypertrophy of the Spleen," p. 707; Petition of Benjamin Edwards Browne, in Loren Schweninger, ed., *The Southern Debate over Slavery*, vol. 1: *Petitions to Southern Legislatures, 1778–1864* (Urbana: University of Illinois Press, 2001), pp. 41–42.

61. Baker, *Homeless, Friendless, and Penniless*, p. 114; S2, vol. 8: Ark., pt. 2, p. 240, and vol. 10: Ark., pt. 5, p. 157, and vol. 14: N.C., pt. 1, pp. 154, 221, and vol. 17: Fla., p. 129.

62. Entries for 10 July 1858 and 29 November 1859, David Gavin Diary, SHC; William L. McCaa, "Observations on the Manner of Living and Diseases of the Slaves on the Wateree River" (Ph.D. diss., University of Pennsylvania, 1823), p. 12; Index for 1856 and Index for 1858, James M. Torbert Diary, pp. 158, 207, typescript copy, ADAH; John I. Garner to James K. Polk, 7 June 1840, in John Spencer Bassett, *The Southern Plantation Overseer as Revealed in His Letters* (New York: Negro Universities Press, 1968), p. 141; Todd L. Savitt, "Patient Letters to an Early Nineteenth Century Virginia Physician," *Journal of the Florida Medical Association* 69 (1982): 691; Fett, *Working Cures*, p. 174. On the resistance of southern white women to attendance at childbirth by male doctors, see McMillen, *Motherhood in the Old South*, pp. 68, 98–99.

63. S2, vol. 8: Ark., pt. 1, p. 319, and pt. 2, p. 328, and vol. 9: Ark., pt. 3, p. 106, and vol. 10: Ark., pt. 5, pp. 137, 244, 257, 301, and vol. 14: N.C., pt. 1, pp. 221, 299; SS1, vol. 6: Miss., pt. 1, p. 23; SS2, vol. 10: Tex., pt. 9, p. 4168.

64. Starr's owner was also his father; Baker and Baker, *WPA Oklahoma Slave Narratives,* pp. 340, 408, 435; Bagwell, *Rice Gold,* p. 127. See also S2, vol. 8: Ark., pt. 1, p. 51, and vol. 15: N.C., pt. 2, p. 270. Hospitals were growing in importance in the North, especially for patients deemed incapable of improving their health at home. See Pernick, *A Calculus of Suffering,* p. 16.

65. S2, vol. 9: Ark., pt. 3, p. 286; E. B. Haskins, "Clinical Observations in Private Practice," *Western Journal of Medicine and Surgery,* 3d ser., 7 (January 1851): 8; entry for 5 November 1857, in Stowe, *A Southern Practice,* p. 321; Baker and Baker, *WPA Oklahoma Slave Narratives,* p. 435.

66. Baker, *Homeless, Friendless, and Penniless,* p. 189; S2, vol. 9: Ark., pt. 3, p. 286; King, *Northern Woman in Plantation South,* p. 114.

67. Pavich-Lindsay, *Anna,* pp. 32n1, 92, 101, 118, 298, 360–361, 362.

68. Ibid., p. 114.

69. On the folk medicine of Euroamericans, see Moss, *Southern Folk Medicine.* On the use of thyme, feverfew, and motherwort, see pp. 208, 184, 195.

70. S2, vol. 10: Ark., pt. 5, pp. 33–35.

71. E. F. Knott, "A Case of Parturition, with Its Complications," *Atlanta Medical and Surgical Journal* 1 (September 1855): 12; Hogg, "Miscellaneous Cases," p. 255.

72. Thomas H. Todd, "On the Use of Cathartics in Retention of the Placenta," *Western Journal of Medicine and Surgery* 7 (May 1843): 349–350 (emphasis added).

73. James S. Dyer, "Abuse of Ergot," *Nashville Journal of Medicine and Surgery* 9 (September 1855): 202–203; A. T. Noe, "Treatment of Dysmenorrhea by Mechanical Dilatation," ibid., 3, no. 4 (1852): 347; Baker and Baker, *WPA Oklahoma Slave Narratives,* p. 66.

74. Editorial, "Practical Suggestions to Young Physicians," *The Stethoscope* 4 (April 1854): 215–216.

75. *Gunn's Domestic Medicine: A Facsimile of the First Edition,* Tennesseeana ed. (Knoxville: University of Tennessee Press, 1986), pp. 305–338; Reynell Coates, *Popular Medicine; or, Family Adviser* (Philadelphia: Carey, Lea, and Blanchard, 1838); Shryock, "Medical Practice in the Old South," p. 174; Michael Tadman, *Speculators and Slaves: Masters, Traders, and Slaves in the Old South* (Madison: University of Wisconsin Press, 1989), p. 128.

76. Philips' notes are in a copy of Samuel Bard, *A Compendium of the Theory and Practice of Midwifery, Containing Practical Instructions for the Management of Women during Pregnancy, in Labour, and in Child-bed,* 4th ed. (New York: Collins, 1817), located in Ruffin, Roulhac, and Hamilton Family Papers,

Records of Ante-Bellum Southern Plantations, Part 7: Alabama, Series J: Selections from the Manuscripts Department, SHC. Bard helped to found what became known as Columbia University College of Physicians and Surgeons.

77. Baker and Baker, *WPA Oklahoma Slave Narratives*, p. 72; S2, vol. 11: Mo., p. 170; letter from Thomas Seddon, 6 April 1822, Letters to Doctor James Carmichael and Son; John I. Garner to James K. Polk, 7 June 1840, in Bassett, *The Southern Plantation Overseer*, p. 141.

78. "An Obstetric Letter," p. 931; Duffy, *Rudolph Matas History of Medicine*, 2: 64–75; Todd, "Use of Cathartics in Retention of Placenta," pp. 349–351. Green singled out a white midwife for criticism, but the majority of midwives who attended slave women were black, and they, too, were disparaged; Rowan Green, "A Shoulder Presentation, and Dissection of the Child," *Nashville Journal of Medicine and Surgery* 15 (July 1858): 29. See also "Transactions of the Medical Society of So. Ca., Oct. 1, 1846," *Southern Journal of Medicine and Pharmacy* 2 (January 1847): 35.

79. T. P. Bailey, "Obstetrical Cases," *Charleston Medical Journal and Review* 15 (September 1860): 599–600, 601.

80. Brickell, "Craniotomy," pp. 329–330; T. P. Crutcher, "Right Occipito Iliac Position and Protracted Labor," *Nashville Journal of Medicine and Pharmacy* 15 (October 1858): 279–280.

81. Hogg, "Miscellaneous Cases," pp. 255–256.

82. Brickell, "Craniotomy," p. 330.

83. Haskins, "Clinical Observations in Private Practice," pp. 8–10; Bailey, "Obstetrical Cases," p. 603. See also B. S. Hopkins, "Excerpts from My Case Book," *Nashville Journal of Medicine and Surgery* 9 (August 1855): 102; "Prof. Cenas' Cases of Difficult Labor," p. 696.

84. S2, vol. 9: Ark., pt. 4, p. 115; SS1, vol. 9: Miss., pt. 4, p. 1467. See also ibid., p. 1801; SS2, vol. 10: Tex., pt. 9, pp. 3998, 4065, 4110; Baker and Baker, *WPA Oklahoma Slave Narratives*, p. 138. On southern midwives in the colonial era, see Kathleen M. Brown, *Good Wives, Nasty Wenches, and Anxious Patriarchs: Gender, Race, and Power in Colonial Virginia* (Chapel Hill: University of North Carolina Press for the Omohundro Institute of Early America, 1996), pp. 97–98, 130, 192, 203, 290. On the situation of mixed-race children who could not be entrusted with knowledge of their fathers, see Marie Jenkins Schwartz, *Born in Bondage: Growing Up Enslaved in the Antebellum South* (Cambridge, Mass.: Harvard University Press, 2000), pp. 44–46.

85. Memorandum Book for Birdfield Plantation, 1857–1859, pp. 21–22, James Ritchie Sparkman Papers, Records of Ante-Bellum Southern Plantations,

Series A, Part 2: Miscellaneous Collections. See also Memorandum Book for Birdfield Plantation, 1850–1857, and Memorandum Book, 1859–1861.

6. Postnatal Complications

1. Todd L. Savitt, "Patient Letters to an Early Nineteenth Century Virginia Physician," *Journal of the Florida Medical Association* 69 (August 1982): 691.

2. John R. Turner, "Plantation Hygiene," *Southern Cultivator* 15 (May–June 1857), in *Advice among Masters: The Ideal in Slave Management in the Old South,* ed. James O. Breeden (Westport, Conn.: Greenwood, 1980), p. 204.

3. Plantation Manual of James H. Hammond of Beach Island, South Carolina, about 1834, Joseph I. Waring Research Files, Waring Historical Library, Medical University of South Carolina, Charleston; Sharla M. Fett, *Working Cures: Healing, Health, and Power on Southern Slave Plantations* (Chapel Hill: University of North Carolina Press, 2002), p. 131.

4. S2, vol. 9: Ark., pt. 3, p. 286; William Ed Grimé, *Ethno-Botany of the Black Americans* (Algonac, Mich.: Reference Publications, 1979), p. 167.

5. S2, vol. 15: N.C., pt. 2, pp. 371, 373. See also T. Lindsay Baker and Julie P. Baker, eds., *The WPA Oklahoma Slave Narratives* (Norman: University of Oklahoma Press, 1996), pp. 81, 141.

6. S2, vol. 14: N.C., pt. 1, p. 447, and vol. 15: N.C., pt. 2, p. 31; SS2, vol. 10: Tex., pt. 9, p. 3970; Wilma King, ed., *A Northern Woman in the Plantation South: Letters of Tryphena Blanche Holder Fox, 1856–1876* (Columbia: University of South Carolina, 1993), p. 114; James E. Bagwell, *Rice Gold: James Hamilton Couper and Plantation Life on the Georgia Coast* (Macon, Ga.: Mercer University Press, 2000), p. 127; Edwin Adams Davis, ed., *Plantation Life in the Florida Parishes of Louisiana, 1836–1846, as Reflected in the Diary of Bennet H. Barrow* (New York: Columbia University Press, 1943), pp. 79, 92, 93, 207, 238, 272.

7. Ronald L. Baker, comp., *Homeless, Friendless, and Penniless: The WPA Interviews with Former Slaves Living in Indiana* (Bloomington: Indiana University Press, 2000), p. 212; Baker and Baker, *WPA Oklahoma Slave Narratives,* p. 81; S2, vol. 8: Ark., pt. 2, p. 15, and vol. 10: Ark., pt. 5, p. 157.

8. George Rosen, *Fees and Fee Bills: Some Economic Aspects of Medical Practice in Nineteenth Century America* (Baltimore: Johns Hopkins Press, 1946), pp. 27, 39; "Tariff of Fees, Etc.," *The Stethoscope* 4 (February–March 1854): 99.

9. Frances Webster to Frances Kirby Smith, 10 August 1851, in Van R. Baker, ed., *The Websters: Letters of an American Army Family in Peace and War, 1836–1853* (Kent, Ohio: Kent State University Press, 2000), pp. 262–263.

10. Thomas H. Todd, "On the Use of Cathartics in Retention of the Placenta," *Western Journal of Medicine and Surgery* 7 (March 1843): 349–351.

11. Henry R. Frost, "Expulsion of a Mass of Hair from the Uterus," *Western Journal of Medicine and Surgery* 6 (September 1842): 218.

12. William M. Boling, "Surgical Cases," ibid., 2d ser., 2 (September 1844): 231–232.

13. E. F. Knott, "A Case of Parturition, with Its Complications," *Atlanta Medical and Surgical Journal* 1 (September 1855): 14–15; M. J. Greene, "A Case of Partial Placenta Previa, Complicated with Transverse Presentation and Rigidity of the Os Uteri," ibid. (June 1856): 593.

14. W. L. Sutton, "Cases of Retained Placenta," *Western Journal of Medicine and Surgery,* 3d ser., 1 (January 1848): 61–70, reprinted from the *Boston Medical and Surgical Journal.*

15. S. Henry Dickson, "Case of Monstrosity," *Southern Journal of Medicine and Pharmacy* 1 (September 1846): 496–497; Charles D. Meigs, *Obstetrics: The Science and the Art* (Philadelphia: Blanchard and Lea, 1863), pp. 337–339; Wooster Beach, *An Improved System of Midwifery* (New York: Charles Scribner, 1853), pp. 115, 142–143. Surgeons in early modern Europe advocated such an approach, although they might induce sneezing or retching to assist the process; Teresa Ortiz, "From Hegemony to Subordination: Midwives in Early Modern Spain," in *The Art of Midwifery: Early Modern Midwives in Europe,* ed. Hilary Marland (New York: Routledge, 1993), p. 106. Today birth attendants wait only about thirty minutes before attempting to remove the placenta manually, less if hemorrhage occurs. Once expelled, the placenta is inspected carefully to ensure that no portion of it or the membranes remains in the uterine cavity. If any part is missing, the attendant explores the uterine cavity manually. Usually an anesthesiologist is called, because severe discomfort characterizes manual removal.

16. L. Faulkner, "Cases from My Note Book and Memory," *New Orleans Medical News and Hospital Gazette* 3 (1 July 1856): 313–314.

17. Todd, "Use of Cathartics in Retention of Placenta," p. 349.

18. Felder, "Adhesion of the Placenta," pp. 72–73.

19. Ibid., pp. 71–72.

20. Ibid., pp. 72–73.

21. On medical experimentation upon slaves generally, see Todd L. Savitt, *Medicine and Slavery: The Diseases and Health Care of Blacks in Antebellum Virginia* (Urbana: University of Illinois Press, 1978), p. 17 and chap. 9 (esp. pp. 293–301); Walter Fisher, "Physicians and Slavery in the Antebellum Southern Medical Journal," *Journal of the History of Medicine and Allied Sciences* 23

(January 1968): 45–47; Weymouth T. Jordan, "Plantation Medicine in the Old South," *Alabama Review* 3 (1950): 85.

22. Sutton, "Cases of Retained Placenta," pp. 64–70.

23. Letter from Arthur Alexander Morson, [18—], Letters to Doctor James Carmichael and Son, Historical Collections at the Claude Moore Health Sciences Library, University of Virginia, http://etext.lib.virginia.edu/healthsci/carmichael/collection.

24. Richard W. Wertz and Dorothy C. Wertz have described puerperal fever as "probably the classic example of iatrogenic disease—that is, disease caused by medical treatment itself." See their *Lying-In: A History of Childbirth in America* (New York: Free Press, 1977), pp. xi, x, 128.

25. "Contagiousness of Puerperal Fever," *Western Journal of Medicine and Surgery,* 2d ser., 5 (March 1846): 245–246; Irvine Loudon, *The Tragedy of Childbed Fever* (New York: Oxford University Press, 2000), pp. 53–57; John Duffy, *From Humors to Medical Science: A History of American Medicine,* 2d ed. (Urbana: University of Illinois, 1993), pp. 126–127.

26. John Duffy, ed., *The Rudolph Matas History of Medicine in Louisiana,* vol. 2 ([Baton Rouge]: Louisiana State University Press, 1962), pp. 68–69; C. R. Harris, "The Epidemic of Puerperal Fever of Mount Solon and Vicinity," *The Stethoscope and Virginia Medical Gazette* 2 (July 1852): 377. For recommended sanitary precautions, see Duffy, *From Humors to Medical Science,* pp. 126–127. Today a continuation of the vaginal discharge that follows childbirth is considered a symptom rather than a cause.

27. John P. Mettauer, "The Prophylactic Treatment of Puerperal Fever," *The Stethoscope and Virginia Medical Gazette* 1 (April 1851): 222–228; Goodridge A. Wilson, "Prophylaxis of Puerperal Peritonitis," ibid. (August 1851): 442–445.

28. John P. Mettauer, "Prophylaxis of Puerperal Peritonitis," ibid. (October 1851): 547–552. Mettauer specifically rejected contagion and communicable disease as responsible for puerperal fever. See idem, "A Case of Puerperal Fever Successfully Treated," ibid. (April 1851): 209.

29. "'Brewers' Yeast in Puerperal Fever,'" *The Stethoscope* 4 (April 1854): 222; Medicus Ransom, "Report on Cases of Child-bed Fever," *Nashville Medical Journal* 16 (February 1859): 114–115, 117.

30. Ransom, "Report on Cases of Child-bed Fever," pp. 114–115, 117.

31. Ibid., p. 115.

32. Ibid., pp. 115–116.

33. Ibid., pp. 116–117.

34. Ibid., p. 117.

35. Ibid., pp. 118–119. Ransom was not the only physician experimenting with veratrum for puerperal fever. See V. H. Taliaferro, "Remarks upon the Medical Properties and Therapeutical Applications of Veratrum Viride," *Atlanta Medical and Surgical Journal* 2 (March 1857): 406.

36. Harris, "The Epidemic Puerperal Fever," pp. 377, 378.

37. Mettauer, "Case of Puerperal Fever Successfully Treated," pp. 205–209.

38. Harris, "The Epidemic Puerperal Fever," pp. 376–377.

39. Mettauer, "Prophylactic Treatment of Puerperal Fever," pp. 222–228; E. B. Haskins, "Clinical Observations in Private Practice," *Western Journal of Medicine and Surgery*, 3d ser., 7 (January 1851): 8–10.

40. Harris, "The Epidemic Puerperal Fever," p. 380.

41. "Second Annual Report to the General Assembly of Kentucky Relating to the Registry and Returns of the Births, Marriages and Deaths, from January 1, 1853, to December 31, 1853," *Western Journal of Medicine and Surgery*, 4th ser., 3 (April 1855): 289. Flawed interpretation of medical statistics was not unusual in the antebellum era. See James H. Cassedy, *American Medicine and Statistical Thinking, 1800–1860* (Cambridge, Mass.: Harvard University Press, 1984). On statistics related to obstetrics, including puerperal fever, see pp. 80–83. On the collection of medical statistics, see also Gerald N. Grob, *Edward Jarvis and the Medical World of Nineteenth-Century America* (Knoxville: University of Tennessee Press, 1978).

42. Boring, "Puerperal Fever—Its Pathology," pp. 148–149; "Close of the Session of the Richmond Medical College," *The Stethoscope and Virginia Medical Gazette* 1 (April 1851): 219. This must have been the Medical College of Virginia at Richmond; "Annual Announcement of Lectures in the Atlanta Medical College for the Session of 1857, with a Catalogue of the Students and Graduates of 1856," *Atlanta Medical and Surgical Journal* 2 (August 1857): n.p.; Roberta O. Burkett, W. A. Sawyer, and W. C. Worthington, comps., *A Bibliography of Inaugural Theses of Graduating Students at the Medical College* (Charleston: Waring Historical Library of the Medical University of South Carolina, n.d.); "Editorial Correspondence," *Atlanta Medical and Surgical Journal* 2 (February 1857): 364–365. Europeans led the search for the cause and cure of puerperal fever. Hungarian physician Ignaz Philipp Semmenlweis in 1847 discovered a cause of puerperal fever when he observed that women in a Vienna lying-in hospital were being infected by physicians who examined them after making pathological dissections. The mortality rate fell after Semmenlweis instituted a policy of handwashing in the hospital; however, the eradication of childbed fevers awaited further developments, and acceptance of his ideas did not occur until after the Civil War. French chemist Louis Pasteur advanced the

cure of childbed fevers when he developed the germ theory, which postulated that infectious diseases are caused by microorganisms (bacteria). English surgeon Joseph Lister applied Pasteur's theory to surgery and demonstrated that an antiseptic agent coupled with heat sterilization could dramatically reduce postoperative deaths from surgery.

43. Steven Weisenburger, *Modern Medea: A Family Story of Slavery and Child Murder from the Old South* (New York: Hill and Wang, 1998), pp. 258–259.

44. W. L. Sutton, "A Case of Infanticide," *Western Journal of Medicine and Surgery*, 3d ser., 11 (January 1853): 28–30.

45. SS1, vol. 9: Miss., pt. 4, p. 1449.

46. Erika L. Murr, ed., *A Rebel Wife in Texas: The Diary and Letters of Elizabeth Scott Neblett, 1852–1864* (Baton Rouge: Louisiana State University Press, 2001), p. 223.

47. Steven Weisenburger discusses Garner's case at length in *Modern Medea*, p. 258. The Savannah *Daily Morning News* in April 1860 carried a story of an attempted suicide by a mother who threw herself and three children down a well. She allegedly explained after her rescue that "she wished to die and didn't want to leave any of her children behind." Quoted in Clarence L. Mohr, *On the Threshold of Freedom: Masters and Slaves in Civil War Georgia* (Athens: University of Georgia Press, 1986), p. 12. I have found no evidence that numerous enslaved women carried out infanticide as some historians have claimed. See Stephanie J. Shaw, "Mothering under Slavery in the Antebellum South," in *Mothering: Ideology, Experience, and Agency*, ed. Evelyn Nakano Glenn, Grace Chang, and Linda Rennie Forcey (New York: Routledge, 1994), p. 248; Darlene Hine and Kate Wittenstein, "Female Slave Resistance: The Economics of Sex," in *The Black Woman Cross-Culturally*, ed. Filomina Chioma Steady (Cambridge, Mass.: Schenkman, 1981), p. 294.

48. Baker and Baker, *WPA Oklahoma Slave Narratives*, p. 392.

49. SS1, vol. 6: Miss., pt. 1, pp. 3–4.

50. Baker, *Homeless, Friendless, and Penniless*, p. 213.

51. S2, vol. 15: N.C., pt. 2, p. 283; SS2, vol. 10: Tex., pt. 9, pp. 4138, 4170.

52. As anthropologist Lucile F. Newman observes, almost all social groups define as "misbegotten" some children because of the "inappropriateness of parentage, pregnancy, number, form, timing, or location of childbearing." The concept of "misbegotten" is not related to biology. See Newman, ed., *Women's Medicine: A Cross-Cultural Study of Indigenous Fertility Regulation* (New Brunswick, N.J.: Rutgers University Press, 1985), p. 3.

53. "Double-Headed Monster," *New Orleans Medical News and Hospital Gazette* 4 (1 May 1857): 129–130; John W. Blassingame, *The Slave Community: Plantation Life in the Antebellum South*, rev. ed. (New York: Oxford University Press, 1979), pp. 41, 45; Charles Joyner, *Down by the Riverside: A South Carolina Slave Community* (Urbana: University of Illinois Press, 1984), p. 138; idem, "The World of the Plantation Slave," in *Before Freedom Came: African-American Life in the Antebellum South*, ed. Edward D. C. Campbell Jr. with Kym S. Rice (Richmond and Charlottesville: Museum of the Confederacy and the University Press of Virginia, 1991), pp. 77, 81. It is difficult to know the emotional toll of such events on parents. Ruth Richardson speculates about the emotional distress presented by grave-robbing on nineteenth-century Englishmen in *Death, Dissection, and the Destitute* (London: Routledge and Kegan Paul, 1987), pp. 78, 322n17.

54. J. E. Manlove, "Remarkable Case of Monstrosity," *Nashville Journal of Medicine and Surgery* 16 (June 1859): 481–483.

55. King, *Northern Woman in Plantation South*, p. 114.

56. J. W. B. Garrett, "Singular Case of Monstrosity," *Western Journal of Medicine and Surgery*, 3d ser., 6 (July 1850): 1–6.

57. J. K. Hamilton, "A Monster," *Atlanta Medical and Surgical Journal*, n.s., 7B (December 1866): 478–480.

58. E. C. Moyer, "Report on a Remarkable Case of Monstrosity, with a Surgical Operation," *Atlanta Journal of Medicine and Surgery* 2 (February 1857): 319.

59. "Medical Items," *Nashville Journal of Medicine and Surgery* 9 (August 1855): 156–165; letter to the editor, ibid., 13 (July 1857): 236–237; letter to Dr. Nelson from A. Munro, January 1855, in "Case of Twin Delivery," *The Stethoscope* 5 (May 1855): 299–300; A. Von Iffland, "Reminiscences of the Siamese Twins," *The Stethoscope and Virginia Medical Gazette* 2 (December 1852): 701–702, which originally appeared in the *Canada Medical Journal*.

60. "Monstrosities," *New Orleans Medical News and Hospital Gazette* 5 (March 1858): 37–38.

61. [P. Claiborne Gooch], "The Carolina Twins," *The Stethoscope and Virginia Medical Gazette* 2 (July 1852): 394.

62. Ibid., pp. 394–395.

63. Ibid., p. 395.

64. "Monstrosities," pp. 38–39.

65. Steven M. Stowe, ed., *A Southern Practice: The Diary and Autobiography of Charles A. Hentz, M.D.* (Charlottesville: University Press of Virginia, 2000), pp. 183, 185, 189, 339–340, 461, 470.

66. M. Emanual, "Case of Malformation of a Child," *The Stethoscope and Virginia Medical Gazette* 1 (August 1851): 474. For another case involving a malformed child born to a white woman, see R. E. Jennings, "A Case of Monstrosity," ibid. (April 1851): 276.

67. Stowe, *A Southern Practice*, pp. 513–514.

68. L. I. Marvin, "A Case of Monstrosity," *Atlanta Medical and Surgical Journal*, n.s., 7B (March 1867): 35.

69. "Catalogue of Drugs, Pharmaceutical Preparations, and Medicinal Wares," p. 21, in *The Stethoscope and Virginia Medical Gazette* 4 (April 1852).

70. Ibid.

71. Michael Sappol, *A Traffic of Dead Bodies: Anatomy and Embodied Social Identity in Nineteenth-Century America* (Princeton: Princeton University Press, 2002), chap. 2, esp. pp. 61–63.

72. Robert L. Blakely and Judith M. Harrington, eds., *Bones in the Basement: Postmortem Racism in Nineteenth-Century Medical Training* (Washington, D.C.: Smithsonian Institution Press, 1997), p. 195; Stowe, *A Southern Practice*, pp. 467–468; Duffy, *From Humors to Medical Science*, p. 132; Kenneth Allen De Ville, *Medical Malpractice in Nineteenth-Century America* (New York: New York University Press, 1990), p. 70; Sappol, *A Traffic of Dead Bodies*, pp. 13, 16, 87, 103, 107; Todd L. Savitt, "The Use of Blacks for Medical Experimentation and Demonstration in the Old South," *Journal of Southern History* 48 (August 1982): 337–338; Deborah Kuhn McGregor, *From Midwives to Medicine: The Birth of American Gynecology* (New Brunswick, N.J.: Rutgers University Press, 1998), pp. 19–20. On opportunities for students to dissect cadavers, see advertisements, *The Stethoscope and Virginia Medical Gazette* 7 (July 1853): n.p.; "Annual Announcement of Lectures in the Atlanta Medical College," *Atlanta Medical and Surgical Journal* 1 (August 1856): n.p.; advertisement, University of Nashville, *The Stethoscope and Virginia Medical Gazette* 1 (August 1851): n.p. African Americans continued to fear the possibility of body snatching by medical students and doctors after emancipation. See Gladys-Marie Fry, *Night Riders in Black Folk History* (Knoxville: University of Tennessee Press, 1975), esp. chap. 6. Blacks and other minority groups (as well as the poor generally) made up a disproportionate number of dissection subjects throughout the United States. The poor were also disproportionately subject to dissection in nineteenth-century Great Britain. See Richardson, *Death, Dissection, and the Destitute*.

73. "The Approaching Meeting of the Medical Society," *The Stethoscope and Virginia Medical Gazette* 3 (March 1853): 154; "Medico-Chirurgical Society of the City of Richmond—First March Meeting," ibid., 4 (April 1853): 231; Savitt, *Medicine and Slavery*, pp. 290, 301–307.

74. Harris, "The Epidemic Puerperal Fever," p. 377; Charles Witsell, "Case of Enormous Polypus of the Uterus Treated with the Muriated Tincture of Iron," *Charleston Medical Journal and Review* 15 (March 1860): 327; T. A. Means, "Diphtheritis or Diphtheritic Sorethroat," *Atlanta Medical and Surgical Journal* 6 (February 1861): 328; James Bolton, "Report of a Fatal Case of Tetanus Following the Ligature of Hemorroids," *The Stethoscope and Virginia Medical Gazette* 1 (December 1851): 662; B. S. Hopkins, "Excerpts from My Case Book," *Nashville Journal of Medicine and Surgery* 9 (August 1855): 102; Fett, *Working Cures*, pp. 154, 156; Maureen McCarthy Capozzoli, "A Rip into the Flesh, a Tear into the Soul: An Ethnography of Dissection in Georgia," in Blakely and Harrington, *Bones in the Basement*, pp. 329–336. Both blacks and whites objected to autopsies, but doctors evidently found it easier to gain access to blacks to autopsy than to whites. In Simpson County, Kentucky, doctors seldom received permission to perform autopsies; only four were conducted from 1852 to 1856, and all of these were on black bodies; J. B. Suddarth, "Physical and Medical Topography, Etc., of Simpson County," *Nashville Journal of Medicine and Surgery* 11 (December 1856): 486. See also "Medico-Chirurgical Society of the City of Richmond—First January Meeting 1853," *The Stethoscope and Virginia Medical Gazette* 3 (February 1853): 108–109.

75. J. O. Sharber, "Death from Exterior Uterine Hemorrhage," *Nashville Journal of Medicine and Surgery* 4 (May 1853): 259–261.

76. Baker and Baker, *WPA Oklahoma Slave Narratives*, p. 91; SS2, vol. 2: Tex., pt. 1, p. 119.

77. Peter R. Reamey, "Post-Mortem Examination of a Case of Tabes-Mesenterica, Etc.," *The Stethoscope and Virginia Medical Gazette* 2 (July 1852): 381.

78. Stowe, *A Southern Practice*, p. 470; S2, vol. 9: Ark., pt. 3, p. 268, and vol. 11: Mo., pp. 246–247; SS2, vol. 2: Tex., pt. 1, p. 276; Charles L. Perdue Jr., Thomas E. Barden, and Robert K. Phillips, eds., *Weevils in the Wheat: Interviews with Virginia Ex-Slaves* (Charlottesville: University Press of Virginia, 1976), p. 342.

79. SS2, vol. 10: Tex., pt. 9, p. 4100.

80. Davis, *Plantation Life in Louisiana*, p. 103; S2, vol. 15: N.C., pt. 2, pp. 218–219; SS2, vol. 10: Tex., pt. 9, pp. 4110, 4318.

81. William L. Andrews, ed., *From Fugitive Slave to Free Man: The Autobiographies of William Wells Brown* (New York: Mentor, 1993), p. 47.

7. Gynecological Surgery

1. D. Warren Brickell, "Vesico-Vaginal Fistula," *New Orleans Medical News and Hospital Gazette* 6 (May 1859): 190–195.

2. E. R. Mordecai, "Vesico-Vaginal Fistula," *New Orleans Medical News and Hospital Gazette* 7 (August 1860): 450–452. Experimentation with surgical procedures on slaves was not limited to women. See Walter Fisher, "Physicians and Slavery in the Antebellum Southern Medical Journal," *Journal of the History of Medicine and Allied Sciences* 23 (January 1968): 45; Todd L. Savitt, "The Use of Blacks for Medical Experimentation and Demonstration in the Old South," *Journal of Southern History* 48 (August 1982): 332–333, 341–342; idem, *Medicine and Slavery: The Diseases and Health Care of Blacks in Antebellum Virginia* (Urbana: University of Illinois Press, 1978), p. 17 and chap. 9, esp. pp. 293–301. On medical experimentation in the late nineteenth and early twentieth centuries, see Susan E. Lederer, *Subjected to Science: Human Experimentation in America before the Second World War* (Baltimore: Johns Hopkins University Press, 1995).

3. N. Bozeman, "Remarks on Vesico-Vaginal Fistule, with an Account of a New Mode of Suture, and Seven Successful Operations," *Louisville Review* 1 (1856): 94–99.

4. John Bellinger, "Operations for the Removal of Abdominal Tumours," *Southern Journal of Medicine and Pharmacy* 2 (May 1847): 242; J. Marion Sims, *The Story of My Life* (New York: D. Appleton, 1884), p. 136; Deborah Kuhn McGregor, *From Midwives to Medicine: The Birth of American Gynecology* (New Brunswick, N.J.: Rutgers University Press, 1998), p. 19.

5. John Duffy, *From Humors to Medical Science: A History of American Medicine,* 2d ed. (Urbana: University of Illinois Press, 1993), pp. 95, 96, 99, 111–112; McGregor, *From Midwives to Medicine,* pp. 19, 51; Martin S. Pernick, *A Calculus of Suffering: Pain, Professionalism, and Anesthesia in Nineteenth-Century America* (New York: Columbia University Press, 1985), pp. 36–58, 108–109, 120–121.

6. W. L. C. Du Hamel, "Anesthetic Agents," *The Stethoscope* 5 (February 1855): 64; Duffy, *From Humors to Medical Science,* p. 112; James S. Olson, *Bathsheba's Breast: Women, Cancer, and History* (Baltimore: Johns Hopkins University Press, 2002), p. 54. On white women's endurance of radical breast extirpation without anesthesia, see pp. 49–49.

7. Pernick discusses attitudes among physicians and white patients in *A Calculus of Suffering,* pp. 62–66, 84.

8. Bozeman, "Remarks on Vesico-Vaginal Fistule," pp. 96, 97, 101. On another operation—this one the removal of a cancerous breast—in which a black woman (possibly free) writhed in pain and tried to get away, see Sharla M. Fett, *Working Cures: Healing, Health, and Power on Southern Slave Plantations* (Chapel Hill: University of North Carolina Press, 2002), p. 147.

9. The enslaved woman's distrust may have stemmed from the doctor's initial belief that Kitty was shamming; S. B. Robison, "Case of Inflammation of the Ovaria," *Nashville Journal of Medicine and Surgery* 3, no. 1 (1852): 77–78.

10. Georgia Writers' Project, *Drums and Shadows: Survival Studies among the Georgia Coastal Negroes* (Athens: University of Georgia Press, 1986), p. 57; SS2, vol. 10: Tex., pt. 9, p. 4319.

11. L. Lewis Wall, "Birth Trauma and the Pelvic Floor: Lessons from the Developing World," *Journal of Women's Health* 8, no. 2 (1999): 152–153; idem, *"Fitsari 'Dan Duniya:* An African (Hausa) Praise Song about Vesicovaginal Fistulas," *Obstetrics and Gynecology* 100 (December 2002): 1328–31; idem, "Dead Mothers and Injured Wives: The Social Context of Maternal Morbidity and Mortality among the Hausa of Northern Nigeria," *Studies in Family Planning* 29 (December 1998): 345. Although Wall reaches his conclusions about obstetric fistula by observing women in today's developing world, his findings offer insight into the childbirth experiences of women in the days before the development of modern obstetrics. On the effects of obstetric fistula see also Sims, *The Story of My Life,* p. 236; F. N. Boney, "Slaves as Guinea Pigs: Georgia and Alabama Episodes," *Alabama Review* 37 (1984): 48–49; McGregor, *From Midwives to Medicine,* pp. 123–124.

12. William N. Morgan, "A Case of Rupture of the Uterus, with Artificial Anus at the Point of Rupture," *Western Journal of Medicine and Surgery,* 2d ser., 2 (December 1844): 498–501; N. Bozeman, "Vesico-Vaginal Fistula, with Laceration of the Anterior Lip of the Cervix Uteri of Nearly Six Years Standing—Cured in Two Weeks," ibid., 4th ser., 4 (September 1855): 234–236.

13. Wall, *"Fitsari 'Dan Duniya,"* pp. 1328–31; idem, "Dead Mothers and Injured Wives," pp. 343–345; idem, "Birth Trauma and the Pelvic Floor," p. 151; James R. Scott, Philip J. Di Saia, Charles B. Hammond, and William N. Spellacy, eds., *Danforth's Obstetrics and Gynecology,* 8th ed. (Philadelphia: Lippincott, Williams, and Wilkins, 1999), p. 764.

14. Wall, "Dead Mothers and Injured Wives," pp. 343, 350; McGregor, *From Midwives to Medicine,* pp. 110, 112.

15. Robert Battey, "Report of a Case of Vesico Vaginal Fistula," *Atlanta Medical and Surgical Journal* 4 (June 1859): 591–594; McGregor, *From Midwives to Medicine,* pp. 120, 218.

16. Episiotomies (incision of the vulva during labor) alleviate the problem of rigid perineums in modern times. A distended bladder can pose a serious problem to the progress of labor. McGregor, *From Midwives to Medicine,* p. 118.

17. Ibid., pp. 110–111, 125. See also Londa Schiebinger, *Nature's Body: Gender in the Making of Modern Science* (Boston: Beacon, 1993), pp. 156–160.

18. "13th Congressional District Meeting," *The Stethoscope and Virginia Medical Gazette* 2 (August 1852): 448; "Editorial Correspondence," *Atlanta Medical and Surgical Journal* 2 (March 1857): 432.

19. McGregor, *From Midwives to Medicine,* pp. 26, 28, 32; Steven M. Stowe, "Seeing Themselves at Work: Physicians and the Case Narrative in the Mid-Nineteenth-Century American South," *American Historical Review* 101 (February 1996): 57, 68; Fett, *Working Cures,* p. 153.

20. McGregor, *From Midwives to Medicine,* pp. 45–46.

21. Ibid., pp. 45–54, 95.

22. Sims, *The Story of My Life,* p. 238–239.

23. J. Marion Sims, *Silver Sutures in Surgery* (New York: Wood, 1858), p. 52; McGregor, *From Midwives to Medicine,* pp. 49–51, 53, 95.

24. Pernick, *A Calculus of Suffering,* p. 156; McGregor, *From Midwives to Medicine,* pp. 49–51, 53, 95. Some people believed that women of mixed race suffered more than others. See ibid., p. 156. Stowe argues that doctors did not include in their narratives of sickness the notion that black women bore the pain of childbirth more easily than white women; "Seeing Themselves at Work," p. 57.

25. Sims, *Silver Sutures in Surgery,* p. 60. On the social isolation of obstetric fistula in a modern-day African community, see Wall, *"Fitsari 'Dan Duniya,"* p. 1329.

26. McGregor, *From Midwives to Medicine,* pp. 59–60; Pernick, *A Calculus of Suffering,* pp. 155–156.

27. Howard L. Holley, *The History of Medicine in Alabama* (Birmingham: University of Alabama School of Medicine, 1982), p. 32; Bozeman, "Vesico-Vaginal Fistula, with Laceration," pp. 234–236. Mattauer received $200 in 1838 for performing the operation on Clark Lunenberg's slave Violet, who remained under his care during July and August 1838; Correspondence, 1825–1853, John Peter Mattauer Papers, Virginia Historical Society, Richmond; John Peter Mattauer, "Vesico-Vaginal Fistula," *Boston Medical and Surgical Journal* 22 (1840): 154–155; McGregor, *From Midwives to Medicine,* p. 62.

28. Bozeman, "Remarks on Vesico-Vaginal Fistule," pp. 86, 94–95, 100–101.

29. McGregor, *From Midwives to Medicine,* pp. 64–66.

30. Comment on the republication of Bozeman's *Louisville Review* article on the subject: "Publications Received," *Atlanta Medical and Surgical Journal* 1 (August 1856): 763–764.

31. Bozeman, "Vesico-Vaginal Fistula, with Laceration," pp. 234–236; idem, "Remarks on Vesico-Vaginal Fistule," p. 98.

32. Battey, "Case of Vesico Vaginal Fistula," pp. 591–594.

33. Joseph W. Smith, "A Case of Spontaneous Discharge of a Urinary Calculus through a Fistulous Opening into the Vagina," *Nashville Journal of Medicine and Surgery* 8 (February 1855): 134–135.

34. W. F. Westmoreland, "Editorial Correspondence," *Atlanta Medical and Surgical Journal* 2 (March 1857): 433.

35. Ibid., pp. 432–433; Charles E. Rosenberg, "Introduction to the New Edition," in *Gunn's Domestic Medicine: A Facsimile of the First Edition*, Tennesseeana ed. (Knoxville: University of Tennessee Press, 1986), p. xvi.

36. "Editorial and Miscellaneous," *Atlanta Medical and Surgical Journal* 2 (July 1857): 703; McGregor, *From Midwives to Medicine*, pp. 62–63.

37. "Vesico Vaginal Fistula," *Atlanta Medical and Surgical Journal* 2 (August 1857): 765; "Operation for Recto-Vaginal Fistula," *New Orleans Medical News and Hospital Gazette* 2 (1 June 1855): 181–184. Doctors in the mid-nineteenth century were moving away from heroic dosing of patients and placing greater faith in the healing power of nature. Although southern doctors clung to heroic practices, they often cited nature as important for the maintenance of women's health. On the increased reliance on nature, see Pernick, *A Calculus of Suffering*, pp. 19–21.

38. Mordecai, "Vesico-Vaginal Fistula"; McGregor, *From Midwives to Medicine*, p. 125.

39. "Proceedings of the Medical Association of the State of Alabama," *Southern Medical Reports* 2 (1850): 325–326.

40. William G. Smith, "Case of Caesarean Operation," *Virginia Medical Journal* 7 (September 1856): 204.

41. Alban S. Payne, "Report of Obstetrical Cases," *The Stethoscope and Virginia Medical Gazette* 3 (April 1853): 203–204.

42. Ibid., p. 204.

43. Ibid., p. 205.

44. Ibid., p. 206.

45. William D. Haskins, "Report of a Case of Doubtful Sex," *The Stethoscope and Virginia Medical Gazette* 1 (February 1851): 99–100; Alice Domurat Dreger, "Doubtful Sex," in *Feminism and the Body*, ed. Londa Schiebinger (New York: Oxford University Press, 2000), pp. 118–151, esp. 135–136. Only recently have surgeons begun to question whether a surgical cure represents the best course of treatment for intersexed individuals. See Mireya Navarro, "When Gender Isn't a Given," *New York Times*, 19 September 2004, sec. 9, pp. 1, 6.

46. Haskins, "Case of Doubtful Sex," p. 101.

47. William M. Broocks, "Report of a Case of Doubtful Sex," *The Stethoscope and Virginia Medical Gazette* 1 (May 1851): 275–276; Savitt, *Medicine and Slavery*, pp. 303–304.

48. Letter from William S. Fife, 26 April 1823, Letters to Doctor James Carmichael and Son, Historical Collections at the Claude Moore Health Sciences Library, University of Virginia, http://etext.lib.virginia.edu/healthsci/carmichael/collection. On the doctor's need to keep secrets, see Steven M. Stowe, *Doctoring the South: Southern Physicians and Everyday Medicine in the Mid-Nineteenth Century* (Chapel Hill: University of North Carolina Press, 2004), pp. 124–127.

49. F. E. H. Steger, "Obstetrical Case," *Nashville Journal of Medicine and Surgery* 9 (August 1855): 104–107; S2, vol. 10: Ark., pt. 6, p. 7. In the North doctors experimented in the Civil War era with genital surgery, both cervical amputation and clitoridectomies, even elytorrhaphy, the latter an attempt to narrow the vagina; McGregor, *From Midwives to Medicine*, pp. 141, 144–149; Roy Porter, *The Greatest Benefit to Mankind: A Medical History of Humanity* (New York: Norton, 1997), p. 35.

50. "Cases Observed by S. Henry Dickson, M.D.," *Southern Journal of Medicine and Pharmacy* 2 (May 1847): 248.

51. Lucile F. Newman, ed., *Women's Medicine: A Cross-Cultural Study of Indigenous Fertility Regulation* (New Brunswick, N.J.: Rutgers University Press, 1985), p. 184.

52. On Nott, see Reginald Horsman, *Josiah Nott of Mobile: Southerner, Physician, and Racial Theorist* (Baton Rouge: Louisiana State University Press, 1987). On Nott and Cartwright, see Savitt, *Medicine and Slavery*, pp. 7–8, 10–11; Stowe, *Doctoring the South*, pp. 129–130, 215–218. On regional medicine, see John Harley Warner, "The Idea of Southern Medical Distinctiveness: Medical Knowledge and Practice in the Old South," in *Sickness and Health in America: Readings in the History of Medicine and Public Health*, ed. Judith Walzer Leavitt and Ronald L. Numbers (Madison: University of Wisconsin Press, 1985), pp, 58, 62, 64; idem, "A Southern Medical Reform: The Meaning of the Antebellum Argument for Southern Medical Education," *Bulletin of the History of Medicine* 57 (1983): 365–373; John O. Breeden, "States-Rights Medicine in the Old South," *Bulletin of the New York Academy of Medicine* 52 (March–April 1976): 348–372, esp. 349–351, 355, and 358; John Duffy, "A Note on Ante-Bellum Southern Nationalism and Medical Practice," *Journal of Southern History* 34 (1968): 266–276.

53. Charles E. Rosenberg, "The Therapeutic Revolution: Medicine, Meaning, and Social Change in Nineteenth-Century America," in *The Therapeutic Revolution: Essays in the Social History of American Medicine*, ed. Morris J. Vogel and Charles E. Rosenberg ([Philadelphia]: University of Pennsylvania Press, 1979), pp. 11, 18–19, 21; H. R. Casey, "Correspondence," *Savannah Journal of Medicine* 1 (September 1858): 207; Steven M. Stowe, "Obstetrics and the Work of Doctoring in the Mid-Nineteenth-Century American South," *Bulletin of the History of Medicine* 64 (winter 1990): 545, 652; E. D. Fenner, "State Medical Society of Louisiana," *Southern Medical Reports* 2 (1850): 296–298; "Negro Hospital," *Charleston Medical Journal and Review* 15 (November 1860): 851.

54. Stowe discusses the tendency of doctors to view white and black bodies interchangeably in "Seeing Themselves at Work," p. 57. See also his *Doctoring the South*. I argue that this tendency was even more pronounced in the case of women's reproductive health. See Pernick, *A Calculus of Suffering*, pp. 132–133. The Thomsonian system of medicine was also universalistic in its treatment system. See ibid., p. 135.

55. E. M. Pendleton, "On the Comparative Fecundity of the Caucasian and African Races," *Charleston Medical Journal and Review* 6 (1851): 355; Duncan Matthews, "The Behavior of the Pelvic Articulations in the Mechanism of Parturition," *The Stethoscope* 5 (February 1855): 105–107; John Duffy, "Sectional Conflict and Medical Education in Louisiana," *Journal of Southern History* 26 (1938): 292.

56. McGregor, *From Midwives to Medicine*, p. 59–60; Sims, *Silver Sutures in Surgery*, pp. 8, 52.

57. McGregor, *From Midwives to Medicine*, pp. 67–68.

58. Pernick, *A Calculus of Suffering*, pp. 40–41; Lederer, *Subjected to Science*.

59. Sally G. McMillen, *Motherhood in the Old South: Pregnancy, Childbirth, and Infant Rearing* (Baton Rouge: Louisiana State University Press, 1990), pp. 16–17; Richard H. Shryock, "Medical Practice in the Old South," *South Atlantic Quarterly* 29 (1930): 168. No medical literature appeared specifically geared to treating the diseases of African Americans, nor did any medical school appoint a professor in this field. And no real evidence exists to indicate that physicians routinely provided different medical treatment to blacks and whites. The "medicine books" kept by many planters rarely distinguished between black and white patients, for example. See Weymouth T. Jordan, "Plantation Medicine in the Old South," *Alabama Review* 3 (1950): 90, 90n26, 92–107.

8. Cancer and Other Tumors

1. Delphy's case is discussed in M. Marsh, "Cancer of the Mammary Gland," *New Orleans Medical News and Hospital Gazette* 7 (May 1860): 174–178.

2. Sharla M. Fett, *Working Cures: Health, Healing, and Power on Southern Slave Plantations* (Chapel Hill: University of North Carolina Press, 2002), pp. 144–145; Steven M. Stowe, "Seeing Themselves at Work: Physicians and the Case Narrative in the Mid-Nineteenth-Century American South," *American Historical Review* 101 (February 1996); Martin S. Pernick, *A Calculus of Suffering: Pain, Professionalism, and Anesthesia in Nineteenth-Century America* (New York: Columbia University Press, 1985), p. 139; Stanley Joel Reiser, *Medicine and the Reign of Technology* (New York: Cambridge University Press, 1978), pp. 2–8.

3. Pernick, *A Calculus of Suffering,* pp. 95–96.

4. Marsh, "Cancer of the Mammary Gland," p. 178.

5. E. Randolph Peaslee, *Ovarian Tumors: Their Pathology, Diagnosis, and Treatment, Especially by Ovariotomy* (New York: D. Appleton, 1872), pp. 237–238.

6. J. F. Peebles, "Spontaneous Recovery from an Ovarian Tumor of Twenty Years Duration," *The Stethoscope and Virginia Medical Gazette* 1 (December 1851): 668.

7. John A. Cotter, "Bloody Vesicle of the Vagina," *Western Journal of Medicine and Surgery,* 2d ser., 7 (April 1847): 367–368; "Polypus Uteri," *New Orleans Medical News and Hospital Gazette* 3 (1 August 1856): 325; R. L. Scruggs, "Medical and Obstetrical Cases," *Western Journal of Medicine and Surgery,* 2d ser., 7 (March 1847): 199–200; Paul R. Eve, "Case of Excision of the Uterus . . . with Remarks by C. D. Meigs," ibid., 3d ser., 6 (November 1850): 401–407.

8. Eve, "Case of Excision of the Uterus"; Henry R. Frost, "Expulsion of a Mass of Hair from the Uterus," *Western Journal of Medicine and Surgery* 6 (September 1842): 218; Walter Fisher, "Physicians and Slavery in the Antebellum Southern Medical Journal," in *The Making of Black America: Essays in Negro Life and History,* ed. August Meier and Elliott Rudwick, vol. 1 (New York: Atheneum, 1969), p. 163; W. A. Brown, "Veratrum Viride: Is It an Abortive?" *Nashville Journal of Medicine and Surgery* 11 (October 1856): 309. Fett discusses issues of consent by slaveholders and slaves in *Working Cures,* pp. 144–147.

9. Alban S. Payne, "Report of Obstetrical Cases," *The Stethoscope and Virginia Medical Gazette* 3 (April 1853): 205; William G. Smith, "Case of Caesarean Operation," *Virginia Medical Journal* 7 (September 1856): 205; John Bellinger, "Operations for the Removal of Abdominal Tumours," *Southern Journal of Medicine and Pharmacy* 2 (May 1847): 242; Peaslee, *Ovarian Tumors,* p. 243.

10. Bellinger, "Operations for Removal of Abdominal Tumours," p. 245.

11. T. Lipscomb [also spelled Lipscomp], "Blighted or False Conception," *Nashville Journal of Medicine and Surgery* 8 (June 1855): 469; "Polypus Uteri," p. 326.

12. Susan Garfinkel, "'This Trial Was Sent in Love and Mercy for My Refinement': A Quaker Woman's Experience of Breast Cancer Surgery in 1814," in *Women and Health in America: Historical Readings,* ed. Judith Walzer Leavitt, 2d ed. (Madison: University of Wisconsin Press, 1999), p. 73; Fett, *Working Cures,* p. 147; James S. Olson, *Bathsheba's Breast: Women, Cancer, and History* (Baltimore: Johns Hopkins University Press, 2002), p. 55.

13. Kenneth Allen De Ville, *Medical Malpractice in Nineteenth-Century America* (New York: New York University Press, 1990), pp. 31, 91, 131.

14. "Medical Etiquette and Professional Rights," *Atlanta Medical and Surgical Journal* 1 (August 1856): 760.

15. Ibid., pp. 759–762.

16. Ibid., p. 759; C. W. Ashby, "Stramonium, as a Remedy for Dysmenorrhea," *Atlanta Medical and Surgical Journal* 1 (March 1856): 393.

17. William D. Haskins, "Report of a Case of Doubtful Sex," *The Stethoscope and Virginia Medical Gazette* 1 (February 1851): 99, 101; Smith, "Case of Caesarean Operation," pp. 2–4.

18. Ashby, "Stramonium, as a Remedy for Dysmenorrhea," p. 393; Bellinger, "Operations for Removal of Abdominal Tumours," p. 242; Steven M. Stowe, ed., *A Southern Practice: The Diary and Autobiography of Charles A. Hentz, M.D.* (Charlottesville: University Press of Virginia, 2000), p. 514; T. F. Craig, "Ovariotomy Successfully Performed, by Dr. John Craig, of Stanford, Kentucky," *New Orleans Medical News and Hospital Gazette* 1 (1 December 1854): 418–420.

19. James Bolton, "A Case of Ovarian and Peritoneal Dropsy," *The Stethoscope and Virginia Medical Gazette* 1 (February 1851): 107–109.

20. *Gunn's Domestic Medicine: A Facsimile of the First Edition,* Tennesseeana ed. (Knoxville: University of Tennessee Press, 1986), pp. 284–286.

21. "Curability of Cancer, and Its Diagnostic by Means of the Microscope," *The Stethoscope* 5 (February 1855): 147–149; A. Richard, "On Discharge of Fluid from the Nipple in Non-Malignant Tumors of the Breast," *New Orleans Medical News and Hospital Gazette* 1 (15 March 1854): 47.

22. "Topical Applications for Tumors of the Breast," *Charleston Medical Journal and Review* 15 (March 1860): 541; "Surgical Operations in Cancerous Diseases," *The Stethoscope and Virginia Medical Gazette* 3 (September 1853): 547; "Curability of Cancer," pp. 147–149.

23. A. G. Grinnan, "Remarks on the Topography and Diseases of Madison County, Virginia," *The Stethoscope and Virginia Medical Gazette* 3 (March 1853): 134; A. S. Helmick, "An Interesting Case in Practice," *The Stethoscope* 5 (December 1855): 717–723; Olson, *Bathsheba's Breast,* pp. 35–36.

24. "Editorial Correspondence," *Atlanta Medical and Surgical Journal* 2 (March 1857): 432, 441; W. F. Westmoreland, "Foreign Correspondence," ibid. (June 1857): 593–597.

25. McDowell's son believed that his father performed the operation thirteen times in all; "Kentucky Surgery," *Western Journal of Medicine and Surgery,* 3d ser., 11 (April 1853): 327–334; Deborah Kuhn McGregor, *From Midwives to Medicine: The Birth of American Gynecology* (New Brunswick, N.J.: Rutgers University Press, 1998), pp. 159–160; Peaslee, *Ovarian Tumors,* p. 241.

26. Samuel Sexton, "A Case of Extra-Uterine Pregnancy, with an Account of the Appearances on Dissection," *Western Journal of Medicine and Surgery* 1 (February 1840): 207–208.

27. "Calcareous Degeneration of the Ovary," *New Orleans Medical News and Hospital Gazette* 5 (February 1858): 746.

28. Thomas E. Massey, "Observations upon Diseases of the Uterus," *The Stethoscope* 5 (February 1855): 167; Juriah Harriss, "What Constitutes Unsoundness in the Negro," *Savannah Journal of Medicine* 1 (January 1859): 294; Walter Johnson, *Soul by Soul: Life Inside the Antebellum Slave Market* (Cambridge, Mass.: Harvard University Press, 1999), p. 127.

29. J. O. Sharber, "Death from Exterior Uterine Hemorrhage," *Nashville Journal of Medicine and Surgery* 4 (May 1853): 259–261; W. K. Bowling, "An Extensive Abdominal Tumor," ibid., 8 (February 1855): 103–104. For a case of a black woman, probably free, who appeared pregnant and about to deliver, see Peebles, "Spontaneous Recovery from Ovarian Tumor," p. 668.

30. Warren Stone, "Observations upon Diseases of the Uterus," *New Orleans Medical News and Hospital Gazette* 1 (1 November 1854): 342; John Duffy, *From Humors to Medical Science: A History of American Medicine,* 2d ed. (Urbana: University of Illinois Press, 1993), p. 101.

31. *Gunn's Domestic Medicine,* pp. 284–286; McGregor, *From Midwives to Medicine,* p. 176; Charles B. Dew, *Bond of Iron: Master and Slave at Buffalo Forge* (New York: Norton, 1994), p. 255.

32. S. B. Robison, "Case of Inflammation of the Ovaria," *Nashville Journal of Medicine and Surgery* 3, no. 1 (1852): 77–78; D. Warren Brickell, "A Case of Pelvic Abscess," *New Orleans Medical News and Hospital Gazette* 5 (March 1858): 10–16; idem, "Pelvic Abscess," ibid. (April 1858): 87–90; "Physico-Medical

Society," ibid., 1 (1 March 1854): 22. See also Stowe, *A Southern Practice,* pp. 345, 348–349.

33. M. M. Pallen, "The Causes of Hemorrhage from the Unimpregnated Uterus," *Atlanta Medical and Surgical Journal* 1 (November 1855): 148–150; "Injection of Ovarian Cysts with Iodine," *The Stethoscope* 5 (February 1855): 120.

34. "Cancer of the Neck of the Uterus," *The Stethoscope* 5 (January 1855): 55–56; "Polypus Uteri," pp. 325–326; Pallen, "Causes of Hemorrhage from Unimpregnated Uterus," pp. 148–150. See also Scruggs, "Medical and Obstetrical Cases," pp. 199–200; Cotter, "Bloody Vesicle of the Vagina."

35. Duffy, *From Humors to Medical Science,* pp. 95–96; Pernick, *A Calculus of Suffering,* pp. 107–108; "Brown on Surgical Diseases of Women," *New Orleans Medical News and Hospital Gazette* 3 (1 May 1856): 237–238; John Travis, "Cancer Cured by an Operation," *Nashville Journal of Medicine and Surgery* 9 (August 1855): 103–104. For reference to a woman whose breast was excised and who lived for some years afterward, see John N. Broocks, "Cases Treated in the Armory and Penitentiary Hospitals, with Remarks," *The Stethoscope and Virginia Medical Gazette* 1 (February 1851): 101.

36. Bellinger, "Operations for Removal of Abdominal Tumours," p. 241; McGregor, *From Midwives to Medicine,* pp. 159–161.

37. Stowe, *A Southern Practice,* p. 346. Frances Walker, a white Virginia woman, underwent blistering for a tumor on her left side, but when that failed she underwent unsuccessful surgery for its removal. See Claudia L. Bushman, *In Old Virginia: Slavery, Farming, and Society in the Journal of John Walker* (Baltimore: Johns Hopkins University Press, 2002), p. 111; Olson, *Bathsheba's Breast,* pp. 33–35.

38. Chas. Witsell, "Case of Enormous Polypus of the Uterus Treated with the Muriated Tincture of Iron," *Charleston Medical Journal and Review* 15 (March 1860): 326–328; Juriah Harriss, "Milk Secreted by Tumors in the Axillae," *Savannah Journal of Medicine* 3 (September 1860): 168, 170.

39. Witsell, "Enormous Polypus of Uterus Treated with Muriated Tincture of Iron," pp. 326–328.

40. McGregor, *From Midwives to Medicine,* p. 175; Travis, "Cancer Cured by an Operation," pp. 103–104. The double incision performed by Travis had remained the standard method of removing a cancerous breast since at least the turn of the century; Kay K. Moss, *Southern Folk Medicine, 1750–1820* (Columbia: University of South Carolina Press, 1999), p. 221.

41. B. W. Avent, "Cancer," *Nashville Journal of Medicine and Surgery* 16 (January 1859): 2–3.

42. "Reviews and Bibliographical Notes," *The Stethoscope and Virginia Medical Gazette* 2 (April 1852): 218–221. The table was published in other places by various doctors beginning in 1845.

43. Peaslee, *Ovarian Tumors*, p. 247.

44. Ibid., p. 249; Pernick, *A Calculus of Suffering*, p. 213.

45. "Surgical Operations in Cancerous Diseases," pp. 545, 547.

46. Eve, "Case of Excision of the Uterus." Eve studied medicine under Meigs. See Howard A. Kelly and Walter L. Burrage, *Dictionary of American Medical Biography* (Boston: Milford House, 1971), p. 142. On the tendency of blacks to be used more readily than whites for experimentation and on the assumption that knowledge gained from the examination of black bodies was applicable to white bodies, see Todd L. Savitt, "The Use of Blacks for Medical Experimentation and Demonstration in the Old South," *Journal of Southern History* 48 (August 1982): 332–333, 341–343.

47. Pernick, *A Calculus of Suffering*, p. 111; Eve, "Case of Excision of the Uterus"; Bellinger, "Operations for Removal of Abdominal Tumours," pp. 243–245.

48. S2, vol. 8: Ark., pt. 2, p. 354. For another former slave who mentioned a white woman's breast cancer, see SS2, vol. 9: Miss., pt. 4, p. 1795.

49. "Calcareous Degeneration of the Ovary," *New Orleans Medical News and Hospital Gazette* 4 (February 1858): 746; J. F. Peebles, "Cases Illustrative of Uterine Pathology," *The Stethoscope and Virginia Medical Gazette* 3 (August 1853): 466–467.

9. Freedwomen's Health

1. Bellamy's remarks here and below are drawn from W. C. Bellamy, "Some Remarks on the Therapeutic Effects of Gossypium as an Emmenagogue and Parturifacient," *Atlanta Medical and Surgical Journal*, n.s., 7B (October 1866): 337–340. Doctors apparently prescribed cotton root after the war to induce or speed labor and to relieve amenorrhea, dysmenorrhea, and scanty menstruation. See William Ed Grimé, *Ethno-Botany of the Black Americans* (Algonac, Mich.: Reference Publications, 1979), p. 122.

2. J. G. Westmoreland, "New Remedies," *Atlanta Medical and Surgical Journal* 8 (August 1867): 248.

3. "Gossypium Herbaccum (Cotton)," ibid., 6 (March 1861): 481.

4. SS1, vol. 9: Miss., pt. 4, p. 1582; Thomas S. Powell, "Extracts from the Introductory Lecture Delivered at the Opening of the Session of the Medical College of Georgia, on the First Tuesday in November 1866," *Atlanta Medical and*

Surgical Journal, n.s., 7B (March 1866): 45 and (July 1866): 212; Joseph Le Cunte, "'On the Law of the Sexes'; or the Production of the Sexes at Will," ibid. (January 1867): 504. Only the Medical College of Virginia stayed open after March 1862; John Duffy, *From Humors to Medical Science: A History of American Medicine,* 2d ed. (Urbana: University of Illinois Press, 1993), p. 158.

5. Dwayne D. Cox and William J. Morison, *The University of Louisville* (Lexington: University Press of Kentucky, 2000), pp. 28–29; *Atlanta Medical and Surgical Journal* 7A (September 1861): 5–8, 51–53, 58–60, 60–61, 62, and (October 1861): 111.

6. Steven M. Stowe, *Doctoring the South: Southern Physicians and Everyday Medicine in the Mid-Nineteenth Century* (Chapel Hill: University of North Carolina Press, 2004), pp. 234, 265–267, 320n11. When the names of blacks appeared in postwar journals, they tended to be of women treated before the war. See for example D. C. O'Keefe, "Dislocation of the Symphysis Pubis during Pregnancy and Parturition," *Atlanta Medical and Surgical Journal,* n.s., 7B (March 1867): 1–11. John Harley Warner discusses the changing nature of medicine in *The Therapeutic Perspective: Medical Practice, Knowledge, and Identity in America, 1820–1885* (Princeton: Princeton University Press, 1997).

7. Stowe, *Doctoring the South,* p. 262; S2, vol. 14: N.C., pt. 1, pp. 61, 62; S. H. Stout, "An Address, Introductory to the Eighth Regular Summer Course of Lectures in the Atlanta Medical College," *Atlanta Medical and Surgical Journal,* n.s., 7B (July 1866): 206; "The Medical Association of Georgia," ibid., 8 (March 1867): 37, 38.

8. Todd L. Savitt, "Politics in Medicine: The Georgia Freedmen's Bureau and the Organization of Health Care," *Civil War History* 28 (1982): 50, 51, 62–63; Randy Finley, "In War's Wake: Health Care and Arkansas Freedmen, 1863–1868," *Arkansas History Quarterly* 51 (summer 1992): 148; Col. E. Whittlesey to Maj. Gen. O. O. Howard, 18 July 1865, LS, July 1865–April 1869, Correspondence, HQ, Office of the Asst. Comr., N.C., Ser. 2446, RG 105.

9. Marshall Scott Legan, "Disease and the Freedmen in Mississippi during Reconstruction," *Journal of the History of Medicine and Allied Sciences* 28 (July 1973): 260; "The Medical Association of Georgia," pp. 37, 38; Dr. Edmund Christian to W. F. DeKnight, Rocky Mount, Franklin Co., Va., 13 September 1866, LR, January 1866–May 1868, Asst. Subasst. Comr., Subordinate Field Offices, Ser. 4257, RG 105; also Endorsement, J. J. DeLamater, 19 September 1866, ibid. The U.S. Congress provided no funding for medical care. On the refusal of private physicians to treat freed people in North Carolina, see Reggie L. Pearson, "'There are Many Sick, Feeble, and Suffering Freedmen': The Freedmen's Bureau's Health-Care Activities during Reconstruction in North

Carolina, 1865–1868," *North Carolina Historical Review* 79 (April 2002): 141–181.

10. James M. Laing to Gen., Atlanta, Ga., 1 October 1867, Annual Reports of the Asst. Comrs., Records of the Comr., Washington HQ, Ser. 32, RG 105; S. P. Anderson to Gen. C. B. Fisk, 16 April 1866, Registered LR, June 1865–April 1869, HQ Office of the Asst. Comr., Tenn., Ser. 3379, RG 105; A. T. Reeve to Brig. Gen. Davis Tillson, 31 January 1866, Unregistered LR, September 1865–January 1869, Correspondence, HQ Office of the Asst. Comr., Ga., Ser. 632, RG 105.

11. SS2, vol. 3: Tex., pt. 2, pp. 570, 851–852; Alan Raphael, "Health and Social Welfare of Kentucky Black People, 1865–1870," *Societas* 2 (spring 1972): 146; Finley, "In War's Wake," p. 148.

12. S2, vol. 11: Ark., pt. 7, p. 94.

13. Temple quoted in Raphael, "Health and Social Welfare of Kentucky Black People," pp. 146, 151; Elizabeth Bethel, "The Freedmen's Bureau in Alabama," *Journal of Southern History* 14 (February 1948): 55.

14. T. K. Leonard, 2 February 1866, LR, June 1865–June 1869, Correspondence, HQ Office of the Asst. Comr., Fla., Ser. 586, RG 105; J. J. Joyce, M.D., to Maj. W [S. G. Williams], 26 November 1866, Unregistered LR, March 1866–December 1868, Asst. Supt. and Asst. Subasst. Comr., Subordinate Field Offices, Alexandria, La., Ser. 1431, RG 105; W. R. Joiner to Capt. White, 30 October 1867, LR, April 1867–July 1868, Subordinate Field Offices, Quitman, Ga., Ser. 988, RG 105. See also Finley, "In War's Wake," pp. 147–148; Circular, J. J. DeLamater, 23 July 1866, LR, June 1865–December 1868, Subordinate Field Offices, Norfolk, Va., Ser. 4153, RG 105.

15. "The Medical Association of Georgia," pp. 38, 41, 45. The meeting occurred on 10 April and not 12 April as stated in this editorial. See *Atlanta Medical and Surgical Journal*, n.s., 8 (April 1867): 87 and (May 1867): 130, 148. R. C. Word, "Obligations of the Public to the Medical Profession," ibid. (June 1867): 149.

16. John E. Tallon to Benjamin F. Flanders, Donaldsonville, 9 January 1864, Incoming Correspondence of the Supervising Special Agent, Benjamin F. Flanders, General Official Correspondence, RG 366: Records of Civil War Special Agencies of the Treasury Department, 3d Agency, National Archives, College Park, Md.; Capt. W. Storer How to Col. O. Brown, 6 November 1865 and 11 December 1865, LS, August 1865–April 1866, Subasst. Comr., Subordinate Field Offices, Winchester, Va., Ser. 4302, RG 105; Circular, J. J. DeLamater, 23 July 1866, LR, June 1865–December 1868, Subordinate Field Offices, Norfolk, Va., Ser. 4153, RG 105; Circular Letter from J. J. DeLamater to Lieut. Robt. Cullen, 23 July 1866, Letters and Orders Received, July 1865–December 1868,

Asst. Subasst. Comr., Subordinate Field Offices, Boydton, Va., Ser. 3897, RG 105. Under some circumstances, taxes were levied on freed people. The Freedmen's Sanitary Commission in Memphis imposed a tax of one dollar on every freed person between the ages of eighteen and sixty in order to establish a hospital. See Special Orders, No. 49, Bvt. Brig. Gen. Benjamin P. Runkle, 13 April 1866, Special Orders and Circulars Issued, October 1865–October 1868, Subasst. Comr. for the Subdistrict of Memphis, Subordinate Field Offices, Memphis, Tenn., Ser. 3523, RG 105.

17. Report of the Asst. Comr. for Tex. for the Year Ending 31 October 1866, in Bvt. Maj. Gen. J. B. Kiddoo to Maj. Gen. O. O. Howard, 31 October 1866, Annual Reports of the Asst. Commissioners, 1866–1868, Records of the Comr., Tex., Ser. 32, RG 105; Col. T. W. Osborn to Dr. T. K. Leonard, 23 February 1866, HQ, LS, September 1865–July 1870, Ser. 582, RG 105; George A. Harmount to Brig. Gen. Wager Swayne, Mobile, Ala., 16 August 1865, Unregistered LR, June 1865–June 1870, Correspondence, HQ Office of the Asst. Comr., Ala., Ser. 9, RG 105; Eric Foner, *Reconstruction: America's Unfinished Revolution, 1863–1877* (New York: Harper and Row, 1988), p. 151. Yet Freedmen's Bureau officials expressed concern about the consequence of physicians' being unable to collect debts; M. R. Hall, n.d., Register of LR, October 1865–May 1869, vol. 1, p. 187, Correspondence, HQ Office of the Asst. Comr., Ga., Ser. 630, and Endorsements Sent, vol. 20, p. 5, Correspondence, HQ Office of the Asst. Comr., Ga., Ser. 628, RG 105.

18. Pearson, "'Many Sick, Feeble, and Suffering Freedmen,'" p. 165; Report of the Asst. Comr. for Tex. for the Year Ending 31 October 1866, Annual Reports of the Asst. Comrs., Records of the Comr., Ser. 32, RG 105. Although the bureau operated from 1865 to 1872, agents grew less willing to intervene in labor disputes after these peak years; Foner, *Reconstruction*, pp. 165–166.

19. Gen. Order No. 12, approved by Louis E. Parsons, Provisional Governor of Ala., 1 September 1865, and by Maj. Gen. C. R. Woods (Dept. of Ala.), 4 September 1865, Gen. Orders, Circulars, and Circular Letters Issued, July 1865–December 1868, Issuances, Ala., Office of Asst. Comr., Ser. 11, RG 105; Chaplain Samuel S. Gardner to Bvt. Col. C. Cadle Jr., 13 December 1865, Unregistered LR, June 1865–June 1870, Correspondence, HQ Office of the Asst. Comr., Ala., Ser. 9, RG 105.

20. Contract between Ephraim and Clary and B. C. Wyly, July 1865, Calhoun Co., Ala., Contracts, Subasst. Comr., Subordinate Field Offices, Jacksonville, Ala., Ser. 137, RG 105; S2, vol. 10: Ark., pt. 6, pp. 155, 179; SS2, vol. 3: Tex., pt. 2, p. 910.

21. Contract between Pettis Smithson and Robert Harvey, 28 December 1865, Records Relating to Complaints and Court Cases, Contracts and Indentures

and Reports and Estimates, Subasst. Comr., Subordinate Field Offices, Farmville, Va., Ser. 3975, RG 105; Contract between William Hamilton and Henry
Miller and Family, 7 January 1867, Contracts, Bills of Lading, Receipts, and
Miscellaneous Records, 1865–1868, Staunton, Va., Ser. 4274, RG 105; Contract
between David S. Johnston and 42 Freed People, 15 July 1865, LR, May
1867–July 1868, Agent, Subordinate Field Offices, Newton, Ga., Ser. 973, RG
105.

22. Contract enclosed in William Lynn to Asst. Comr., Ala., 27 May 1866,
Unregistered LR, Correspondence, HQ, Office of the Asst. Comr., Ala., Ser. 9,
RG 105; Contract between Thomas Henderson and Ginetta Howard, Jenny
Howard, and Mary Susan Howard, 15 December 1865, Labor Contracts, Sep-
tember 1865–March 1867, Supt., Subordinate Field Offices, Alexandria, Va.,
Ser. 3870, RG 105; Contract between R. H. Griffin and Nathan, Sarah Ann,
and Family, 17 June 1865 and Contract between Miles W. Abernathy and Pene-
lope, 19 July [1865], Contracts, June–December 1865, Subasst. Comr., Subor-
dinate Field Offices, Jacksonville, Ala., Ser. 137, RG 105; Contract between
Edward H. Turner and Eliza Pinkwood, 11 November 1865, Labor Contracts,
September 1865–March 1867, Supt., Subordinate Field Offices, Alexandria,
Va., Ser. 3870, RG 105. On the custom of slaves' cultivating patches of land, see
Ira Berlin and Philip D. Morgan, eds., *Cultivation and Culture: Labor and the
Shaping of Slave Life in the Americas* (Charlottesville: University Press of Vir-
ginia, 1993).

23. Contract between W. C. Penick and Asberry Penick et al., 1 June 1865,
Unregistered LR, June 1865–June 1870, HQ, Office of the Asst. Comr., Ala.,
Ser. 9, RG 105; Contract between H. R. Felder and Eighteen Freed People, 2
January 1867, Labor Contracts and Miscellaneous Court Papers, 1866–1868,
Agent, Subordinate Field Offices, Perry, Ga., Ser. 985, RG 105; Contract
between McQueen McIntosh and 47 Freed People, 8 July 1865, Reports Sent to
the Asst. Comr. and Contracts, 1865–1868, Agent, Subordinate Field Offices,
Bainbridge, Ga., Ser. 784, RG 105; McQueen McIntosh to the Georgia's Freedmen's Bureau Asst. Comr., 6 December 1865, Unregistered LR, September
1865–January 1869, Correspondence, HQ, Office of the Asst. Comr., Ga., Ser.
632, RG 105; SS2, vol. 10: Tex., pt. 9, pp. 4221–22, 4241. On North Carolina
contracts, see Pearson, "'Many Sick, Feeble, and Suffering Freedmen,'"
pp. 166–170.

24. Contract between Littleton Flippo and Polly Minor, 15 January 1866, Letters and Orders Received, July 1865–December 1868, Asst. Subasst. Comr.,
Subordinate Field Offices, Boydton, Va., RG 105.

25. Contract between S. T. Lucas and Hetty Conquest, 15 January 1865, Contracts, 1866, Asst. Subasst. Comr., Subordinate Field Offices, Drummondtown,

Va., Ser. 3962, RG 105; Contract between L. C. Williamson and Sallie Pettegrew, 11 July 1865, Contracts and Indentures, 1865–1867, Subasst. Comr., Subordinate Field Offices, Lynchburg, Va., Ser. 4081, RG 105; Contract between Mary H. Ford and Netty Ann Webb, 13 July 1865, Contracts, July–October 1865, Asst. Supt., Subordinate Field Offices, Petersburg, Va., Ser. 4221, RG 105.

26. Contract between Benjamin F. Pope and Dulcena, 3 August 1865, Labor Contracts, August 1865, Subordinate Field Office, Ashville, Ala., Ser. 72, RG 105.

27. W. King, "Regulation of Labor for Freedmen, Who Are Possessed of No Visible Means of Support for Themselves and Families," 9 November 1865, Circulars and Circular LR, June 1865–December 1868, Issuances, HQ, Office of the Asst. Comr., Ala., Ser. 15, RG 105; Contract between James H. Fletcher and Patsy Teackle, 10 January 1865, Office of the Supt. of Labor, Labor Contracts, 1864 and 1865, Dept. of Negro Affairs, Subordinate Field Offices, Fort Monroe, Va., Ser. 4111, RG 105; Contract between Miles W. Abernathy and Wesley, 25 July [1865], Contracts, June–December 1865, Subasst. Comr., Subordinate Field Offices, Jacksonville, Ala., Ser. 137, RG 105; Contract between T. T. Treadway and Freedmen, 1 January 1866, Records Relating to Complaints and Court Cases, Contracts and Indentures, and Reports and Estimates, 1865–1868, Subasst. Comr., Subordinate Field Offices, Farmville, Va., Ser. 3975, RG 105; Contract between E. R. Flewellen and Alfred Walker et al., 11 February 1867, Indentures, Contracts and Leases of Land Received, 1865–1868, Supt. of the Western District, Subordinate Field Offices, Salisbury, N.C., Ser. 2848, RG 105.

28. Contract between R. S. Foster and Twenty-four Freedpeople and Contract between Tom Fleming and Seventeen Freedpeople, n.d., Reports, Contracts, Indentures, and Proceedings of Freedmen's Court, 1865–1868, Asst. Supt., Subordinate Field Offices, Fredericksburg, Va., Ser. 3997, RG 105; Contract between S. T. Lucas and Hetty Conquest.

29. Contract between James E. Waddy and Freedmen, 10 January 1867, and Brien Maquire to Gen. Tillson, 10 January 1867, Unregistered LR, September 1865–January 1869, Correspondence, HQ, Office of the Asst. Comr., Ga., Ser. 632, RG 105.

30. Contract between H. H. Haddock and Jim Sharpe et al., 1 January 1867, Labor Contracts and Miscellaneous Court Papers, 1866–1868, Agent, Subordinate Field Offices, Perry, Ga., Ser. 985, RG 105; Contract between Clark Anderson and Co., and Freed People, 9 January 1866, Miscellaneous Records, 1862–1869, Other Records, Office of the Asst. Comr., Ga., Ser. 654, RG 105.

31. Contract between Clark Anderson and Co., and Freed People, 9 January 1866.

32. Quoted in Deborah Gray White, *Ar'n't I a Woman? Female Slaves in the Plantation South* (New York: Norton, 1985), p. 139.

33. S2, vol. 8: Ark., pt. 1, p. 71, and vol. 14: N.C., pt. 1, pp. 391–392; SS2, vol. 3: Tex., pt. 2, pp. 789, 943; Report of the Asst. Comr. for Tex. for the Year Ending 31 October 1866.

34. A. C. Swartzwelder to Bvt. Maj. Gen. C. B. Fisk, 18 January 1866, Registered LR, June 1865–April 1869, HQ Office of the Asst. Comr., Tenn., Ser. 3379, RG 105; Savitt, "Politics in Medicine," p. 57. See also SS1, vol. 9: Miss., pt. 4, p. 1704.

35. Contract between H. H. Haddock and Jim Sharpe et al., 1 January 1867.

36. Affidavit, Anderson Garret, 17 July 1866, LR, September 1865–April 1869, Correspondence, HQ Office of the Asst. Comr., Ga., Ser. 631, RG 105; S. Crawford to Bt. Maj. Gen. D. Tillson, 24 Sept. 1866, Register of Complaints, July–November 1867, Supt. and Agent, Subordinate Field Offices, Lewisville, Ark., Ser. 362, RG 105.

37. Affidavit, Isham Crowell [June 1867], and Charles Raushenberg to Bvt. Lt. Col. O. H. Howard, 6 June 1867, LR, 1867–1868, Agent, Subordinate Field Offices, Albany, Ga., Ser. 700, RG 105.

38. Affidavit, Isham Crowell [June 1867].

39. Jacqueline Jones, *Labor of Love, Labor of Sorrow: Black Women, Work, and the Family from Slavery to the Present* (New York: Basic Books, 1986), chap. 2, esp. pp. 46, 58, 60–61.

40. Ira Berlin et al., eds., *Free at Last: A Documentary History of Slavery, Freedom, and the Civil War* (New York: New Press, 1992), p. 244; S2, vol. 8: Ark., pt. 1, pp. 146, 174, and pt. 2, p. 320, and vol. 9: Ark., pt. 3, p. 343; SS2, vol. 3: Tex., pt. 2, p. 581, and vol. 9: Tex., pt. 8, pp. 3863–64.

41. SS1, vol. 9: Miss., pt. 4, p. 1615; SS2, vol. 3: Tex., pt. 2, pp. 757–758, 778.

42. SS1, vol. 8: Miss., pt. 3, p. 959; John E. Tallon to Benjamin F. Flanders, Donaldsonville, 9 January 1864, Incoming Correspondence of the Supervising Special Agent, General Official Correspondence, RG 366; Report of the Asst. Comr. for Tex. for the Year Ending 31 October 1866; Legan, "Disease and Freedmen in Mississippi," p. 260; S2, vol. 10: Ark., pt. 5, pp. 182–183. Some freed people sought medical training for former slaves; Heather Andrea Williams, *Self-Taught: African American Education in Slavery and Freedom* (Chapel Hill: University of North Carolina Press, 2005), p. 77.

43. John Strain to Gen. Swayne, 28 October 1866, Unregistered LR, ser. 9, Ala. Asst. Comr., RG 105. No record of a reply has been found. I am grateful to Steven F. Miller for bringing this letter to my attention. W. R. Joiner to Capt. White, 30 October 1867, LR, April 1867–July 1868, Subordinate Field Offices, Quitman, Ga., Ser. 988, RG 105; Contract between McQueen McIntosh and 47 Freed People, 8 July 1865. Former slaves also wanted to ensure that any doctors appointed by the Freedmen's Bureau met their approval. See Petition of Hamilton Brown et al., 29 April 1867, Registered LR, July 1865–October 1870, Correspondence, HQ, Office of the Asst. Comr., S.C., Ser. 2922, RG 105; Petition of Benjamin Capers et al. [July 1867] and S. B. Thompson to M. K. Hogan, 20 July 1867, ibid.

44. Raphael, "Health and Social Welfare of Kentucky Black People," p. 146.

45. Some of the freed people suffered from more than one illness. One of the children was a girl. The diagnosis of worms suggests that most of the males were children. John E. Tallon to W. H. Wilder, 16 [no month] 1863, Incoming Correspondence of the Supervising Special Agent, Benjamin F. Flanders, General Official Correspondence, RG 366.

46. The apparent purpose of the shooting was to warn former slaves away from political activities; S2, vol. 8: Ark., pt. 2, p. 108. North Carolina doctor quoted in Pearson, "'Many Sick, Feeble, and Suffering Freedmen,'" pp. 150–151; John E. Tallon to Benjamin F. Flanders, Donaldsonville, 9 January 1864; Jerry Bryan Lincecum, Edward Hake Phillips, and Peggy A. Redshaw, eds., *Gideon Lincecum's Sword: Civil War Letters from the Texas Home Front* (Denton, Tex.: University of North Texas Press, 2001), pp. 3, 32, 42–43, 49–50, 343, 362; Legan, "Disease and Freedmen in Mississippi," p. 260; Onnie Lee Logan, *Motherwit: An Alabama Midwife's Story* (New York: Dutton, 1989), p. 58.

47. Cox and Morison, *The University of Louisville*, p. 29; Savitt, "Politics in Medicine," p. 63.

48. James F. Brooks, *Captives and Cousins: Slavery, Kinship, and Community in the Southwest Borderlands* (Chapel Hill: University of North Carolina Press, 2002); Kathleen M. Brown, *Good Wives, Nasty Wenches, and Anxious Patriarchs* (Chapel Hill: University of North Carolina Press, 1996).

49. SS1, vol. 6: Miss., pt. 1, p. 61; SS2, vol. 3: Tex., pt. 2, pp. 893–896.

50. S1, vol. 17: Fla., p. 87; S2, vol. 9: Ark., pt. 3, pp. 302–304, and vol. 10: Ark., pt. 6, p. 236, and vol. 14: N.C., pt. 1, p. 6, and vol. 10: Ark., pt. 2, p. 927; SS1, vol. 9: Miss., pt. 4, pp. 1816, 1818; SS2, vol. 1: Ala., Ariz., Ark., and Other Narratives, pp. 274, 275, 317, and vol. 2: Tex., pt. 1, p. 201, and vol. 3: Tex., pt. 2, pp. 875, 927; Newbell Niles Puckett, *Folk Beliefs of the Southern Negro* (New York: Negro Universities Press, 1968), chap. 2; David Brown, "Conjure/

Doctors: An Exploration of a Black Discourse in America, Antebellum to 1940," *Folklore Forum* 23 (1990): 3–46.

51. SS2, vol. 10: Tex., pt. 9, p. 4319; D. E. Cadwallader and J. F. Wilson, "Folklore Medicine among Georgia's Piedmont Negroes after the Civil War," *Georgia Historical Quarterly* 49 (1965): 217, 220, 221, 223, 224n5, 226n75; Cindy Belew, "Herbs and the Childbearing Woman: Guidelines for Midwives," and Laurel Lee, "Introducing Herbal Medicine into Conventional Health Care Settings," both in *Journal of Nurse-Midwifery* 44 (May/June 1999): 231–252 and 253–266 respectively.

52. T. Lindsay Baker and Julie P. Baker, eds., *The WPA Oklahoma Slave Narratives* (Norman: University of Oklahoma Press, 1996), p. 385; Robert Wright to Unknown, 20 September 1869, Case Files of Pension Claims, Claims Division, Subordinate Offices, Md. and Del., Ser. 2002, RG 105; S2, vol. 10: Ark., pt. 5, p. 82; Pearson, "'Many Sick, Feeble, and Suffering Freedmen,'" p. 169.

53. S2, vol. 15: N.C., pt. 2, p. 353.

54. S2, vol. 8: Ark., pt. 1, pp. 239, 344, and pt. 2, p. 282, and vol. 10: Ark., pt. 5, pp. 33, 34; SS1, vol. 6: Miss., pt. 1, p. 267.

55. S2, vol. 8: Ark., pt. 1, p. 344, and vol. 9: Ark., pt. 4, p. 139, and vol. 10: Ark., pt. 6, p. 295, and vol. 11: Ark., pt. 7, p. 149. See also SS1, vol. 9: Miss., pt. 4, p. 1883.

56. S2, vol. 8: Ark., pt. 1, p. 196; SS2, vol. 1: Ala., Ariz., Ark., and Other Narratives, p. 270; Susan L. Smith, "White Nurses, Black Midwives, and Public Health in Mississippi, 1920–1950," in *Women and Health in America: Historical Readings,* ed. Judith Walzar Leavitt, 2d ed. (Madison: University of Wisconsin Press, 1999), p. 445. Not until the 1950s did the number of physician-assisted births begin to rise appreciably.

Index